Whiplash Injuries

Dario C. Alpini • Guido Brugnoni
Antonio Cesarani
Editors

Whiplash Injuries

Diagnosis and Treatment

Second Edition

Springer

Editors
Dario C. Alpini
ENT-Otoneurology Service
IRCCS "Don Carlo Gnocchi" Foundation
Milan
Italy

Guido Brugnoni
Italian Academy of Manual Medicine
Italian Institute for Auxology
Milan
Italy

Antonio Cesarani
Department of Clinical Sciences and Community Health
University of Milan
Milan
Italy

Audiology Unit
IRCCS "Ca' Granda" Ospedale Maggiore Policlinico
Milan
Italy

ISBN 978-88-470-5789-0 ISBN 978-88-470-5486-8 (eBook)
DOI 10.1007/978-88-470-5486-8
Springer Milan Heidelberg New York Dordrecht London

Printed on acid-free paper

Springer is part of Springer Science+Business Media (www.springer.com)

Foreword

I have dedicated my early researches to the study of learning disturbances and behavioral disorders in childhood, especially with regard to autism. The focus of my study was on the correlation between posture, that is the language of the body, and mental health. During my fellowship at Stanford University in the 1970s, I developed the idea that measurement of postural control might be the best way to investigate cognitive functions. The basic posture of the human being is upright bipedalism; maintaining dynamic equilibrium of the body, which is like an inverted pendulum on a relatively restricted base area, is an evolutionary phenomenon directly linked to high-level cognitive development. In adulthood, maintaining stance is perceived to be easy, at least under normal conditions on steady surfaces, but it actually requires a very high level of sensorimotor control to allow a low-effort antigravitary alignment of the different parts of the body.

One of the major positive aspects of an upright position is the possibility of having an improved perception of the environment. In the horizontal plane, the atlanto-occipital joint enables a wide range of head movement, thus allowing the eyes to explore further. The relatively limited support base allows the body to turn rapidly in order to control the environment behind us. In the vertical plane, the lumbosacral spine allows the extension of the head and the trunk in order to explore the environment over our head. Thus, the human posture is an evolution from the quadrupedal motion, offering tremendous possibilities exploring the environment along the three space axes.

The posturographic equipment I developed in the 1970s I called tetra-ataxiometry because it records simultaneously the pressures exerted on the ground by the four supports: right and left toes and right and left heels. It also allows investigating how the free movement of the neck during rotation, extension, and flexion influences the control of the upright position. In other words, the equipment lets us to investigate how abilities that were specific to human beings correlated with motor programs specific to quadrupeds. In the phylogenesis, bipedal posture was relatively recently implemented on quadrupedal motor control, and this can be retraced by observing how a child fights against the force of gravity in the early years of life.

This concept explains the pathogenesis of whiplash associated disorders (WADs) that frequently cause impairments not proportionate to the intensity of the impact. The relatively low energy transferred to the body during an accident specifically affects the two most phylogenetically recent parts of the body – the atlanto-occipital joint and the lumbosacral spine – thus limiting the ability of the body to rotate the head and to extend the head and the trunk. In other words, the whiplash effect makes the human body akin to that of primates. This probably reveals the biological and social importance of WADs.

This second edition is primarily based on the evolutionary concepts of the vestibular system, originating in quadrupeds and advanced in bipeds. The vestibular system supports, in an entirely unique way, perceptual orientation, dynamic body stabilization, retinal image stabilization, and autonomic nervous functions.

This book discusses the different aspects of whiplash, a particular kind of trauma that has a significant impact on the body as a whole. In WADs, pain is an important aspect, but it is only one of the effects, with functional ones being more prevalent. This book is therefore particularly interesting and complete as it focuses both on the painful and the functional aspects of WADs.

Prof. Reuven Kohen-Ratz,
Professor Emeritus of Special Education – Hebrew
University of Jerusalem
Jerusalem, Israel

Preface to Second Edition

The incidence of whiplash injuries has been estimated to be 1/1,000 people per year in the Western world. Chronic spine pain and associated symptoms following whiplash injury cause severe individual burdens of disease and high costs of healthcare systems at least in the Western countries (with the exception of Lithuania and Greece due to specific approach of health system and insurance companies to whiplash associated disorders in these countries).

The first edition of this book was prepared one year before that the Quebec Task Force (QTF) presented the first classification of whiplash associated disorders (WADs). QTF guidelines are still widely accepted both for diagnosis and treatment.

Furthermore, evidence based medicine (EBM) became more and more important in these last 10 years in leading clinicians toward the most effective approach to diseases and disorders, including WADs. However, whiplash mechanism is so complicated to lead to complex disturbances that very frequently they are very difficult to simplify into EBM tracks.

The term "whiplash" dates back to 1928, when the American physician H.E. Crowe used it in a symposium of traffic accidents held in San Francisco. Crowe did not refer to the injury as such, but as the motion of the head and neck that underwent in conjunction with a collision.

The interaction between the accident and the human body is not simply a mechanic interaction. In contrast to mechanical systems in which component parts interact linearly to produce a predictable output, the components of complex systems interact nonlinearly over multiple scales and produce unexpected results. The output of mechanical systems can be controlled by manipulating each one of its parts, while the output of complex systems is dynamic, behaving differently according to initial conditions and feedback. This is the case of whiplash and WADs.

In order to minimize the risk of long-term problems among people with acute whiplash injury, concurrently acute stress disorder (ASD) and/or posttraumatic stress disorder (PTSD) should be diagnosed and adequately treated.

For the above complex reasons, we thought to be necessary an updating of the first edition that takes into account the different challenges to whiplash, the most updated EBM diagnostic and therapeutic indications, and the evolution of QTF guidelines.

More specifically, in this edition, the Editors tried to include all the pathological effects of whiplash and not just the traditional neck and spine effects. The leading idea of this book is the conception of whiplash as a trauma of the body as a whole, obviously with different impact on the different parts of the body. The second leading idea is that the effects of whiplash are substantially unpredictable per se and thus a brain damage has to be expected just like a temporo-mandibular joint disorder or low back pain.

Some problems have been encountered in updating the chapter dedicated to medico-legal aspects. Various studies on how possible insurance compensation may influence the course of whiplash injuries have produced diverging results. Generally, however, there is no evidence indicating any significant difference in the results between those who have applied for such compensation and those who have not.

Furthermore, a common legal procedure about compensation of whiplash injuries in the different countries of the Western world is lacking. For these reasons we focused on management and treatment of patients disorders, but we avoided to include a chapter about medico-legal aspects of WADs.

Finally, we can state that the spirit of this second edition is paying our attention to collect in this book *What's new – What else besides pain – What to do* for patients affected with WADs.

Dario C. Alpini
Guido Brugnoni
Antonio Cesarani

Milan
Milan, Italy
November 2013

Preface to First Edition

This book is based on the proceedings and discussions of a closed workshop held in Santa Margherita Ligure in January 1995.

It was an original scientific experience: no public was admitted. For 3 days the main contributors of this book remained closed in a wonderful hotel.

At the same hotel in the 1930s, Guglielmo Marconi performed his first experiments with radio waves. The hotel was therefore an ideal place, although the problems we discussed were not so "revolutionary" like Marconi's experiments.

On these days round tables, we performed highly restricted meetings on specific topics and presentation of selected papers, only for very few persons, were performed.

Discussions were on definition, ethiopathogenesis, physiopathology, clinical and instrumental evaluations, and medicolegal and therapeutic aspects of whiplash injuries.

All the attendants tried to report and discuss personal experiences and ideas in order to compare them.

All the discussions were especially aimed to prepare the chapters you will read in this book.

We returned to our homes very tired, but very rich in our minds. We really hope that after reading this book you will be as tired as rich.

We are very grateful to Pharmacia, who supported the closed workshop and the preparation of this publication.

Antonio Cesarani
Dario C. Alpini

Milan, Italy

Contents

Whiplash: An Interdisciplinary Challenge

1

A. Cesarani, C.F. Claussen, and D.C. Alpini

Definitions of whiplash syndrome are controversial. Generally speaking, the syndrome comprehends symptoms following a traffic accident, usually a rear-end collision. These symptoms are varied and variably combined:

- Orthopedic, such as neck pain and functional limitation of cervical movements
- Neurological, such as paresthesias
- Audiological, such as tinnitus and hypoacousia
- Otorhinolaryngological, such as dysphagia and dysphonias
- Equilibriometric, such as vertigo and dizziness
- Odontoiatric, such as disturbances of occlusions and temporomandibular joint pain
- Neuropsychological, such as anxiety and attentional disturbances

The term whiplash was used for the first time in 1928 and included several mechanisms. For example, the kinematics of the head-neck movements are different in rear-end collisions than in side collisions, and it is different for the driver rather than the passenger. It is also different if the subjects wore safety belts or not.

Thus, the first challenge is definition. In this book, whiplash injury can be defined as a noncontact quick (« 50 ms) acceleration-deceleration head-neck trauma [1–3].

A. Cesarani
Department of Clinical Sciences and Community Health,
University of Milan, Milan, Italy

Audiology Unit, IRCCS "Ca' Granda" Ospedale Maggiore Policlinico, Milan, Italy
e-mail: antonio.cesarani@unimi.it

C.F. Claussen
Neurootologic and Equilibrium Society (NES), Bad Kissingen, Germany
e-mail: claussensology@gmx.de

D.C. Alpini (✉)
ENT-Otoneurology Service, IRCCS "Don Carlo Gnocchi" Foundation, Milan, Italy
e-mail: dalpini@dongnocchi.it

D.C. Alpini et al. (eds.), *Whiplash Injuries*,
DOI 10.1007/978-88-470-5486-8_1, © Springer-Verlag Italia 2014

Table 1.1 Abbreviated injury score (AIS)

AIS-Code	Injury
0	No injury
1	Minor
2	Moderate
3	Serious
4	Severe
5	Critical
6	Maximum
9	Not further specified (NFS)

The different combinations of symptoms lead to different syndromes so described in the literature: cervical syndrome, traumatic cervical syndrome, cervico-cephalic syndrome, and cervicobrachial syndrome.

Generally, all syndromes are characterized by a plethora of functional symptoms and lack of sufficient objective morphological findings. Either for diagnosis or for therapy, different specialists and examinations are usually necessary; however, visit to different specialists usually leads to different "specialized" diagnosis and treatments.

The second challenge is gathering documentation of the functional and morphological basis for the patient's complaints. Documentation is indispensable for medicolegal expertise and/or for treatment planning.

Due to the complexity and the wide differences of the legal system regarding insurances' approach to WAD, this reedition explains how to document WAD in patients but not how to use this documentation for medicolegal expertise. In this way, medicolegals of the different countries can adapt our information in their specific field of application.

Since a patient's complaint is caused by the trauma that lasts for months and can persist for years, the third challenge is an interdisciplinary approach to the treatment in order to avoid chronic impairment and over specialized therapy.

Whiplash injuries vary from minor to severe. They can be classified according to the Abbreviated Injury Score (Table 1.1). Generally, the evolution of whiplash is divided into three phases:

1. The onset phase, involving local reactions with release of neuromediators such as serotonin, histamine, bradykinin, and classical inflammation [4]
2. The recovery phase, locally characterized by synthesis of new collagen fibers
3. The remodelling phase, in which the neck and the body modify their positions and movement strategies in order to restore normal daily life activities

During whiplash, the kinematics of the cervical spine is completely disrupted (Fig. 1.1). During the impact, the vertebrae do not reciprocally move harmonically such as during physiological antero- and retroflexion of the neck. Whiplash is characterized by transient, but not always temporary, reciprocal inversions of the different cervical segments [5–7]. For example, in the last phase of anteroflexion, inversions in segments CI–C2 and CO–Cl have been observed, while in the second phase of retroflexion, an inversion of the segment CO–Cl happens [8, 9]. The reciprocal inversions lead to ligament and soft tissue lesions, with a segmental

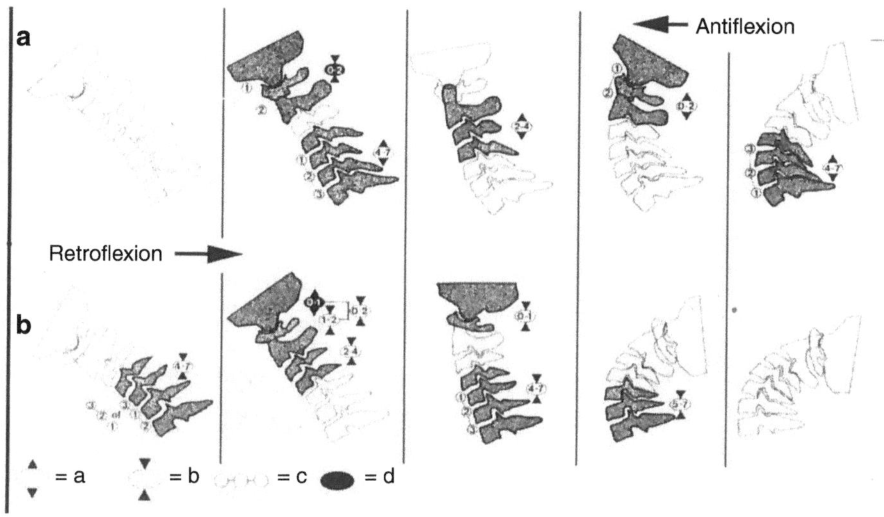

Fig. 1.1 Modification of reciprocal positions of cervical spine segments during antero-(**a**) and retroflexion (**b**) in whiplash mechanisms. In the initial phase of anteroflexion Cl–C2 and CO–C2 invert their position (**a**). In the second phase of retroflexion, inversion of CO–Cl is observed. a: flexion; b: extension; c: sequence; d: inversion symptoms

dysregulation causing a specific activation of nociceptive inputs and consequent somatomotor and sympathetic-motor dysfunctions [1]. The nociceptive inputs, via interneurons and alpha-motoneurons, provoke a dysregulation of motoneurons for the flexors and extensors leading to an asymmetrical hypertonus. The latter [10, 11] is generally observed in the trapezius and sternocleidomastoid with consequent compression of the accessorius nerve, and in scaleni with compression of the brachial plexus, responsible for paresthesias. The dysregulation of the orthosympathetic cervical system causes activation of vasoconstrictive subsystems, not always localized to the involved segments. Vasoconstriction induces dystrophic impairment contributing to the cervicofacial and cervicobrachial symptoms.

The ganglion cervicalis superius is localized at the CI–C4 segment and innervates the neck and upper respiratory and digestive tracts [12].

The cervicobrachial sympathetic complex from C5 to Th1, along with the postganglionate synapses in the cervical medius ganglion (C5–C6) and inferius (C7–C8), innervates the medium parts of the respiratory and digestive tracts.

Cervico- and craniospinal injuries during acceleration-deceleration lead to head/neck proprioception disruption causing transient, sometimes permanent, abnormal proprioceptive information regarding the reciprocal position of the neck, head, and trunk. In Fig. 1.2, the so-called spinocerebello-vestibulospinal circuitry is shown. General proprioception information (from muscles, ligaments, and joints) is integrated and elaborated in the cerebellum together with special proprioception information from maculae and cristae. From the cerebellum, efferent pathways return to spinal motoneurons through another elaboration in the vestibular nuclei (with special regard to the lateral Deiter's nucleus) [13–16].

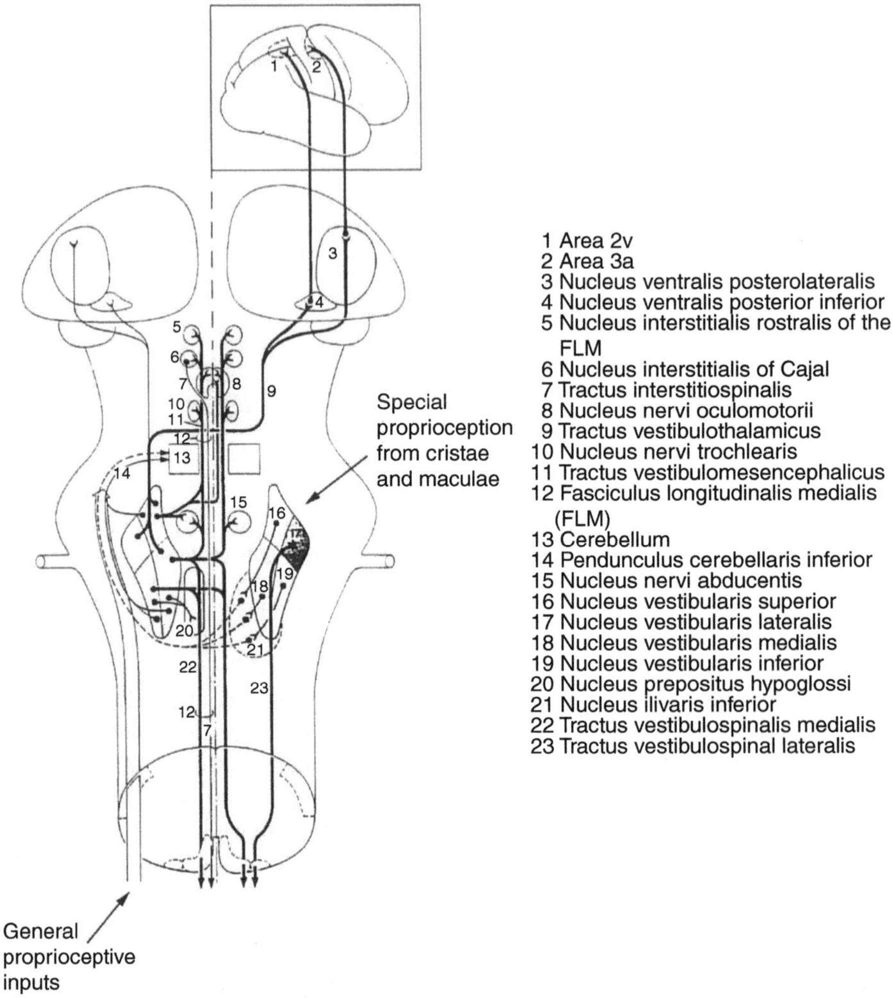

Fig. 1.2 The connections of the vestibular system: efferent connections of the vestibular nuclei and the spinocerebello-vestibulospinal circuitry

This circuitry is the anatomo-neurophysiological basis needed to understand why an apparent segmental injury often becomes an injury of the whole individual. Equilibrium disorders can be directly caused by perturbation of the integration of general and special proprioception due to abnormal peripheral inputs from the neck or for central dysfunction, particularly of the brainstem [17–20].

Whiplash is a true head trauma even if there is no contact of the head with an object. Cerebral contusions or intracranial bleeding are extremely rare, but abducens mono and bilateral palsy [21] and laryngeal palsy have been described [22]. Neurovegetative symptoms and affective-cognitive symptoms are as frequent as in post-commotional syndromes and are characterized by hyperesthetic emotional and neuroasthenic symptoms including tinnitus, dysphasia, nausea, unsteadiness, and vertigo [23–29].

True neuropsychological disorders are frequent after whiplash. Typically, especially 6–8 months after the trauma, psychological symptoms appear: restlessness, nervousness, anxiety, emotional instability, difficulties in concentration, and depression. In 15–25 %, this neuropsychological syndrome can evolve chronically and can be misdiagnosed as an "indemnity syndrome." Experimental postmortem studies showed focal contusions in frontal and temporal cortex, corpus callosum, subcortical structures, diencephalon, and subdural and subarachnoid microbleeding as consequences of sudden angular accelerations. Rarely, alterations are macroscopic, while generally, microscopic lesions have been revealed [30–33].

One of the central networks involved in post-whiplash disorders is the ascending reticular activating system (ARAS). Experimental studies showed involvement of the ARAS especially for transitory accelerations. In Ommaya's hypothesis [34, 35], the centripetal forces during acceleration-deceleration lead to an abnormal stretching of the cerebrum with, furthermore, a sudden transient increase of the pressure of the cerebrospinal fluid [36]. In this hypothesis, whiplash provokes a commotio cerebri with potential injuries of temporal cortex, amygdala, hippocampus, medial temporal cortex, corpora mamillaria, medial thalamus, basal nuclei, prefrontal cortex, and retrosplenial cingulate cortex. All these structures may be involved in the genesis of neuropsychological symptoms [2, 37, 38].

The cerebral effects of whiplash have been studied also by electroencephalography (EEG). After a period ranging from 1 to 9 years in patients with a chronic whiplash syndrome, EEG alterations have been observed with percentages ranging from 30 to 49 %.

Glucose cerebral metabolism has been investigated by positron-emission tomography (PET) [39], and alterations have been shown in the frontal and temporal cortex and in nucleus caudatus. Lesions of frontal cortex are responsible for attentional disorders.

Pathogenesis of otoneurological disorders is still debated and includes the following explanations:

- Mechanical compression with dynamic stenosis of the vertebral artery
- Sympathetic abnormal stimulation
- Proprioceptive disorders especially from the cervical and lumbar regions [40, 41]
- Central vestibular system disorder

Probably, equilibrium disorders derive from different combinations of different mechanisms. The kinematics of the acceleration-deceleration are different, for example, for the driver, who usually opposes the trauma by means of his/her arms on the wheel, and the passenger, who usually receives, completely and passively, the impact forces. Differences can be observed if patients did or did not wear safety belts during the impact: with safety belts the movement of the head and the neck is not sagittal but torsional with the first dorsal vertebra as fulcrum. The sense of the torsional component is different: clockwise for the passenger, counterclockwise for the driver. Furthermore, the impact is rarely caused by a perfect sagittal rear-end collision, while very often, the impact causes a rotational acceleration of the car. Torsional and angular accelerations cause microlesions in different parts of the brain, and this can lead to different combinations of signs and symptoms in the so-called whiplash syndrome [42].

Torsional and rotational acceleration-deceleration can lead to cranio-mandibular dysfunctions, too. Computer simulations [43] showed an initial derangement of condylus position with a myogenic secondary reaction during hyperextension and consequent modification of the condylus position. During hyperflexion, the retropositioning of the condylus leads to a compression of the posterior ligament rich in vessels and proprioceptors [44–47].

Following whiplash either for mechanical lesions of cervical dynamic or for central dysfunctions, some modifications of patient posture are usually observed [48]: the head modifies its position according to an antalgic flexion; the head reduces its rotational and lateroflexion movements. During subject movements, the rotation of the body is along the trunk and not the neck, the trunk is ipsilaterally rotated with respect to the side of the lesion, the pelvis is rotated according to head antalgic position, and the position of center of gravity (CoG) is modified. In the months following the trauma, erector paravertebral muscles become hypotonic, and the prevalence of flexors induces a forward displacement of the CoG facilitating forward falling. Rotation of the trunk increases unsteadiness, and forward CoG displacement provokes a relative flexion of the legs to oppose falling and derangement of normal ankle and hip strategies. In fact, Equitest shows a prevalence of ankle strategies and delayed motor control test latencies either in backward or in forward translations.

From a cybemetic point of view, equilibrium disorders are provoked by distortion and desynchronization of the proprioceptive chain:

- Modification of the proprioceptive cervical inputs to the vestibular nuclei and reticular formation
- Desynchronization between special vestibular inputs and general cervical inputs regarding head position and movement
- Modification of the cervico-spinal reflexes

If desynchronizations of proprioceptive signals "force" the limits of the patient's equilibrium system calibration (see Chap. 29), the system is not able to adapt and it becomes dysfunctional: vertigo and dizziness appear.

Thus, the fourth challenge is correct treatment of an apparently localized injury that causes a systemic dysfunction. The treatment must be planned on the basis of an accurate functional local and systemic diagnosis. In the acute phase, treatment is aimed at reducing the impairment that is principally caused by local dysfunction. In the immediate post-acute phase, impairment is due to the dysregulation of somatic and vegetative reflexes at the involved spinal segment level. This dysregulation, if not correctly treated, can lead to the so-called chronic phase of segmental impairment. Further evolution of the syndrome includes non-segmental dysregulation: primary damage induces secondary damage. The chronic syndrome can lead to disability with motor dysfunction of the patient, usually combined with vertigo and dizziness. Rarely, motor dysfunction leads to social handicap with working and/or attending to normal daily life activity.

Rehabilitation is generally the treatment of choice either in acute or in chronic syndromes, and it is usually combined with drugs [49] and with both physical [50–54] and instrumental therapies. Rehabilitation is aimed either at the treatment of the spine or at ataxia and motor uncoordination. In the chronic phase, rehabilitation must also include instruction for ergonomic daily life activities [55, 56].

References

1. Foreman SM, Croft AC (1988) Whiplash injuries. The cervical acceleration/deceleration syndrome. Williams & Wilkins, Baltimore
2. Jenkins A et al (1986) Brain lesions detected by magnetic resonance imaging in mild and severe head injuries. Lancet 23:445–446
3. McKenzie JA, Williams JF (1975) The effect of collision severity on the motion of the head and neck during "whiplash". J Biomech 8:257–259
4. Dooms GC et al (1985) Mr imaging of intramuscular hemorrhage. J Comput Assist Tomogr 9:908913
5. White AA III, Panjabi M (1978) Clinical biomechanics of the spine. Lippincott, Philadelphia
6. Wilmink JT, Penning L (1987) Rotation of the cervical spine. A CT study in normal subjects. Spine 12:732–738
7. Wismans JSHM et al (1986) Omni-directional human head-neck response. In: 30th Stapp Car Crash conference proceedings, San Diego, SAE paper 861893. Society of Automotive Engineers, Warrendale
8. Wike BD (1967) The neurology of joints. Ann R Coll Surg Engl 41:2550
9. Wyke BD (1979) Neurology of cervical joints. Physiotherapy 65:72–76
10. Hinoki M, Kurosawa T (1964) Note on vertigo of cervical origin. Pract Otol (Kyoto) 57:10–20
11. Hinoki M (1985) Vertigo due to whiplash injury: a neurotological approach. Acta Otolaryngol Suppl 419:9–29
12. Miura Y, Tanaka M (1970) Disturbances of the venous system in the head and neck regions in rabbits with whiplash injury. Brain Nerve Inj (Tokyo) 2:217–223
13. Drukker J, van der Wal JC (1990) Centrai verbindingen van het vestibulaire apparaat. In: Fischer AJEM, Oosterveld WJ (eds) Duizeligheid en Evenwichtsstoomissen. Data Medica, Utrecht, pp 29–45
14. Drukker J, Jansen JC (1975) Compendium anatomie. De Tijdstroom, Lochem
15. Igarashi M et al (1972) Nystagmus after experimental cervical lesions. Laryngoscope 2:1609–1621
16. Ikeda K, Kobayashi T (1967) Mechanisms and origin of so-called whiplash injury. Clin Surg 22:1655–1660
17. Dichgans J et al (1974) The role of vestibular and neck afferents during eye-head coordination in the monkey. Brain Res 71:225–232
18. Doerr M et al (1984) Eye movements during active head turning with different vestibular and cervical input. Acta Otolaryngol 98:14–20
19. Doerr M et al (1991) Tonic cervical stimulation: does it influence eye position and eye movements in man? Acta Otolaryngol 111:2–9
20. Gray LP (1956) Extralabyrinthine vertigo due to cervical muscle lesions. J Laryngol Otol I70:352–361
21. Shifrin LZ (1991) Bilateral abducens nerve palsy after cervical spine extension injury. Spine 16:374–375
22. Helliwell M et al (1984) Bilateral vocal cord paralysis due to whiplash injury. Br Med J 6:1876–1877
23. Dikmen S' et al (1986) Neuropsychological and psychological consequences of minor head injury. J Neurol Neurosurg Psychiatry 49:1227–1232

24. Merskey K (1984) Psychiatry and the cervical sprain syndrome. Can Med Assoc J 1: 1119–1121
25. Miller Fisher C (1982) Whiplash amnesia. Neurology 32:667–668
26. Olsnes BT (1989) Neurobehavioral findings in whiplash patients with long-lasting symptoms. Acta Neurol Scand 80:584–588
27. Rowe MC, Carlson C (1980) Brainstem auditory evoked potentials in post-concussion dizziness. Arch Neurol I37:670–683
28. Rubin W (1973) Whiplash with vestibular involvement. Arch Otolaryngol 97:85–87
29. Winston KR (1987) Whiplash and its relationship to migraine. Headache 27:452–457
30. Sa H et al (1988) Whiplash syndrome: fact or fiction? Orthop Clin North Am 19:791–795
31. Hodgson SP, Grundy M (1989) Whiplash injuries: their long-term prognosis and its relationship to compensation. Neuro Orthop 7:88–91
32. Miller H (1961) Accident neurosis. Br Med J 1:919–925
33. Zomeren AH, Brouwer WH (1990) Attentional deficits after closed head injury. In: Deelman BG et al (eds) Traumatic brain injury: clinical, social and rehabilitational aspects. Swets & Zeintlinger, Amsterdam/Lisse, pp 33–48
34. Ommaya AK et al (1968) Whiplash and brain damage. JAMA 204:75–79
35. Ommaya AK (1988) Mechanisms and preventive management of head injuries: a paradigm for injury control. In: 32nd annual proceedings of Association of the Advancement of Automobile Medicine, Seattle, WA, Sept 12–14 1988
36. Swenson MY et al (1990) Transient pressure changes in the spinal canal under whiplash motion. Report R-008. Department of Injury Prevention, Chalmers University of Technology, Gothenburg
37. Hofstad H, Gjerde IO (1985) Transient global amnesia after whiplash trauma. J Neurol Neurosurg Psychiatry 48:956–957
38. Kischka U et al (1991) Cerebral symptoms following whiplash injury. Eur Neurol 31:136–140
39. Humayun MS et al (1989) Local cerebral glucose abnormalities in mild closed head injured patients with cognitive impairments. Nucl Med Commun 10:335–344
40. Thodem U, Mergner T (1984) Effects of proprioceptive inputs on vestibulo-ocular an vestibulospinal mechanisms. Prog Brain Res 76:109–119
41. Ushio N et al (1973) Studies on ataxia of lumbar origin in cases of vertigo due to whiplash injury. Agressologie 14:73–82
42. Campana BC (1988) Cervical hyperextension injuries and low back pain. In: Rosen P (ed) Emergency medicine, vol I. CV Mosby, Philadelphia, pp 799–817
43. Kronn E (1990) A study on the incidence of temporomandibular dysfunction due to internal derangement in patients who have suffered from a whiplash injury. Dublin School of Physiotherapy, Dublin
44. Eckerdahl O (1991) The petrotympanic fissure: a link connecting the tympanic cavity and the temporomandibular joint. Cranio 9:15–21
45. Lader E (1983) Cervical trauma as a factor in the development of TMJ dysfunction and facial pain. Cranio 1:86–90
46. McGlone R et al (1988) Trigeminal pain due to whiplash injury. Injury 19:366
47. Roydhouse RH (1973) Whiplash and temporomandibular dysfunction. Lancet 1394–1395
48. McElhaney JH et al (1976) Handbook of human tolerance. Report Japan Automobile Research Institute Inc, Yataba-Chuo, Tsukuba
49. Vink R et al (1988) Treatment with the thyrotropin-releasing hormone analog CG 3703 restores magnesium homeostasis following traumatic brain injury in rats. Brain Res 460:184–188
50. McKinney LA (1989) Early mobilisation and outcome in acute sprains of the neck. Br Med J 299:1006–1008
51. Mealy K et al (1986) Early mobilisation of acute whiplash injuries. Br Med J 292:656–657
52. Odent M (1975) La réflexotherapie lombaire. Nouv Presse Med 4:26

53. Rydevik B, Szpalaski M, Acbi M, Gunzburg R (2008) Whiplash injuries and associated disorders: new insights into an old problem. Eur Spine J 17:359–416
54. Seletz E (1958) Whiplash injuries: neurophysiological basis for pain and methods used for rehabilitation. JAMA 168:1750–1755
55. Fitz-Ritson D (1990) The chiropractic management and rehabilitation of cervical trauma. J Manipulative Physiol Ther 13:17–25
56. Foley-Nolan D et al (1990) Post whiplash dystonia well controlled by TENS: case report. J Trauma 30:909–910

Part I

General Aspects

Epidemiology of Whiplash-Associated Disorders

2

F. Ioppolo and R.S. Rizzo

Until recently, there was no consensus on the definition of whiplash. According to the Quebec Task Force (QTF) on whiplash-associated disorders (WAD), "whiplash is an acceleration-deceleration mechanism of energy transfer to the neck. It may result from rear-end or side-impact motor vehicle collisions, but can also occur during diving or other mishaps. The impact may result in bony or soft-tissue injuries (whiplash-injury), which in turn may lead to a variety of clinical manifestations called Whiplash-Associated Disorders."[1] Patients with whiplash can be classified by the severity of signs and symptoms: Grade 0 means no complaints or physical signs; Grade 1 indicates neck complaints (such as pain, tenderness, and stiffness) but no physical signs; Grade 2 indicates neck complaints and musculoskeletal signs (such as a decreased range of motion or muscle weakness); and Grade 3 and Grade 4 indicate neck complaints and, respectively, neurological signs (such as sensory deficit) or fracture or dislocation.

The incidence of whiplash injury varies between different parts of the world, with rates as high as 70 per 100,000 inhabitants in Quebec [1], 106 per 100,000 in Australia [2], and 188–325 per 100,000 inhabitants in the Netherlands [3]. Versteegen also reported a sharp increase in whiplash injuries from 1989 to 1995 in the Netherlands, in conjunction with a more or less stable pattern of seat belt use [4].

F. Ioppolo (✉)
Department of Physical Medicine and Rehabilitation,
"Sapienza" University,
Piazzale Aldo Moro 5, 00185 Rome, Italy
e-mail: francescoioppolo@yahoo.it

R.S. Rizzo
Department of Physical Medicine and Rehabilitation,
"Sapienza" University,
Piazzale Aldo Moro 5, 00185 Rome, Italy

Physical Medicine and Rehabilitation Unit,
Nomentana Hospital, Largo Berloco 1, Fonte Nuova,
Rome 00010, Italy

D.C. Alpini et al. (eds.), *Whiplash Injuries*,
DOI 10.1007/978-88-470-5486-8_2, © Springer-Verlag Italia 2014

Moreover, Versteegen et al. identified patients who complained of neck pain after having been involved in a traffic accident and gone to an emergency room. Over a 20-year period, they found a tenfold increase in such visits, from an average annual incidence of 3.4 visits per 100,000 inhabitants (1970–1974) to 40.2 visits per 100,000 (1990–1994) [5].

Richter reported an increase of whiplash injuries in drivers injured in motor vehicle collisions in Hanover, Germany; these went from less than 10 % in 1985 to more than 30 % in 1997 [6].

The cumulative incidence of patients seeking healthcare for whiplash arising from a road traffic accident has increased during the last 30 years to recent estimates of >3/1,000 inhabitants in North America and Western Europe [7] and between 1.0 and 3.2/1,000 inhabitants in Sweden [8].

A 1983–1984 hospital-based study from the UK (which included persons going to the hospital for evaluation of WAD symptoms) reported an annual incidence of WAD of 27.8 (95%CI 23.6–32.6) per 100,000 inhabitants [9]. In the UK, insurance statistics indicate that 300,000 patients present per annum with whiplash-associated disorders [10].

With annual North American incidence rates estimated to be between 70 and 329 per 100,000 people [1, 11], whiplash injuries are the most common injury following a motor vehicle collision [4, 12]. Indeed, in 2000, whiplash was the most common emergency room-treated motor vehicle injury in the USA [4]. In the Canadian province of Saskatchewan, 83 % of traffic injury claims were for whiplash during 1994–1995, giving an annual incidence of 677 insurance claims per 100,000 adult population [13].

Incidence data for WAD are based mainly on study settings such as emergency room visits and insurance injury claims.

In literature, there are no published studies regarding the Italian epidemiology of WAD. Thus, data collection comes from the "Casellario Centrale Infortuni," which includes data on damage to the person with particular reference to those covered by "RC Auto" insurance [14].

Specifically, in 2009, there were 491,736 reports made to the CCI, 355,334 of which involved the cervical rachis. Of these latter, 218,754 qualify for definition as whiplash. Whiplash represented 44.5 % of all accidents.

In 2010, there was a notable decrease in the overall number of accidents and cases of whiplash. There were 130,433 cases of whiplash, which represents 42.8 % of all accidents.

2.1 Factors Associated with WAD

One potentially important factor for risk of WAD is the severity of impact, but no method exists to assess this in a standardized way. However, various preventive devices have a protective effect in passenger cars in rear-end collisions [7].

Although it seems that females are at slightly greater risk of WAD, the evidence of gender as a risk factor for seeking healthcare or making a claim for WAD is not consistent [15, 16].

Younger persons (aged 18–23) seem to be at greater risk of making insurance claims and/or being treated for WAD [13].

There is some evidence that neck pain before a collision might be a risk factor for acute neck pain after a rear-end collision [17]. Today, there are no scientifically admissible studies examining the effect of psychological, social, genetic, and cultural factors in the onset of WAD after traffic collision [7].

2.2 Prognosis

The Quebec Task Force states that whiplash injuries have favorable prognosis and their conclusion is that the 87 % and the 97 % of the patients recovered (recovery is defined by authors as cessation of time-loss compensation) from their injury at 6 and 12 months after the vehicle collision, respectively. Statement and conclusion are questionable. Whether these patients still had pain or discomfort and needed medical care, it was not reported. A review contradicted the QTF's conclusions that most whiplash injuries were short-lived [18]. These authors concluded that between 14 and 42 % of the whiplash patients developed chronic complaints (longer than 6 months) and that 10 % of those had constant severe pain. Internationally, the proportion of chronic complaints varies between 2 and 58 % [19, 20], but lies mainly between 20 and 40 %. Other studies observed that the proportion of patients who report pain and disability 6 months after the accident varies between 19 and 60 % [21, 22].

Various studies of how possible insurance compensation may influence the course of WAD have produced diverging results, but according to Jansen et al. [23], there is no evidence indicating any significant differences between those patients who have applied for such compensation and those who have not.

Regarding the economic cost due both to management of whiplash disorders and time off work, epidemiological results are limited, but it could be estimated as $3.9 billion in the USA and €10 billion in Europe in a year [24].

References

1. Spitzer WO, Skovron ML, Salmi LR, Cassidy JD, Duranceau J, Suissa S et al (1995) Scientific monograph of the Quebec Task Force on Whiplash Associated Disorders: redefining 'whiplash' and its management. Spine 20(8 Suppl):8S–58S
2. Miles KA, Maimaris C, Finlay D, Barnes MR (1988) The incidence and prognostic significance of radiological abnormalities in soft tissue injuries to the cervical spine. Skeletal Radiol 17:493–496
3. Wismans KSHM, Huijkens CG (1994) Incidentie en prevalentie van het 'whiplash'-trauma. TNO report 94. R.B.V.041. TNO Road-Vehicle Research Institute, Delft
4. Versteegen GJ, Kingma J, Meijler WJ et al (2000) Neck sprain after motor vehicle accidents in drivers and passengers. Eur Spine J 9:547–552
5. Versteegen GJ, Kingma J, Meijler WJ et al (1998) Neck sprain in patients injured in car accidents: a retrospective study covering the period 1970–1994. Eur Spine J 7:195–200

6. Richter M, Otte E, Pohlemann T et al (2000) Whiplash-type neck distortion in restrained car drivers; frequency, causes and long-term results. Eur Spine J 9:109–117
7. Holm LW, Carroll LJ, Cassidy JD et al (2008) The burden and determinants of neck pain in Whiplash associated disorders after traffic collisions, results of the Bone and Joint Decade 2000–2010 Task Force on Neck pain and its Associated Disorders. Spine 33(4 Suppl):S52–S59
8. Jansen GB, Edlund C, Grane P et al (2008) The Swedish Society of Medicine and the Whiplash Commission Medical Task Force. Whiplash injuries: diagnosis and early management. Eur Spine J 17(Suppl 3):S359–S418
9. Otremski I, Marsh JL, Wilde BR et al (1989) Soft tissue cervical spinal injuries in motor vehicle accidents. Injury 20:349–351
10. Burton K (2003) Treatment guidelines: is there a need? In: Proceedings of Whiplash Conference 2003, Bath, England, 6–8 May. Lyons Davidson Solicitors, Bristol
11. Quinlan KP, Annest JL, Myers B, Ryan G, Hill H (2004) Neck strains and sprains among motor vehicle occupants – United States, 2000. Accid Anal Prev 36:21–27
12. Berglund A, Alfredsson L, Jensen I, Bodin L, Nygren A (2003) Occupant-and crash-Related factors associated with risk of whiplash injury. Ann Epidemiol 13:66–72
13. Cassidy JD, Carroll LJ, Côté P et al (2000) Effect of eliminating compensation for pain and suffering on the outcome of insurance claims for whiplash injury. N Engl J Med 342: 1179–1186
14. Il Casellario Centrale Infortuni, Rapporto Statistico (2011) http://casellario.inail.it/repository/ContentManagement/information/N115396216/RapportoStatisticoCasellario2011.pdf
15. Bjornstig U, Hildingsson C, Toolanen G (1990) Soft-tissue injury of the neck in a hospital based material. Scand J Soc Med 18:263–267
16. Bring G, Bjornstig U, Westman G (1996) Gender patterns in minor head and neck injuries: an analysis of casualty register data. Accid Anal Prev 28:359–369
17. Obelieniene D, Schrader H, Bovim G, Miseviciene I, Sand T (1999) Pain after whiplash: a prospective controlled inception cohort study. J Neurol Neurosurg Psychiatry 66(3):279–283
18. Barnsley L, Lord S, Bogduk N (1994) Whiplash injury: clinical review. Pain 58(3):283–307
19. Coté P, Cassidy JD, Carroll L, Frank JW, Bombardier C (2001) A systematic review of the prognosis of acute whiplash and a new conceptual framework to synthesize the literature. Spine 26:E445–E458
20. Scholten-Peeters GGM, Verhagen AP, Bekkering GE, van der Windt DAWM, Barnsley L, Oostendorp RAB et al (2003) Prognostic factors of whiplash-associated disorders: a systematic review of prospective cohort studies. Pain 104:303–322
21. Freeman MD, Croft AC, Rossignol AM (1998) Whiplash associated disorders: refining whiplash and its management. The Quebec Task Force. Spine 23:1043–1049
22. Stovner LJ (1996) The nosologic status of the whiplash syndrome: a critical review based on a methodological approach. Spine 21:2735–2746
23. Jansen GB, Edlund C, Grane P, Hildingsson C, Karlberg M, Link H, Måwe U, Portala K, Rydevik B, Sterner Y, Swedish Society of Medicine; Whiplash Commission Medical Task Force (2008). Whiplash injuries: diagnosis and early management. The Swedish Society of Medicine and the Whiplash Commission Medical Task Force. Eur Spine J 17 (Suppl 3):S355–S417
24. Eck JC, Hodges SD, Humphreys SC (2001) Whiplash: a review of a commonly misunderstood injury. Am J Med 110:651–656

Functional Anatomy 3

C.L. Romanò, A. Mondini, S. Brambilla, and F. Ioppolo

The anterior faces of the cervical column is composed by a median portion made of the overlapping of the vertebral bodies which include the intervertebral disks on top of the bodies. This median portion is at first narrowed on the top (15 mm) and is progressively broadened toward the bottom, reaching 25–30 mm at the last cervical metamer.

The superior vertebral plate of the vertebral bodies that go from C3 to C7 ends laterally with two osseous raised portions directed toward the top, called unciform processes or uncus. These are included with the corresponding incisions on the lateral inferior side of the above vertebral body, functionally behaving like true articulations (Von Luschka articulations) that limit the lateral slant movement of the head.

Laterally, in correspondence of the top half of the vertebral bodies, the reliefs of the transverse processes can be noticed, and they end laterally with their anterior tuberculum. Of the latter, the C6 is called Chassaignac's tuberculum and represents an important surgical traceable point, since it is more neatly developed in respect to the others (Fig. 3.1) [1, 2].

The intertransversal foramina are found in the middle of the transverse processes and give way to the vertebral arteries which penetrate in most cases in C6, with its veins, the vegetative nerve, and the rachis nerve.

C.L. Romanò
Center of Reconstructive Surgery and Osteoarticular Infection,
IRCCS "Galeazzi" Orthopedic Institute, via R. Galeazzi, 4,
20161 Milan, Italy

A. Mondini • S. Brambilla
"G. Pini" Orthopedic Institute, Via Rugabella 4,
20122 Milan, Italy

F. Ioppolo (✉)
Department of Physical Medicine and Rehabilitation,
"Sapienza" University, Piazzale Aldo Moro 5,
00185 Rome, Italy
e-mail: francescoioppolo@yahoo.it

D.C. Alpini et al. (eds.), *Whiplash Injuries*,
DOI 10.1007/978-88-470-5486-8_3, © Springer-Verlag Italia 2014

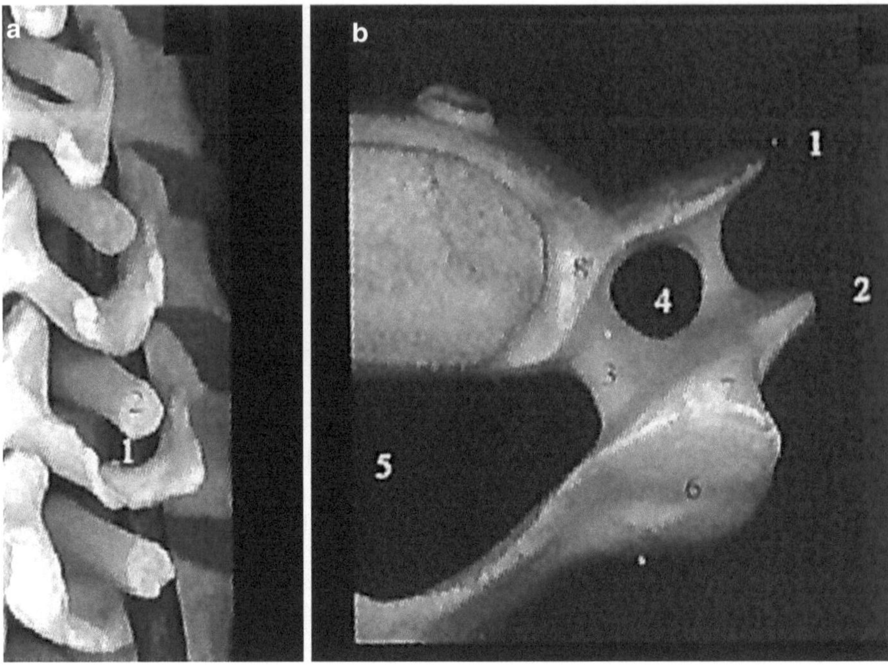

Fig. 3.1 (**a**) Lateral view: vertebral artery (1) and rachis nerve (2) passing by the conjugate foramen. (**b**) Transversal section: intertansversal foramen (4). Anterior tuberculum (1); posterior tuberculum of the transverse process, peduncle (3); spinal channel (5); articular mass (6) with the superior articular facet (7); uncus (8)

The posterior faces shows the reliefs of the spinal apophysis from C2 to C6 on the median line, and both sides of the spinal apophysis extend to two osseous plates that end on both sides: the first paramedian includes the series of the vertebral laminae, lightly oblique externally, interrupted transversally by the narrow depression of the interlaminar spaces. The second lateral side is formed by the overlapping of the zygapophyseal articular processes and extends itself to the frontal plane for a median width of 15 mm.

The external border of this side is easily found because it is blunt and sticks out like a step [3].

A cavity separates the medial borders from the plane of the laminae: it represents an important surgical traceable point because in front of it passes the vertebral artery (Fig. 3.2).

Viewed in the lateral projection, the cervical column shows an anterior portion formed by the alignment of the vertebral bodies, the intervertebral disks, two series of reliefs of the transverse processes, and by a series of articular processes. The latter are piled on top of others to form the overall posterior articulations, characterized by an articular oblique interline, below and behind, forming an angular variation of 30–50° from the horizontal line. This inclination makes the superior articular process of each vertebra lay on a more anterior plane, with respect to the inferior articulation of the same vertebra. The inferior articular process of a vertebra overlaps on the superior articular process of the vertebra underneath (Fig. 3.3).

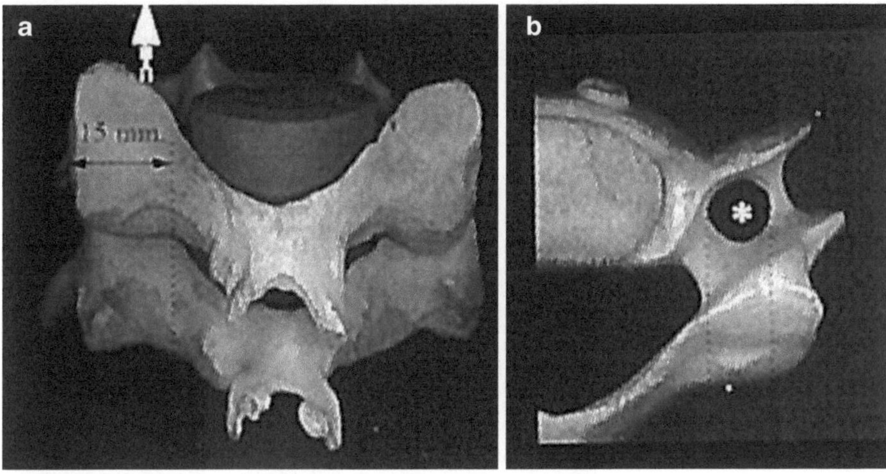

Fig. 3.2 (**a**) Posterior view: the articular mass has a mean width of 15 mm; a sulcus (*dotted line*), well appreciable at surgery, separates the articular mass from the lamina; the *white arrow* shows the projection of the vertebral artery. (**b**) Transversal section: the *dotted line* shows the projections or the intertransversal foramen (*asterisk*) on the articular mass

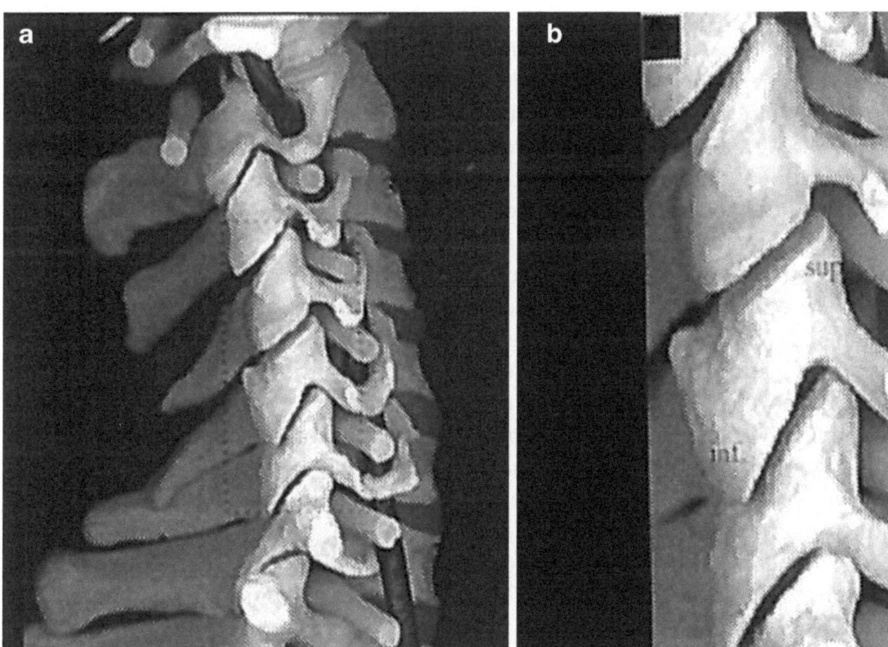

Fig. 3.3 (**a**) Lateral view: the articular mass are superimposed to form the plane of the posterior zygapophyseal joints. (**b**) Detail of the zygapophyseal joint with their obliqueness ranges from 30 to 50° with respect to the horizontal plane

The transverse processes are inserted in front of the articular columns via the connecting roots: an anterior one to the side of the vertebral body and the other one posterior to the side of the articular columns, forming a cavity in front and out of the

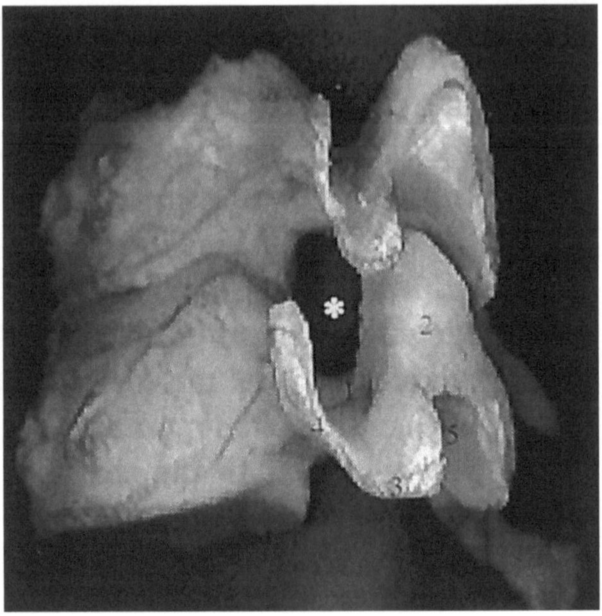

Fig. 3.4 Conjugate foramen (*asterisk*). *(1)* peduncle; (2) articular mass; (3) transverse process; (4) anterior tuberculum; (5) posterior tuberculum

conjugate foramen, through which the nerve roots abandon the rachis. The conjugate foramen is delimited superiorly and inferiorly by the peduncles in the anterior part, by the half inferior-posterior portion of the vertebral body, the lateral-posterior faces of the intervertebral disk and the unciform processes and in the posterior portion by the posterior articulation, reinforced on the anterior faces by the yellow ligament. It lies on a mildly oblique plane 20° below the horizontal plane, in front and out about 30° of the frontal plane. It has median dimensions of 12 mm in height, 6 mm in width, and from 6 to 8 mm in height (Fig. 3.4) [4, 5].

These dimensions are influenced by the movements of the rachis; in fact, the conjugate foramina are open during flexion, lateral angulation, and rotation movements on the opposite side. They close during extension, lateral angulation, and rotation movement on the same side. The horizontal or transverse section includes the vertebral cavity, anteriorly delimited by the laminae and yellow ligaments, laterally by the articular mass and by the peduncles. The vertebral foramen in the inferior cervical rachis assumes a grossly triangular form with blunted angles; the dimensions present great individual variability in the transverse and posterior diameter. The figures at both ends of anthropometric studies vary from 19 to 29 mm in the transverse sense from C3 to C7 and from 10 to 19 mm in the anteroposterior sense from C3 to C7 [6].

The peduncles constitute osseous bridges that connect the vertebral bodies and the articular mass; their distribution is along an oblique axis directed anteriorly and medially with an angle of about 20°. On the cross section, they have an oval form with an axis of 10 by 7 mm. Because of the small dimensions and the tight connection close to the vertebral artery with the nerve root in the cervical rachis, the peduncles are not considered to be good joining structures, rather the articular mass is preferred [7].

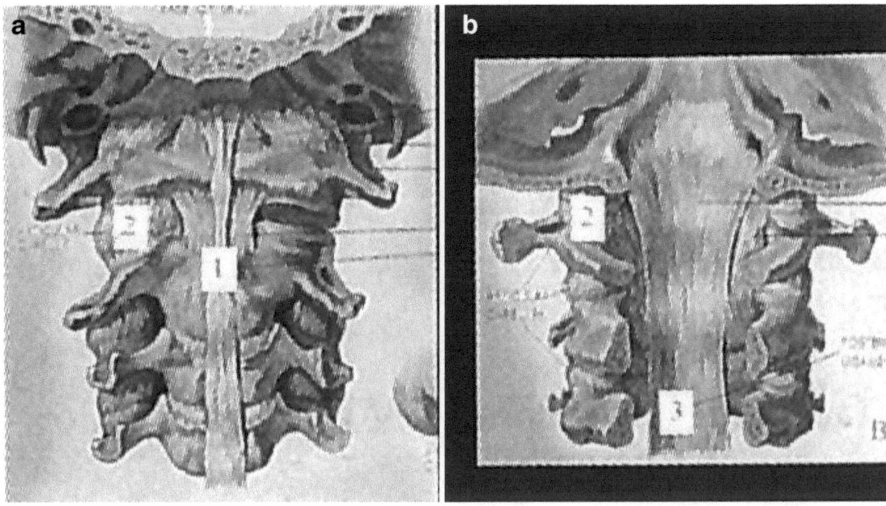

Fig. 3.5 (**a**) Frontal view: anterior longitudinal ligament *(J)* and zygapophyseal joints (2). (**b**) Posterior view: after removal of posterior arch: posterior longitudinal ligament (3)

The cervical metamers are joined together with the capsular ligament, essential for vertebral stability [8, 9]. The anterior longitudinal ligament is a thin ribbonlike translucent structure that without interruption extends itself on to the anterior faces of the vertebral bodies. It is intimately connected to the vertebral limitants and to the intervertebral disk, tightly adhering to the fibers of the annulus fibrosus and to a lesser degree with the central portion of the vertebral body, resulting less extent in width (Fig. 3.5). The annulus fibrosus appears tightly connected to the cartilage of the vertebral plates in the peripheral part, practically in continuity with the anterior and posterior longitudinal ligament [10, 11]. The posterior longitudinal ligament is a ribbonlike structure that extends itself along the posterior faces of the vertebral bodies, connected to the limitants and to the disk but separated from the central concave portion of the vertebral body. Its transverse extension becomes smaller from top to bottom, thereby increasing its width, which is always greater than that of anterior longitudinal ligament (which reaches 3 mm). It limits the flexion of the rachis and the movement of the vertebral bodies, protecting the spinal cord from herniations of the discal material in a median position, while laterally leaving a breach for releasing the discal material in the connecting channel.

The articular capsules are made of dense fibrous tissue tightly attached to the osseous ends that extend horizontally for 5–7 mm. The capsular ligaments have fibers that are orthogonal faces, and this allows some degree of controlled movement. When the articular faces are in the neutral position, the fibers are more relaxed. At the limit of their articular excursion, the fibers are tenser, due to their orientation, limiting movement to a maximum of 3 mm with respect to the neutral position. Even the orientation of the articular faces allows flexion of the column (a controlled flexion) because it limits the outward anterior skid.

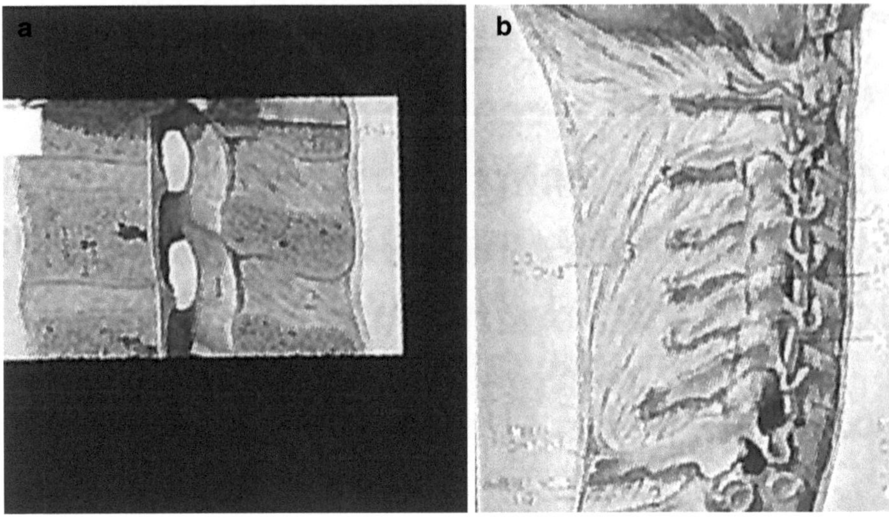

Fig. 3.6 (**a**) Lateral view: yellow ligaments *(J)* and interspinal ligaments (2). (**b**) Bilateral view: supraspinous ligaments connect two spinal apophyses crossing each other on the median line

Without the articular faces, the flexion is diminished, but an outward anterior skid is seen, leading to an instability which is important to preserve in the posterior approaches of the cervical column [12, 13].

The yellow ligaments represent the means of interlaminar union (Fig. 3.6) and are tied from half of the inner faces of the above lamina to the topmost third of the external faces of the lamina from below and included for the most part in the vertebral channel. Normally, the elasticity does not allow an introflexion, an impingement inside of the spinal channel during extension. Their hypertrophy, calcification, or loss of elasticity due to degenerative factors can cause a dynamic stenosis with compression of the spinal marrow. The interspinous ligaments are tied between two spinal processes in an oblique and posterior direction; the supraspinous ligaments are the continuation of the nuchal ligaments; they connect the apex of the spinal apophysis crossing on the median line.

The cervical rachis includes nervous and vascular structures that are vitally important, and since the latter are strictly bounded to the rachis, they can be destroyed during traumatic events [14, 15].

The spinal cord is in the center of the vertebral body, enveloped by three membranes (dura mater, pia mater, and arachnoid) that form the dural sac, which is suspended by the dentate ligaments, bathed in the cephalorachidian fluid. The marrow is an elastic structure that allows itself to adapt to various movements. During extension, it shortens itself and shows plicae on the surface. During flexion movements, it elongates and its surface becomes smooth. The nerve roots take their origin from the spinal cord with an anterior motor branch and the sensory posterior branch. They go through a first and then a second extradural tract, starting from the opening of the conjugation channel. The posterior root forms an ovoidal swelling within the channel: the spinal ganglion. This forms an anastomosis with the anterior root, forming the spinal nerve, which divides into its two anterior and posterior branches at the exit from the conjugate channel forming the brachial plexus.

Dissection in vertebral and carotid arteries is uncommon, and the incidence of cervical vascular dissection after whiplash trauma is not known even if widely accepted that indirect neck trauma-like manipulations could be a cause of vertebral dissection.

The vertebral artery [16] generally takes its origin from the subclavian artery and penetrates into C6 and goes to C1, passing through the corresponding transverse foramina. During its intrarachidial passage, it is enveloped by a sympathetic nervous plexus and by a venous plexus. Both of these structures are strictly bonded to the periosteum of the transverse foramina and are intimately attached to the nerve roots at the cross-point outside of the conjugate channel [17]. The symptoms of vertebral artery dissection are neck pain and signs of ischemia in the posterior cranial fossa.

Another aspect to be considered about functional anatomy of the neck is the role of venous vertebral plexus in drainage of cerebral venous blood [18].

The cerebrospinal venous system is a three-dimensional structure that is often asymmetric and considerably represents a more variable pattern than the arterial anatomy. The intracranial venous system is mainly composed of parenchymal veins draining into the dural sinuses. The former can be subdivided into two systems:

1. The superficial (cortical) system reaches dural sinuses by cortical veins and drains blood mainly from cortex and subcortical white matter
2. The deep cerebral venous system (DCVS) is composed by the internal cerebral veins, the basal vein of Rosenthal, and the great cerebral vein of Galen and their tributaries, and drains the deep white and gray matter surrounding the lateral and third ventricles.

The cerebral veins collect blood into the dural sinuses and in turn redirected toward the main extracranial venous outflow routes: the internal jugular veins (IJVs) and the vertebral veins (VVs) system. The anatomical pathways of jugular drainage are well established. The main jugular blood drainage pathway leads from the transverse sinuses via the sigmoid sinuses into the IJVs, which meet the superior vena cava via the brachiocephalic vein (Fig. 3.7) [19].

The VVs system is a freely communicating, valveless system present throughout the entire spinal column and may be divided into an internal intraspinal part, the epidural veins and an extraspinal paravertebral part. The system communicates with the deep thoracic and lumbar veins, intercostal veins, azygous vein (AZ), and hemiazygos veins. The AZ represents the final collector of such an enormous plexus and in turn drains into the superior vena cava, as well as into the inferior vena cava, via the anastomosis of the hemiazygos veins with the left renal vein.

The blood leaves the brain by using the back propulsion of the residual arterial pressure (vis a tergo), complemented by anterograde respiratory mechanisms (vis a fronte). The latter consists of the thoracic pump increased venous outflow during inspiration, thanks to increased thoracic negative pressure, which improves the aspiration of blood toward the right atrium. In addition to vis a tergo and vis a

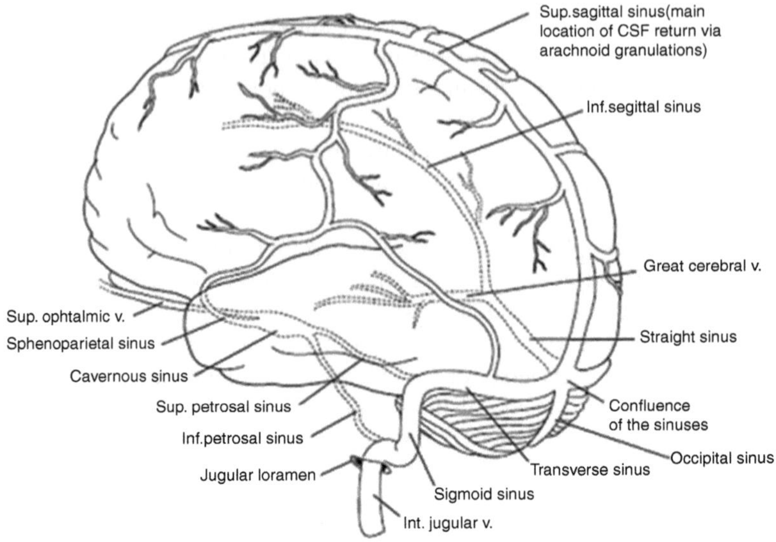

Fig. 3.7 Venous drainage system from the brain to the neck. Internal jugulars vein are the main way of cerebral venous blood in supine position, while when sitting or standing, they collapse and the main way of cerebral drainage is through vertebral plexus (not represented) along all the spine

fronte, postural mechanisms play a main role in ensuring a correct cerebral venous return. Several studies of healthy volunteers demonstrated that the pattern of cerebral venous drainage changes, even under physiological conditions, depending on the body position:

- In the prone position, the outflow through the IJVs is favored
- The supine posture favors cerebral venous outflow through the IJVs
- Passing to the upright position transfers most of the encephalic drainage to the VVs

It has been reported that flow is monodirectional in the IJVs/VVs. Flow is always increased by the activation of the pump asking the subject to breath. Blood flow velocity in the cervical veins is increased by activation of the thoracic pump. Temporary outflow block can be seen in the cervical veins in healthy subjects, but never reported in all the postural and respiratory conditions.

References

1. Roy-Camille R (1988) Rachis cervical inferieur. Sixiemes journèes d'orthopedie de la Pitiè. Masson, Paris
2. Tominaga T, Dickman CA, Sonntag VKH, Coons S (1995) Comparative anatomy of the baboon and the human cervical spine. Spine 20:131–137
3. Swartz EE, Floyd RT, Cendoma M (2005) Cervical spine functional anatomy and the biomechanics of injury due to compressive loading. J Athl Train 40(3):155–161
4. Jaumard NV, Welch WC, Winkelstein BA (2011) Spinal facet joint biomechanics and mechanotransduction in normal, injury and degenerative conditions. J Biomech Eng 133(7):071010

5. McLain RF (1994) Mechanoreceptor endings in human cervical facet joints. Spine 19: 495–501
6. Bogduk N, Mercer S (2000) Biomechanics of the cervical spine, I: normal kinematics. Clin Biomech (Bristol, Avon) 15:633–648
7. White AA, Panjiabi MM (1990) Clinical biomechanics of the spine. JB Lippincott, Philadelphia
8. Ivancic PC, Coe MP, Ndu BM, Tominaga Y, Carlson EJ, Rubin W, Panjabi MM (2007) Dynamic mechanical properties of intact human cervical spine ligaments. Spine J 7(6): 659–665
9. Hollinshead WH (1965) The anatomy of the spine: points of special interest to orthopaedic surgeons. J Bone Joint Surg Am 47A:209
10. Halliday DR, Sullivan CR, Hollinshead WH, Bahn RC (1964) Torn cervical ligaments: necropsy examination of normal cervical region. J Trauma 4:219
11. Cusick JF, Yoganandan N, Pintar F, Myklebust J, Hussain H (1988) Biomechanics of cervical spine facetectomy and fixation techniques. Spine 13:808–881
12. Penning L (1995) Kinematics of cervical spine injury: a functional radiological hypothesis. Eur Spine J 4:126–132
13. Ono K, Kaneoka K, Hattori S, Ujihashi S, Takhounts EG, Haffner MP, Eppinger RH (2003) Cervical vertebral motions and biomechanical responses to direct loading of human head. Traffic Inj Prev 4(2):141–152
14. Kaneyama T, Hashizume Y, Ando T, Takahashi A (1994) Morphometry of the normal cadaveric cervical spinal cord. Spine 19:2077–2081
15. Okada Y, Ikata T, Katoh S, Yamada H (1994) Morphologic analysis of the cervical spinal cord, dural tube, and spinal canal by magnetic resonance imaging in normal adults and patients with cervical spondylotic myelopathy. Spine 19:2331–2335
16. Vaccaro AR, Ring D, Scuderi G, Garfin S (1994) Vertebral artery location in relation to the vertebral body as determined by two-dimensional computed tomography evaluation. Spine 19:2637–2641
17. Yukawa Y, Kato F, Suda K, Yamagata M, Ueta T (2012) Age-related changes in osseous anatomy, alignment, and range of motion of the cervical spine Part I: radiographic data from over 1,200 asymptomatic subjects. Eur Spine J 4:347–351
18. Schaller B (2004) Physiology of cerebral venous blood flow: from experimental data in animals to normal function in humans. Brain Res Rev 46:243–260
19. Zamboni P, Consorti G, Galeotti R (2009) Venous collateral circulation of the extracranial cerebrospinal outflow routes. Curr Neurovasc Res 3:204–212

Kinematics and Dynamics of the Vehicle/Seat/Occupant System Regarding Whiplash Injuries

4

P.L. Ardoino and F. Ioppolo

4.1 Introduction

Whiplash injuries continue to have significant societal cost; however, the mechanism and location of whiplash injury is still under investigation. Predicting neck response and injury resulting from motor vehicle accidents is essential to improving occupant protection. Recently, the upper cervical spine ligaments, particularly the alar ligament, have been identified as a potential whiplash injury location [1].

4.2 Accident Typology at the Origin of the Whiplash

From accident analysis, it has been noticed that neck injuries are mostly caused by rear-end collisions: in a Dutch study conducted in the 1980s [2], neck injuries made up 51.6 % of all the lesions found in the drivers of cars involved in rear-end collisions (Table 4.1); in a Japanese study conducted at the beginning of the 1990s [3], the neck injury percentage in rear-end collisions increased to 80 %.

A second characteristic of neck injuries is their low seriousness degree: the abovementioned Japanese study [3] showed that during a rear-end collision, 93 % of the injuries are classified as AIS 1 level according to the Abbreviated Injury Scale [4]. As far as neck is concerned, in almost all cases, the AIS 1 level indicates a

P.L. Ardoino
FIAT Auto SpA, Technical Office,
Technical Coordination/Legal Safety, Orbassano (TO), Italy

F. Ioppolo (✉)
Department of Physical Medicine and Rehabilitation,
"Sapienza" University, Piazzale Aldo Moro 5,
00185 Rome, Italy
e-mail: francescoioppolo@yahoo.it

D.C. Alpini et al. (eds.), *Whiplash Injuries*,
DOI 10.1007/978-88-470-5486-8_4, © Springer-Verlag Italia 2014

Table 4.1 Distribution of injuries by body region for several collision types, driver only [1]

Main group	Lateral collisions	Front to front	Rear collisions	Total (including other types)
1 Skull and brain	23.7	20.0	14.4	22.2
2 Face	11.2	21.1	7.2	16.1
3 Neck	4.4	3.7	51.6	6.9
4 Thorax	20.2	16.9	6.8	16.5
5 Abdomen	2.6	2.3	0.4	2.3
6 Back	2.4	1.3	4.0	2.4
7 Pelvis	5.0	1.3	0.4	2.0
8 Arms	16.0	13.6	7.2	14.2
9 Legs	14.5	19.8	6.0	17.3
Total (%)	100	100	100	100

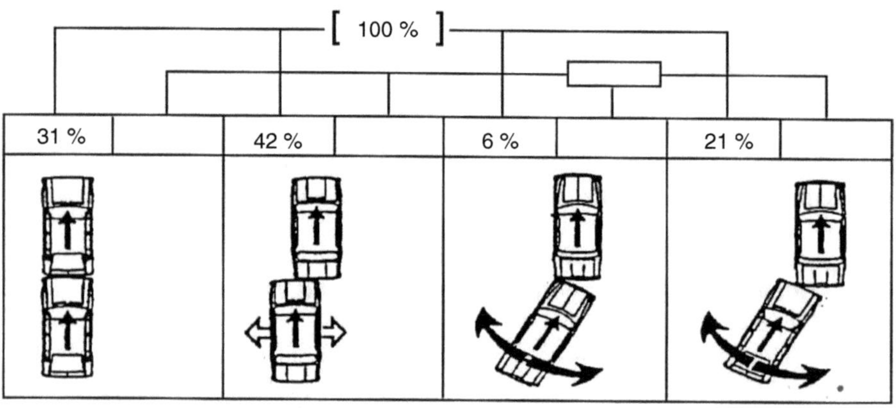

Fig. 4.1 Distribution of the rear accidents with injured occupants by impact type [4]

cervical rachis strain without any evidence of anatomical lesions. The same trend is emphasized in a study conducted in Germany [5] on a sample of about 10,500 car collisions.

With regard to the rear-end collision typology, in the abovementioned German study [4], center and offset crashes make up about 73 % of all the rear-end collisions (Fig. 4.1); only 27 % present an angled direction.

It is necessary to point out that in low-impact speed offset crashes, the off-centering does not produce notable rotations in the hit vehicle, as it is regularly noticed in damageability tests with off-center crashing barriers and above 20 km/h crash speeds.

On the basis of what has been said above, we can conclude that, in almost all cases, whiplash injuries happen in a low speed impact rear-end collision, in which the speed variation takes place on the longitudinal axis of the vehicle.

Fig. 4.2 Injury mechanism in whiplash

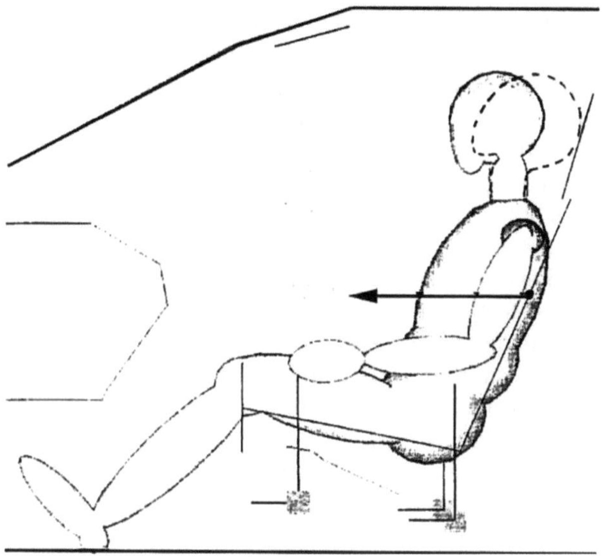

4.3 Whiplash Injury Mechanism

In a rear-end collision, the chest is pushed forwards by the seatback; the burden on the neck results from the strength of inertia that works through the center of gravity of the head in a front-back direction; in this case, the neck injury mechanism is one of hyperextension and tension ("traction" in mechanical terminology) of the cervical rachis (Fig. 4.2). It should be pointed out that not all hyperextension/tension injury mechanisms are caused by whiplash.

Chronic radicular symptoms have been documented in whiplash patients, potentially caused by cervical neural tissue compression during an automobile rear crash. Simulated rear crashes with whiplash protection system (WHIPS) and active head restraint (AHR) have been compared to those obtained with no head restraint (NHR) with the aim to determine how whiplash may induce neural space narrowing of the lower cervical spine [6, 7]. Average peak canal and foramen narrowing could not be statistically differentiated between WHIPS, AHR, and NHR. While lower cervical spine cord compression during a rear crash is unlikely in those with normal canal diameters, it has been demonstrated [8] that foraminal kinematics is sufficient to compress spinal ganglia and nerve roots. Disc strains are highest in the C4-C5-C6 segments.

4.4 Technical and Structural Limits

The technical norms now in force in Europe prescribe that the seatback must be able to withstand the application of a static moment of 53 (m daN). Even though from a theoretical point of view it is not possible to define a dynamic stress that is equivalent to the static one, on the basis of experimental data and for normal seats with 50 % male anthropometric characteristics, we can consider that such a burden corresponds to the capacity to withstand the chest's inertia load in a rear-end collision between vehicles of equal mass with a closure speed of about 35 km/h.

Ignoring the retaining action of the headrest, we can deduce that speed variations of the vehicle higher than 18 km/h the seatback can rotate backwards absorbing part of the chest kinetic energy; these phenomena in fact limit both the angle of rotation of the head and the value of the extension moment.

The technical norms assure that the headrest withstands additional loadings compared to the seatback.

We can therefore conclude that the crash that must be considered is a rear-end one at AV < 18 km/h with a longitudinal movement of the passenger compartment.

Review of whiplash injury mechanisms and effects of anti-whiplash systems, including active head restraint (AHR) and Whiplash Protection System (WHIPS), investigated whether seat design and biomechanical knowledge of proposed whiplash injury mechanisms translates to understanding outcomes of rear crash occupants. In fact, in attempt to reduce whiplash injuries, some newer automobiles incorporate anti-whiplash systems such as AHR or WHIPS. During a rear crash, mechanically based systems activate by occupant momentum pressing into the seatback, whereas electronically based systems activate using crash sensors and an electronic control unit linked to the head restraint.

Biomechanical studies of simulated rear crashes have been performed using human volunteers, mathematical models, crash dummies, whole cadavers, and hybrid cadaveric/surrogate models. They indicated that AHR and WHIPS reduce the potential for some whiplash injuries but did not completely eliminate the risk of injury.

Epidemiological outcomes indicate reduced whiplash injury claims or subjective complaints of crash-related neck pain between 43 and 75 % due to AHR and between 21 and 49 % due to WHIPS as compared to conventional seats and head restraints [9], concluding that energy-absorbing seats aim to reduce occupant loads and accelerations, whereas AHRs aim to provide early head support to minimize head and neck motions. Continued objective biomechanical and epidemiological studies of anti-whiplash systems together with industry, governmental, and clinical initiatives will ultimately lead to reduced whiplash injuries through improved prevention strategies [10].

Some differences have been observed [11] regarding gender-based whiplash effects in the dynamic response for the females with respects to the males in volunteer experiments. In fact the peak head acceleration in the posterior-anterior direction was higher and occurred earlier for the females than for the males. These experiments could be used in developing and evaluating a female dummy model for rear-impact safety assessment in order to design gender-specific protective systems.

4.5 Phases of the Collision

A stereotypical kinematic and neuromuscular response has been observed in human subjects exposed to rear-end impacts [6]. Combined with various models of injury, these response data have been used to develop anti-whiplash seats that prevent whiplash injury in many, but not all, individuals exposed to a rear-end crash. Understanding of the occupant kinematics and neuromuscular responses, combined with data from various seat-related interventions, have shown that differential motion between the superior and inferior ends of the cervical spine is responsible for many whiplash injuries. The number of whiplash injuries not prevented by current anti-whiplash seats suggests that further work remains, possibly related to designing seats that respond dynamically to the occupant and collision properties.

Neck muscles alter the head and neck kinematics during the interval in which injury likely occurs, even in initially relaxed occupants. It remains unclear whether muscle activation mitigates or exacerbates whiplash injury. If muscle activation mitigates injury, then advance warning could be used to help occupant tense their muscles before impact. Alternatively, if muscle activation exacerbates whiplash injury, then a loud preimpact sound that uncouples the startle and postural components of the muscle response could reduce peak muscle activation during a whiplash exposure [12, 13].

Generally speaking, rear-end collision is characterized by three different phases [14]:

- First phase: crash between the vehicles until the struck one assumes the speed variation (AV) due to the impact conditions.
- Second phase: interaction between the seat and its occupant.
- Third phase: loadings on the occupant; the three phases surely are linked and temporarily, partially overlapping.

4.5.1 First Phase

Regardless of the initial speed of the two vehicles, the struck one in this phase assumes a speed variation that is a function of the masses of the vehicles, their closure speed, and the spring restitution coefficient; the analytic expression of the speed variation of the vehicle that is hit is the following:

$$\Delta V\mathrm{A} = \frac{M\mathrm{A} \times M\mathrm{B}}{M\mathrm{A} + M\mathrm{B}} (V\mathrm{A} - V\mathrm{B})(1 + \mathrm{e})$$

where:
A = struck vehicle
B = striking vehicle
V = speed at the impact
ΔV = speed variation
M = mass
e = spring restitution coefficient
(VA − VB) = closure speed

Higher or lower stiffness of the vehicles brings a different degree of deformation and therefore influences the duration of the collision and the values of average acceleration, but does not modify the extent of the variation in speed.

4.5.2 Second Phase

The variations in motion of the hit vehicle are also those of the fastening of the seat to the body shell; the seat, mostly the seatback, is the element through which the occupant adapts its motion situation to the final one of the hit vehicle.

In a rear impact, the seatback is the actual restraint system of the occupant, just as the seatbelt is in a frontal impact.

It is important to point out that the fact of wearing the seat belt does not influence the kinematics and the dynamics of the occupant during a lengthwise rear-end collision; the only function of the seat belt in this particular case is to hold the occupant once the crash is over.

Recently Viano et al. [15] analyzed matched rear sled tests with all belts to seat (ABTS) and conventional seats from the same vehicle model to determine differences in BioRID IIg dummy responses. The BioRID IIg rear-impact dummy was placed on ABTS or conventional seats and subjected to 10 m/h rear sled tests using the Insurance Institute for Highway Safety (IIHS) whiplash assessment protocol. Measurements in the dummy included head and pelvis triaxial accelerations, T1 and L1 biaxial accelerations, and upper and lower neck triaxial forces and moments. High-speed video captured the dummy and seat kinematics during seat loading and rebound into the lap-shoulder belts. Four vehicles were used with conventional and ABTS seats in the same model. They were the 2007–2008 Chrysler Sebring, 2006 Ford F-150, 2005–2007 Saab 9–3, and 2006–2007 BMW 3 series.

Authors noticed that the upper neck tension was 44 % higher and the lower neck extension moment was 102 % higher and that the Saab 9–3 responses were lower than the 3 other vehicles for both the conventional and ABTS seats. There was less rearward shear and extension of the neck in the Saab seats. In conclusion, the tests show that ABTS seats involved significantly higher neck tensions, rearward shear forces, and extension moments than matched conventional seats. Overall, ABTS seats applied more load on the head and spine, had less control of neck kinematics, and had higher risks for whiplash and more severe injury than conventional seats in the same vehicle model.

Two characteristics of the seat influence the stress transfer from the vehicle to the occupant: (1) the seat foam which cushions the stresses, filters, and further offsets the small transversal and rotational movements of the vehicle; (2) the elasticity of the seatback structure which obviously acts only in situations which do not exceed the structural limits indicated before.

The relative head/headrest position plays a basic role in the extensional traction movement of the neck and therefore in limiting the whiplash injuries.

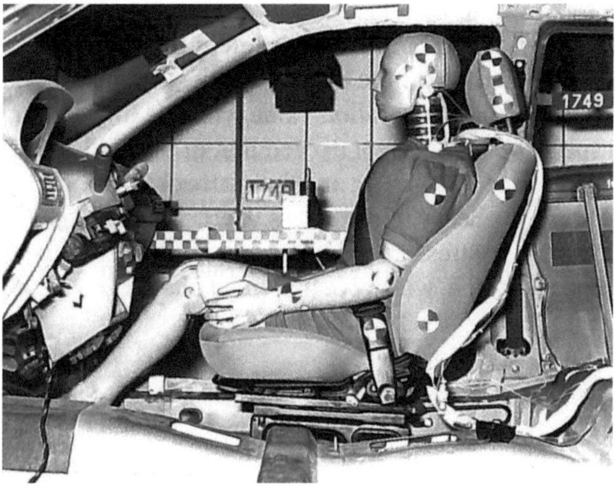

Fig. 4.3 Rear-impact simulation. Test configuration

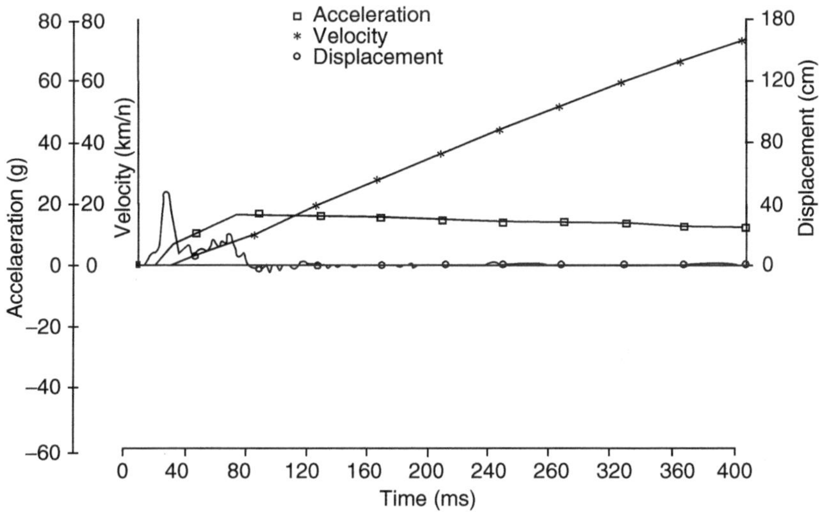

Fig. 4.4 Time histories of the passenger compartment

4.5.3 Third Phase

The human body is an articulated system of body segments which are submitted to external loads, applied mainly through the seat, and they interact among themselves. In order to analyze the stresses on the single-body segments, an experimental rear-end collision test has been carried out on a crash simulator with the previously described conditions (Fig. 4.3).

A 17 km/h variation in speed has been applied to the passenger compartment with an acceleration curve corresponding to a rear-end collision with a rigid moving barrier and, therefore, a particularly severe one (Fig. 4.4) segments.

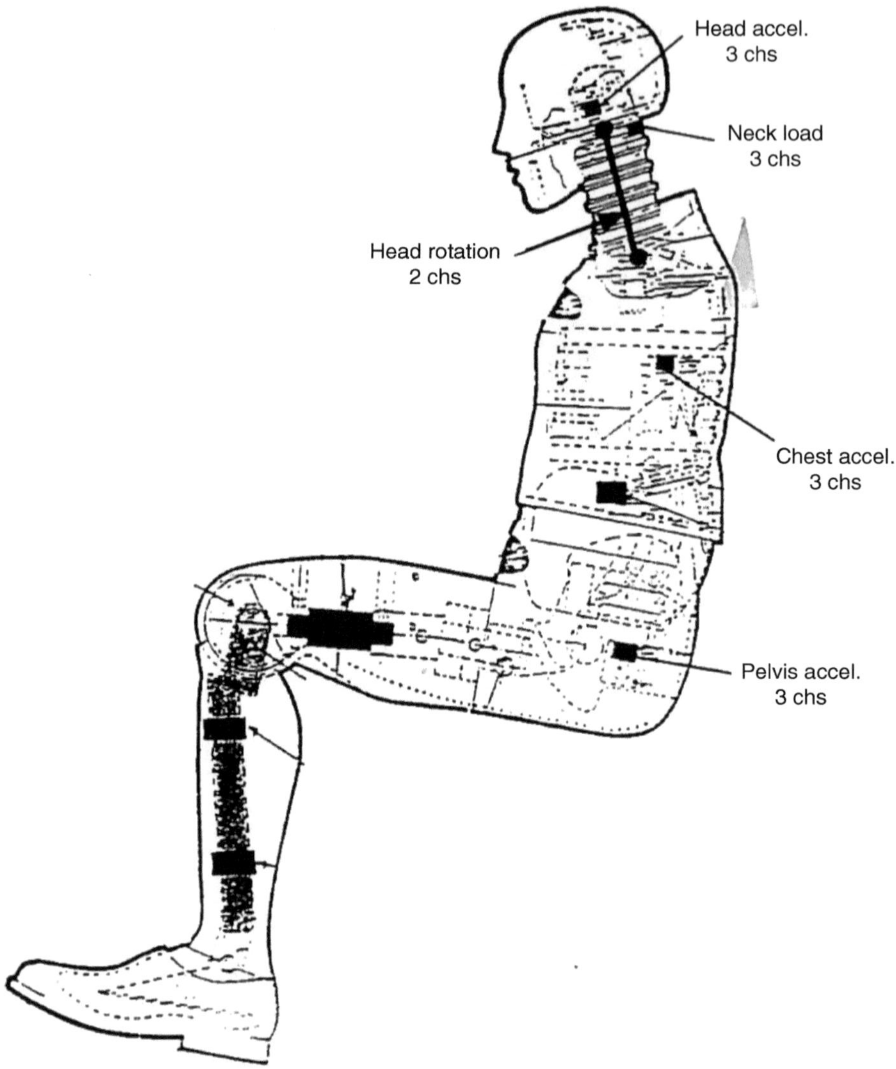

Fig. 4.5 Hybrid III instrumentation

A Hybrid III dummy has been used in the front passenger position, provided with the necessary instruments in order to obtain (Fig. 4.5): (1) the pelvis, chest, and head accelerations; (2) the axial loads (compression and traction), the moments (flexion and extension), and the shear force on the neck; (3) the rotation of the head with regard to the basis of the neck.

Figure 4.6 shows the time histories (acceleration, velocity, displacement) of the occupant's pelvis, chest, and head in the direction of the applied forces that, in this particular case, were horizontal-longitudinal.

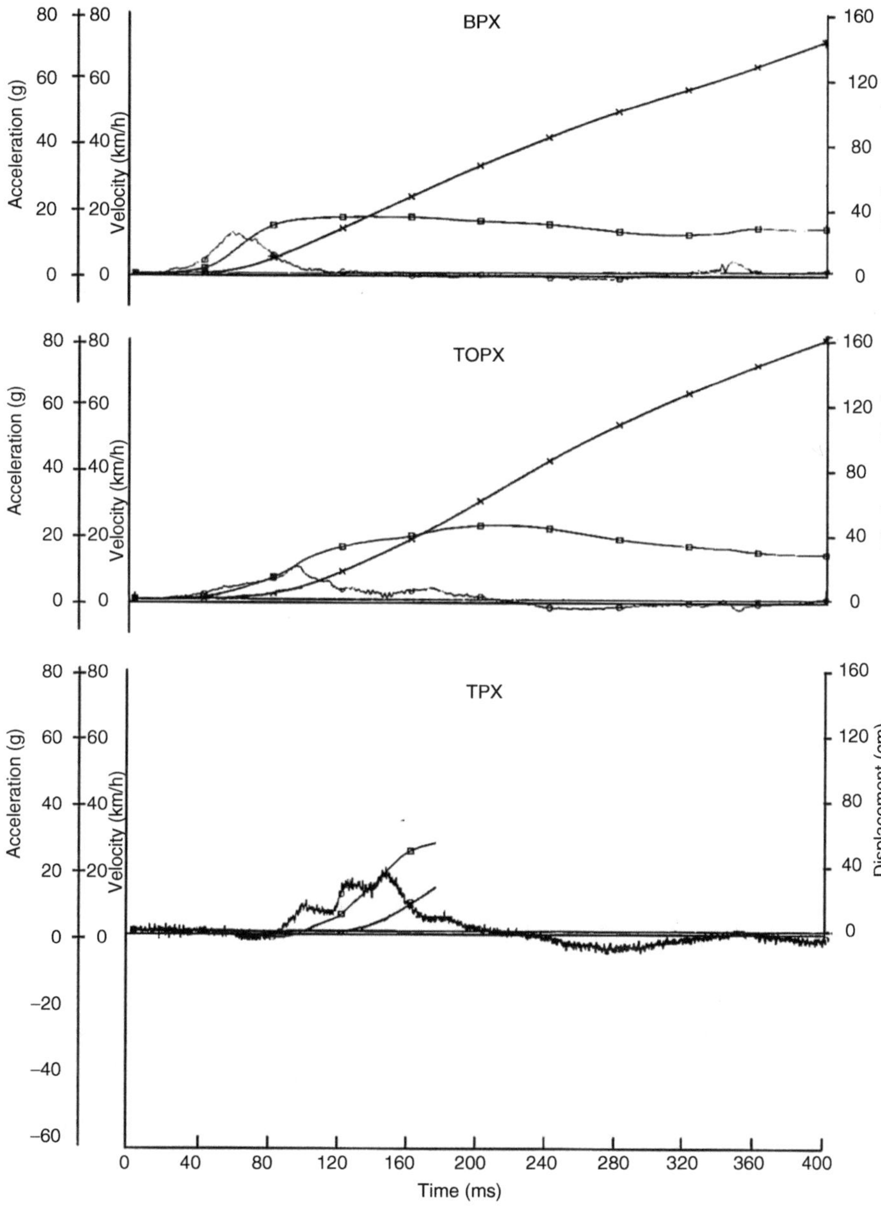

Fig. 4.6 Pelvis, chest, head time histories

It is necessary to point out that the head's speed and displacement values above 130 ms do not correspond to the actual values of the speed and displacement components along the *X*-axis, due to the rotation of the head.

It is therefore evident that the stresses on the three-body segments have different values and are transmitted in different times.

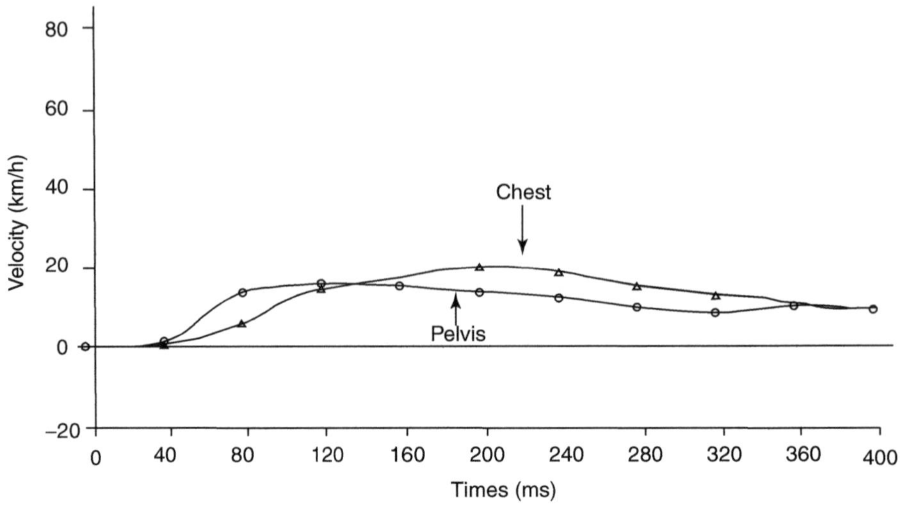

Fig. 4.7 Pelvis, chest velocity vs time

The pelvis compared to the chest is subject to a stress that is shorter lasting, with an average acceleration value which is higher, but it has a variation in speed which does not exceed that of the vehicle (17 km/h); this means that, at pelvis level, the seat and the seatback cushion the crash and do not elastically return energy to the pelvis itself.

The duration of the stress on the chest is longer due to the spring restitution of the seatback which, with a coefficient of about a 0.3, brings the chest's variation in speed to about 23 km/h.

Regarding the head, though we do not have the exact value of the variation in speed along the horizontal-longitudinal axis, we have noticed a higher stress degree in terms of both mean acceleration and variation in speed.

The head's increase in speed variation compared to that of the chest is mainly due to the neck's spring restitution.

It should be noted that all the recorded acceleration values are at least one order of magnitude below the human tolerance levels universally accepted in the biomechanic field for these body segments. The fact, which is also emphasized by the accident analysis, that in rear-end collisions of this severity no pelvis, chest or head injuries occur, does not alter the significance of the dynamic and kinematic trends of the system which are the input conditions for the analysis of stresses on the neck. The overlapping of the pelvis and chest speed curves (Fig. 4.7) shows how, in the time interval between 80 and 200 ms, the variation in speed between chest and pelvis passes from about –10 to +7 km/h.

The same behavior has been noticed between head and chest (Fig. 4.8). Regarding stresses on the neck (moments and axial loads) (Fig. 4.9), we noticed a time correspondence with the acceleration of the head; the same can be said for the rotation of the head with regard to the basis of the neck. The head acceleration and speed

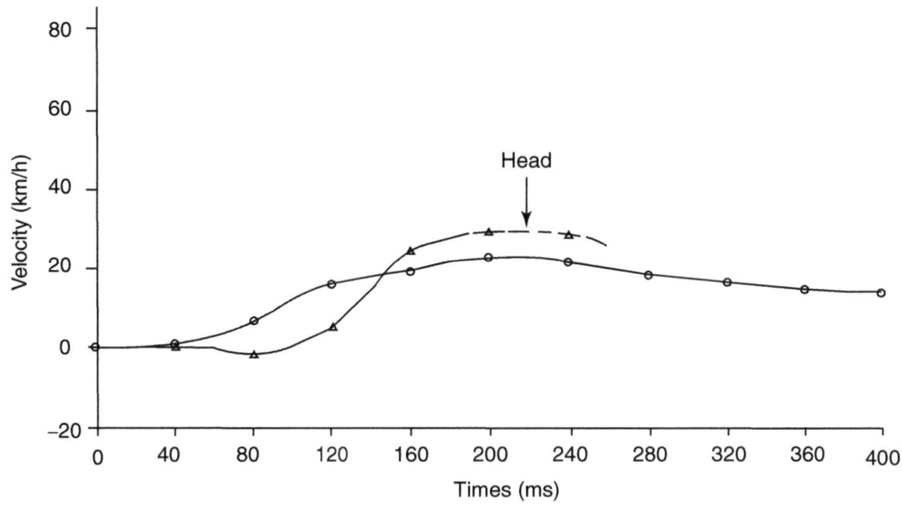

Fig. 4.8 Chest, head velocity vs time

curves (Fig. 4.6) show, at about 80 ms, a small backward movement of the head, due to the lever effect of the pelvis, chest, and seatback, to which a small bending moment value corresponds (Fig. 4.9).

There is a question whether the standing or seated pelvis should be used in Hybrid III dummy evaluations of seats and belt restraint systems in severe rear impacts. Viano and Parenteu performed [12] sled tests in a belted standing and seated Hybrid III dummy. The head, chest, and pelvis were instrumented with triaxial accelerometers and the upper and lower neck, thoracic spine, and lumbar spine had transducers measuring triaxial loads and moments. Belt loads were measured. In 40 km/h sled tests, the dummy motion and excursion were essentially similar with the standing and seated pelvis. The similarities included the lap belt interaction with the pelvis and the leg movement upward flexing the hip joint. Overall, similar biomechanic and kinematic responses were found, including the pelvic acceleration, spinal forces, and moments. For the lower speed tests at 10, 16, and 24 km/h, the motion sequence was also similar with the two different pelvises, including the upward movement of the legs as the seat was loaded and rebound kinematics. The biomechanical responses were similar. The seated pelvis involves only a small portion of the upper leg molded into the vinyl skin of the pelvis and does not limit leg rotation at the hip joint. Furthermore, lap belt loads were minimal during the rearward movement of the dummy. In conclusion, tests showed no significant difference in occupant kinematics or biomechanical responses between the standing and seated pelvis in rear sled tests.

By examining Figs. 4.6 and 4.9, the following can be noted:

- The chest starts its forward movement, pushed by the seatback, at about 50 ms.
- The rotation of the head starts at about 90 ms.
- The head's center of gravity starts to shift forwards at about 120 ms.

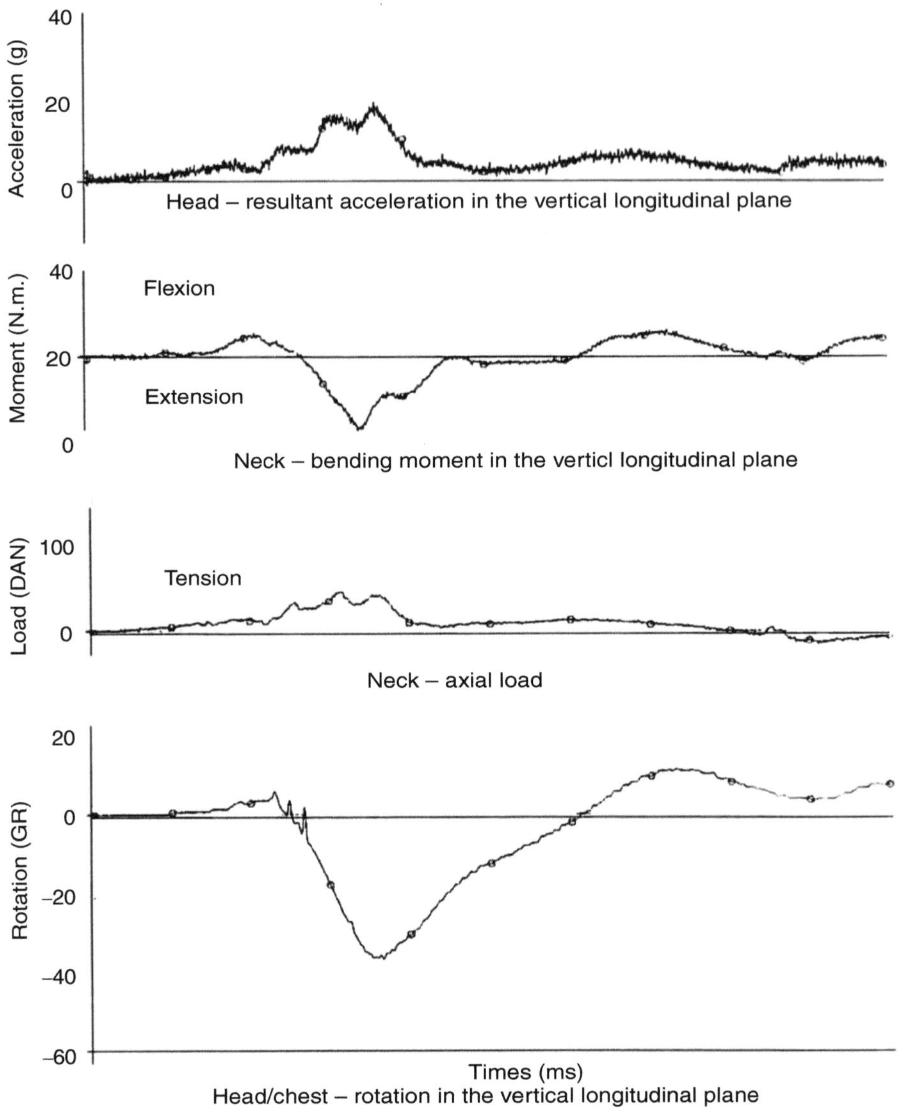

Fig. 4.9 Head and neck loadings

- The maximum stresses on head and neck occur at about 150 ms. Based on what was mentioned above, it is clear that the neck – the link between chest and head – is stressed in different ways during the crash (Fig. 4.10):
  - Between 50 and 90 ms, the chest moves forwards and the head stays in its rest position; the neck is essentially subject to small shear strains.
  - Between 90 and 120 ms, the forward movement of the chest continues; the head rotates due to the fact that the neck is subject to the application of an extension moment.

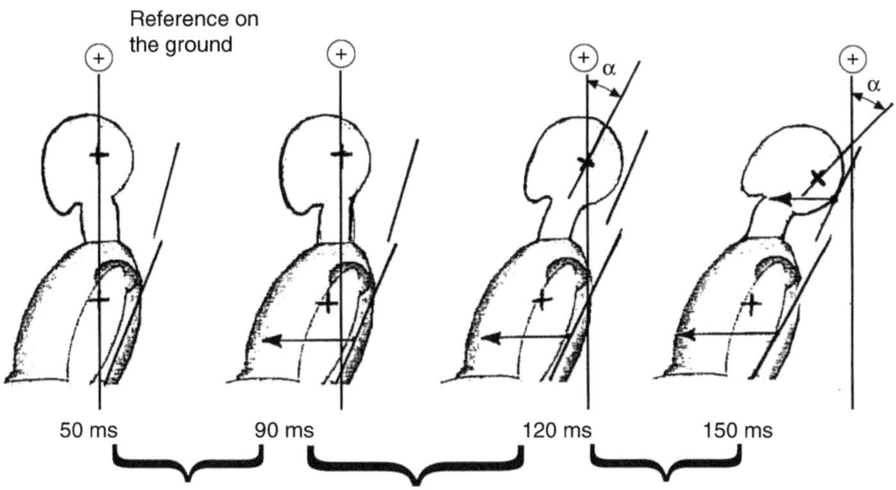

Fig. 4.10 Neck loadings and kinematics

- Between 120 and 150 ms, the head continues to turn and also moves forwards pulled by the neck and pushed by the headrest. In this phase, the neck is subject to the largest stress of extension moment and traction force and whiplash injuries occur.

Notice how, up to 200 ms (Fig. 4.6), and therefore after the largest stresses on the neck have taken place, the occupant is in contact with and is meanwhile pushed by the seatback; the seat belt up to now has not exercised any restraining action and cannot therefore alter in any way the kinematics and dynamics of the occupant.

On the basis of existing biomechanically based research [16], the following occupant-related characteristics can influence the response of the cervical spine during automotive rear impacts:

- Anatomical dimensions of the cervical spine
- Head-neck and cervical spine orientation at the time of impact
- Facet joint orientation
- Neck muscle size and orientation

The response of the cervical spine to rear impacts can be described using biomechanical concepts, but occupant-related factors can influence injury susceptibility and biomechanically related researches outline the method by which those factors affect the overall head-neck and cervical spine response in such a way.

4.6 Angled Rear-End Collisions

Regardless of the kind of rear-end collision, it is the seat which induces the stresses on the occupant. In the case of mainly centered-angled rear-end collisions (Fig. 4.11), which means angles not larger than 15–20°, the seat moves towards the occupant

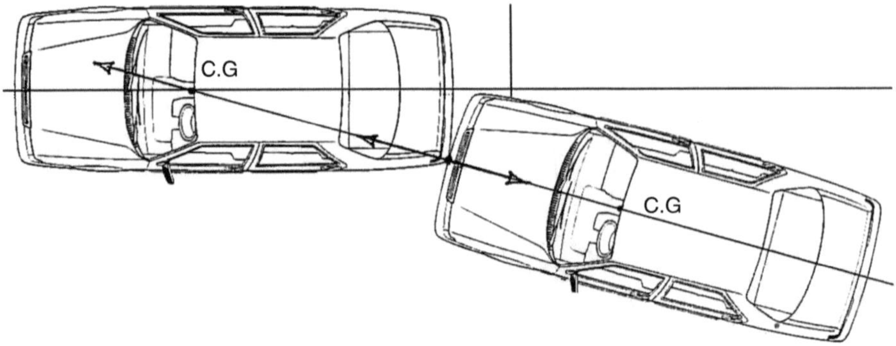

Fig. 4.11 Centered-angled-rear collision; *CG* center of gravity

along the collision direction, and the stress components along the longitudinal axis represent about 95 % of the total stress.

The neck injury mechanism is always an extension and tension one. In the worst case, the movement occurs on a vertical plane tilted about 15–20° with regard to the vertical longitudinal plane. In this case, due to the small size of the angle, the human tolerance values in terms of extension moment and traction force could slightly differ from those universally accepted in the biomechanic field for longitudinal loads.

In the remaining kinds of offset-angled rear-end collisions, the rotation of the hit vehicle dominates; the vehicle/occupant interaction does not take place solely through the seat, and therefore the whiplash stress on the neck is unlikely to occur.

4.7 Out-of-Position Whiplash

Particular attention should be paid to the whiplash that occurs when the occupant is out of position; for example, just think what the neck injury mechanism could be if the stresses described above were applied to a head that initially is rotated around its vertical axis of about 60°.

Very little knowledge is available on the human tolerance and on the biomechanics of the rotated neck in the rear impact; nevertheless, an injured out-of-position occupant should show an asymmetric lesion or symptomatology.

The necks of the current dummies do not allow us to study the injuries that could result in these situations of asymmetric and compound stresses; in fact, their biofidelity is limited to the longitudinal vertical plane, and the neck structure is symmetric with regard to any plane that passes through its vertical axis.

Conclusions

Automotive rear impacts are mechanical events and the response of the human head-neck complex can be thought of in biomechanical terms.

Rear-impact collisions at low speed are a leading cause of economic costs among motor vehicle accidents. Dummy tests focused on occupant position may lead to development of specific tools aimed to reduce whiplash effects on the head, the neck, and the trunk, both in drivers and passengers.

References

1. Ivancic PC, Xiao M (2011) Understanding whiplash injury and prevention mechanisms using a human model of the neck. Accid Anal Prev 43(4):1392–1399
2. Van Kampem LTB (1993) Hoofdsteunen in personenauto's. Institute for Road Safety Research (SWOV), Leidschendam, Netherlands
3. Koshiro Ono (1993) Influences of the physical parameters on the risk to neck injuries in low impact speed rear-end collisions. Proceedings of IRCOBI, Conference
4. Association for the Advancement of Automotive Medicine, Committee on Injury Scaling. The Abbreviated Injury Scale—1990 Revision (AIS-90). Des Plains, IL: Association for the Advancement of Automotive Medicine; 1990
5. Verband HUK (1994) Fahrzeugsicherheit 90. Verband HUK, Munchen
6. Siegmund GP (2011) What occupant kinematics and neuromuscular responses tell us about whiplash injury. Spine 36(25 Suppl):S175–S179
7. Tencer AF, Mirza S, Bensel K (2002) Internal loads in the cervical spine during motor vehicle rear-end impacts: the effect of acceleration and head-to-head restraint proximity. Spine 27(1):34–42
8. Ivancic PC (2012) Cervical neural space narrowing during simulated rear crashes with anti-whiplash systems. Eur Spine J 21(5):879–886. Epub 2012 Jan 24
9. Panzer MB, Fice JB, Cronin DS (2011) Cervical spine response in frontal crash. Med Eng Phys 33(9):1147–1159. Epub 2011
10. Fice JB, Cronin DS (2012) Investigation of whiplash injuries in the upper cervical spine using a detailed neck model. J Biomech 45(6):1098–1102
11. Carlsson A, Linder A, Davidsson J, Hell W, Schick S, Svensson M (2011) Dynamic kinematic responses of female volunteers in rear impacts and comparison to previous male volunteer tests. Traffic Inj Prev 12(4):347–357
12. Viano DC, Parenteau CS (2011) BioRID dummy responses in matched ABTS and conventional seat tests on the IIHS rear sled. Traffic Inj Prev 12(4):339–346
13. Ivancic PC (2011) Does knowledge of seat design and whiplash injury mechanisms translate to understanding outcomes? Spine 36(25 Suppl):S187–S193
14. Arregui-Dalmases C, Pozo ED, Lessley D, Barrios JM, Nombela M, Cisneros O, De Miguel JL, Seguí-Gómez M (2011) Driving position field study, differences with the whiplash protocol and biomechanics experimental responses. Ann Adv Automot Med 55:71–79
15. Viano DC, Parenteau CS, Burnett R (2012) Influence of standing or seated pelvis on dummy responses in rear impacts. Accid Anal Prev 45:423–431. Epub 2011 Nov 21
16. Stemper BD, Pintar FA, Rao RD (2011) The influence of morphology on cervical injury characteristics. Spine 36(25 Suppl):S180–S186

Whiplash Lesions: Orthopedic Considerations

5

E. Meani, S. Brambilla, A. Mondini, C.L. Romanò, and F. Ioppolo

5.1 Introduction

Whiplash usually stands for a syndrome characterized by a soft tissue lesion of the neck (muscles, ligaments, capsules, intervertebral disk, spinal marrow, nerve roots, veins and arteries, sympathetic system).

Normally though, this term is used in a broader way to define the majority of traumatic events that involve the cervical rachis following street accidents. In this context, whiplash does not represent a clinical syndrome, but rather comprises a group of pathological entities that are extremely different in their entity, prognosis, and treatment.

5.2 Clinical Course

In an acute phase right after the trauma, the symptomatology is characterized by pain in the cervical and occipital areas, with the addition of the scapular girdle and the dorsal region; the tendency is to reach a peak in the following hours and days

E. Meani • C.L. Romanò
Center of Reconstructive Surgery and Osteoarticular Infection, IRCCS "Galeazzi" Orthopedic Institute, Via R. Galeazzi 4, 20161 Milan, Italy

S. Brambilla • A. Mondini
"G. Pini" Orthopedic Institute, Via Rugabella 4, 20122 Milan, Italy

F. Ioppolo (✉)
Department of Physical Medicine and Rehabilitation, "Sapienza" University, Piazzale Aldo Moro 5, 00185 Rome, Italy
e-mail: francescoioppolo@yahoo.it

D.C. Alpini et al. (eds.), *Whiplash Injuries*,
DOI 10.1007/978-88-470-5486-8_5, © Springer-Verlag Italia 2014

with establishment of a muscular contracture of the paravertebral muscles (trapezius muscle and the long muscles of the back).

These symptoms are totally aspecific and are mostly all present in the traumatic affections of the rachis; there is no relationship between the extent of the symptomatology and the gravity of the lesions [1].

Normally, in the acute phase, no signs of involvement of the myeloradicular structures of the rachis are present. If these signs were evident, they indicate a lesion of the soft tissues and the osteoarticular structures.

The symptomatic pain can completely resolve itself in a variable period of time from the traumatic event or it can become chronic. The clinical course is worsened with symptoms such as headache, nausea, tinnitus, lack of concentration, photophobia, retro-orbital pain, anxiety, depression, easy irritability, sleep disturbances, and dysesthesias of the upper limbs. Carrol et al. [2] in a prospective cohort study design, through a self-reported scale which investigated pain, depression, anxiety, fear, anger, and frustration, showed that pain-related frustration was the most intense. Only 3 % of the cohort reported having no pain-related frustration, and 4 % reported no pain-related anxiety. Their findings suggest that it may be beneficial for health care providers to address emotional status related to pain in the first few weeks after a whiplash injury.

Neck pain is determined by contracture of the paravertebral cervical muscles and is accompanied by a limitation of the articular excursion; the most involved muscles (sternocleidomastoid, scalene, trapezius, long neck muscles) can determine lesions that go from simple stretching to rupture with the formation of intrafascicular hematomas. The same stretching lesions can also involve the anterior and posterior long ligaments. Less frequent are cleavages and lacerations of the annulus fibrosus, separation of the somatic limiting of the cartilaginous plate, and lesions that can predispose to discal degeneration, which contributes to prolonging the symptomatic pain.

With some frequency, pain in the interscapular and high dorsal regions has been reported, expression of the myofascial lesions of the trapezius, rhomboid, levator of the scapular muscles, and large dentate muscle.

If the brachial pain and paresthesias are not tied to an irritative-compressive factor of the nerve roots (discal protrusion, stenosis of the conjugate channel, compression of a fractured articular apophysis), they do not generally present with a precise metameric distribution and remain difficult to interpret, even if they have been indicated as a possible cause of lesions associated with the brachial plexus or with a thoracic outlet syndrome.

Widespread hyperalgesia in chronic whiplash-associated disorders have been showed by Lemming et al. [3] that investigated deep tissue pain hyperalgesia in women using computerized cuff pressure algometry and hypertonic saline infusion. They demonstrated a widespread hyperalgesia with facilitation of temporal summation outside the primary pain area, suggesting involvement of central sensitization.

Headache in the occipital area is a common symptom; generally, it is due to a painful muscular spasm of the semispinal muscles and rectus muscles of the head and neck, or splenius muscle, or to stretching or laceration of the nuchal ligaments [4]. Often, in association, there is a neuralgia of Arnold's large occipital nerve.

The retro-orbital pain and the reading fatigue that are often included in the complaints of patients with whiplash injuries could be tied to a proprioception problem of the paravertebral muscles, with major involvement of the intrinsic oculomotor system.

5.3 Diagnosis

Due to the aspecificity of the clinical picture, it is necessary to recur to a radiographic examination in a patient suffering from traumatic injury of the spine. Recent studies evidenced morphological changes (atrophy and fatty degeneration) of neck muscles in whiplash-associated disorders (WAD) highlighted emerging evidence for the pathophysiological mechanisms behind muscle degeneration and their potential role in the transition from acute to chronic pain [5].

Magnetic resonance imaging (MRI) can be regarded as the gold standard for muscle imaging. There is emerging evidence to highlight in vivo features of neck muscle degeneration in patients with chronic WAD and the temporal development of such acute changes after trauma. However, the precise underlying mechanisms for such changes and their influence on functional recovery after whiplash remain largely unknown, even if current evidence from structural MRI-based studies demonstrates the widespread presence of fatty infiltrates in neck muscles of patients with chronic whiplash. Such findings have not shown to feature in patients with chronic insidious onset neck pain, suggesting traumatic factors play a role in their development. Recent studies have revealed that the muscle fatty infiltrates manifest soon after whiplash but only in those with higher pain, disability, and symptoms of post-traumatic stress disorder. The possibility that such muscle changes are associated with a more severe injury, including poor functional recovery, remains the focus of current research efforts.

Under an orthopedic point of view, the first step is X-ray diagnosis, at least for the acute cases in emergency room; it should include, apart from the classical frontal and lateral projections, the oblique and transoral projections, all easily performable exams in an emergency room. Fundamentally important is good execution and interpretation of the above exams: the lateral projection assesses alignment of the vertebral bodies (anterior and posterior somatic lines), the normal orientation of the articular faces, and the absence of fanning of the spinal apophysis [6].

The anterior-posterior projection is used to evaluate the correct alignment of the spinal apophysis, the peduncles, and the normal position of the vertebral bodies and the articular mass (Fig. 5.1).

In case of abnormal position of the vertebrae in these two standard projections, it is good to recur to the oblique projections, especially in cases that too often are thought to be partial dislocations. The oblique projections can better point out the posterior articular structures, the peduncles, and the normal conformation and dimension of the conjugate foramina (Fig. 5.2) [7, 8].

Furthermore, it is necessary to remember that at the moment of the trauma, an extensive antalgic muscular contraction can hide a grave lesion of the capsular,

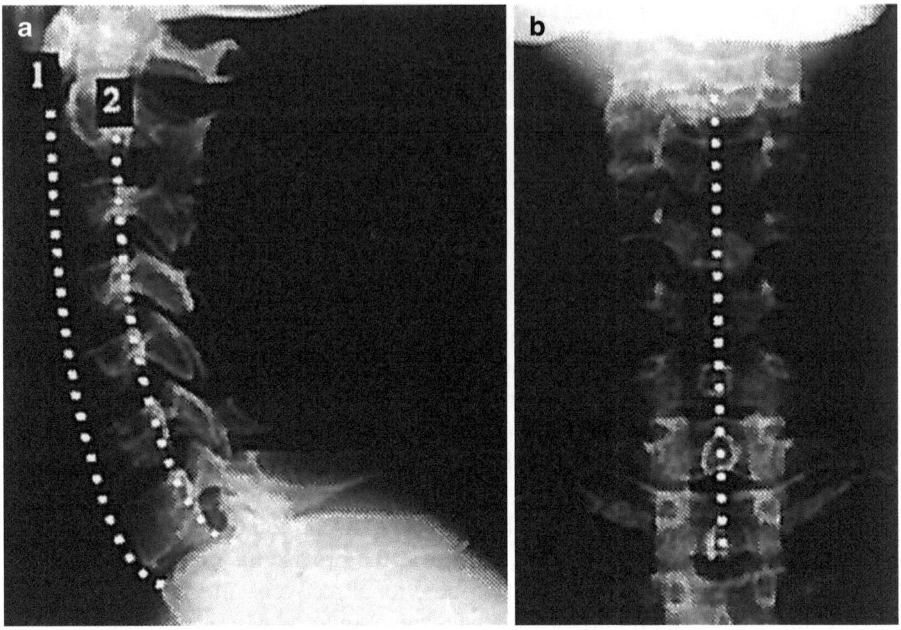

Fig. 5.1 (**a**) Lateral view: dashed line shows the normal position of the vertebral bodies (*1*) and correct alignment of the peduncles and articulator mass (*2*). (**b**) Anteroposterior view: dashed line shows the correct alignment of the spinal apophysis and normal position of vertebral bodies

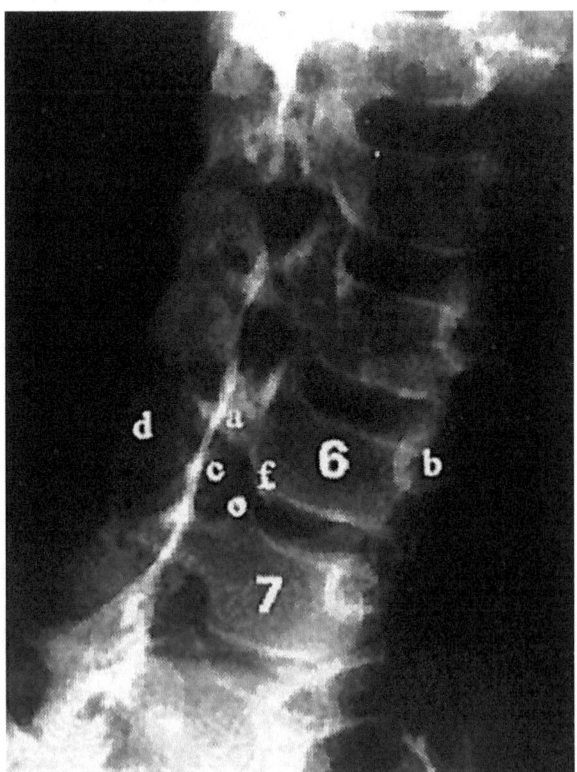

Fig. 5.2 Oblique view

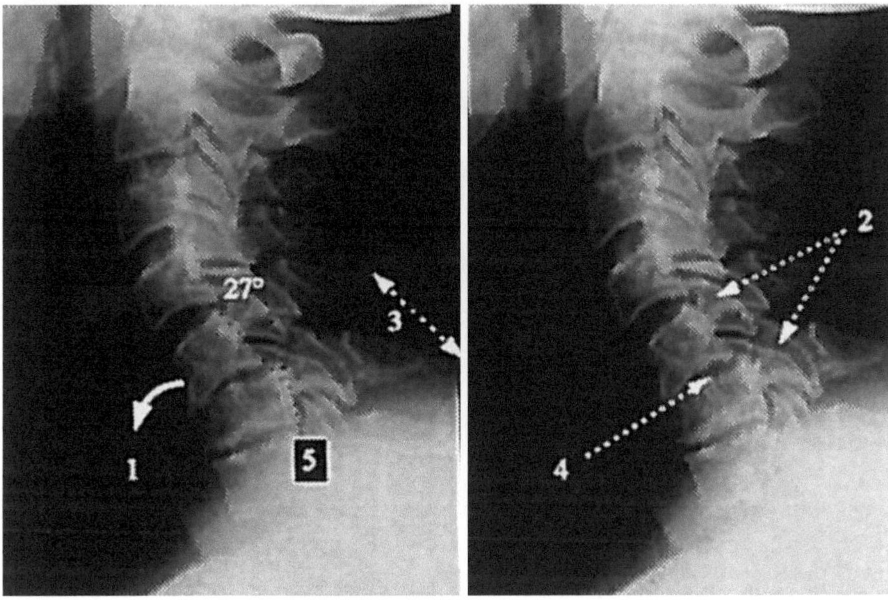

Fig. 5.3 Severe whiplash trauma

disk, ligament structures (severe sprain). However, this will eventually become clear with execution of radiographs in the lateral projection in maximal flexion and extension positions [9].

Pressure pain threshold (PPT) could provide additional prognostic ability to predict short-term outcomes in people with acute whiplash, but it has yet to be explored in people with acute (of less than 30 days in duration) whiplash-associated disorder. PPT measured at a site distal to the injury is the most parsimonious predictor of short-term neck-related disability score, and it represents promising addition to assessment of traumatic neck pain even if neither age nor PPT at the local site is able to explain significant variance of results [10].

Dynamic radiographs will evaluate signs of vertebral in stability that consist [11] of (1) anterolisthesis of a vertebral body with respect to the one underneath and >3 mm, (2) loss of contact and alignment of the zygapophyseal articular surfaces >50 %, (3) increase of the interspinal distance with respect to the upper or lower metamers (fanning), (4) elective discal kyphosis, and(5) angulation of the posterior somatic wall ~15° (Fig. 5.3).

The simultaneous presence of "at least three of" the above radiographic signs suggests a severe sprain, an instable lesion that implies a surgical type of treatment.

A partial dislocation or a lesion that in the lateral projection points out a mild anterior sliding of a vertebral body with respect to the one underneath cannot be underestimated, because it is often tied to an unilateral lesion (fracture or dislocation of a articular apophysis, pillar fracture); the rotation type implies a mild skid in an anteroposterior sense. In this case, even if the standard projection can point out a correct

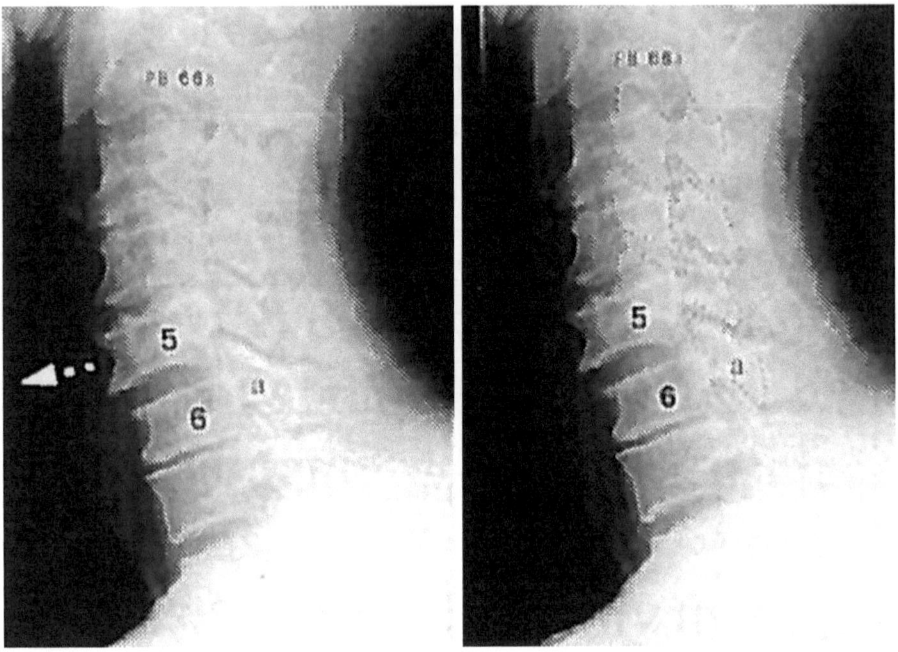

Fig. 5.4 In the lateral view, the articular mass is usually shown as one image as the articular apophyses are superimposed on each other. In this case of unilateral fracture-dislocation of C6, the articular mass present a double profile due to the rotational component. The arrow shows the mild shift typical for unilateral lesions

diagnosis (loss of an alignment of the spinal apophysis in the frontal projection; doubling of the articular apophysis silhouette in the lateral projection), the oblique projections eliminate all doubts and indicate correct treatment (Fig. 5.4) [12, 13].

In the unilateral fractures, there is an eventual decomposition of the articular apophysis and its rime (frequently the top ones), or in case of dislocation, there is a stenosis in the conjugate foramina and loss of the normal alignment of the zygapophyseal articular surfaces (Fig. 5.5).

In the pillar fracture of the facial mass, the characteristic sign is the horizontalization of the articular mass This happens because this peculiar cervical rachis lesion is characterized by two rimes of fracture: the anterior one in the peduncle and the posterior one within the laminae that isolate the articular mass, which is completely torn off and can rotate downward and forward, losing its normal oblique position in the lateral projection (Fig. 5.6).

The CT scan in this case will better evidence the two rimes of fracture, while in unilateral lesions it will confirm the diagnosis and show other lesions such as lamina fractures, not well distinguished with traditional radiology (Fig. 5.7) [9]. Magnetic resonance imaging (MRI) is especially indicated in patients who show persisting algesic symptomatology with radiation to the upper limb and with paresthesias, even if the metameric distribution is not precise.

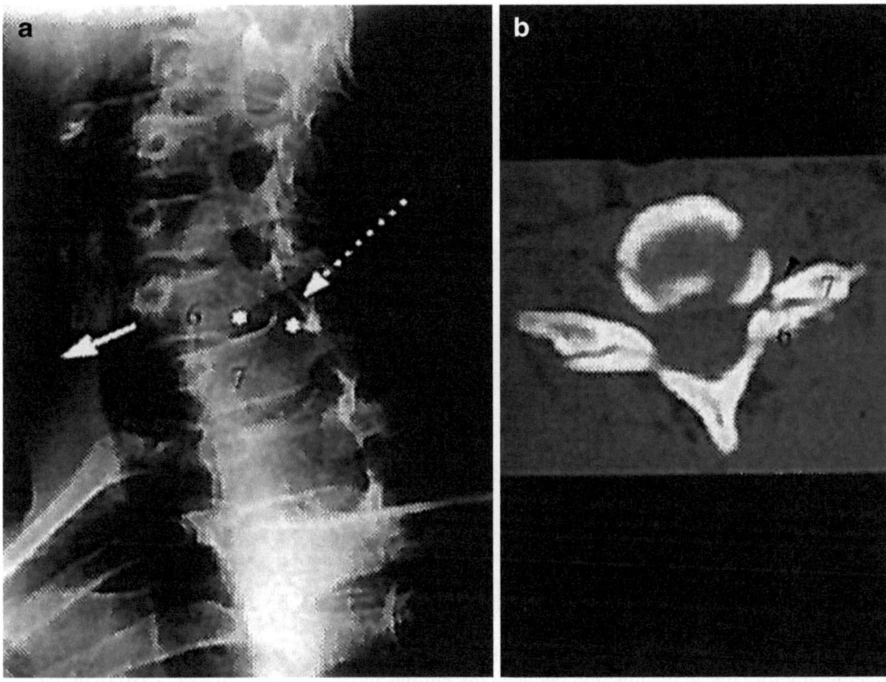

Fig. 5.5 (**a**) Unilateral fracture-dislocation C6–C7. The *arrow* shows the absence of normal alignment of zygapophyseal articular surfaces. The asterisks show the altered relationship between uncus and the semilunar facet. (**b**) The CT scan points out the stenosis of the conjugate channel (*arrow*)

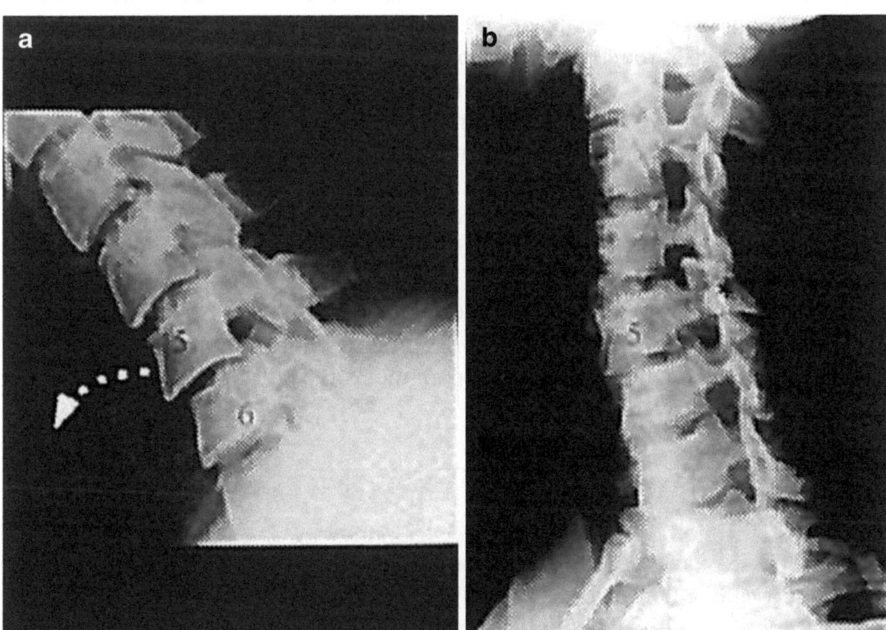

Fig. 5.6 Fracture of the articular mass of C5. (**a**) Lateral view, showing a mild sliding of C5 over C6. (**b**) Oblique view: the articular mass of C5 (*asterisk*) is anteriorly and downward rotated, narrowing the conjugate foramen of C4–C5

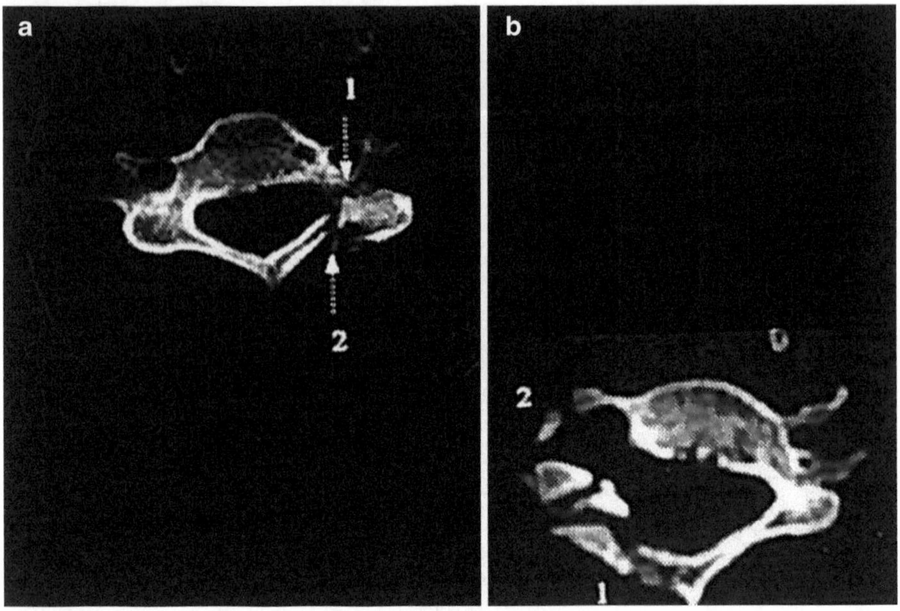

Fig. 5.7 (**a**) Fracture of the articular mass. The CT scan shows the fracture of the peduncle (1) and a second fracture line at the junction between the lamina and the articular mass (2). (**b**) In unilateral lesions the CT scan can show associated lesions, like fracture of the lamina (1) and (2) of the transverse process

MRI allows to demonstrate rupture of the anterior longitudinal ligament, osteochondral detachments of the vertebral plate, cleavages of the annulus fibrosus, separation of the intervertebral disk from the vertebral plate, and, frequently, discal protrusion.

Radiological findings associated with poor recovery following whiplash injury remain elusive [14]. Muscle fatty infiltrates in the cervical extensors occur soon following whiplash injury and suggest the possibility for the occurrence of a more severe injury with subsequent post-traumatic stress disorders (PSTD) in patients with persistent symptoms. MFI in the cervical extensors on MRI in patients with chronic pain have been observed. According to Elliot et al. (2011) [15], MFI values increased in moderate/severe group and were significantly higher in comparison to the recovered and mild groups at 3 and 6 months. They did not find differences in MFI values between the mild and recovered groups. Initial severity of PTSD symptoms mediated the relationship between pain intensity and MFI at 6 months.

5.4 Treatment

The initial phase of treatment of mild distortional forms of whiplash involves immobilization with a rigid or Philadelphia-type collar for a period of time not less than 2 weeks.

From a pharmacological point of view, the patient will benefit from the administration of analgesics (NSAIDs), myorelaxants (more efficient if with central action), and anti-vertigo drugs. With the removal of the orthopedic support, it will be important to restore muscular tone to guarantee correct posture and kinematics of the cervical column: this is possible with physical training and stretching.

There are few diagnostic tools for chronic musculoskeletal pain as structural imaging methods seldom reveal pathological alterations. Linnman et al. (2012) [16] visualized inflammatory processes in the neck region by means of positron-emission tomography using the tracer C-D-deprenyl, a potential marker for inflammation in 22 patients with enduring pain after a rear-impact car accident (whiplash-associated disorder grade II). They showed that patients, with respect to controls, displayed significantly elevated tracer uptake in the neck, particularly in regions around the spinous process of the second cervical vertebra, suggesting that whiplash patients have signs of local persistent peripheral tissue inflammation, which may potentially serve as a diagnostic biomarker.

It is useful to combine gymnastics with physiokinetic therapy, massage therapy, TENS, and ultrasound, which all have analgesic action. Vertebral manipulation is still controversial, particularly in elderly subjects in whom degenerative alterations of the cervical rachis are present, due to the risk of permanent neurologic lesions.

In a later phase, the persisting algesic symptomatology in some patients can be relieved by the infiltration of steroid compounds in the posterior articular facies, possibly associated with local anesthetics.

Noninvasive treatment is normally undertaken in the true forms of whiplash or in mild traumatic sprain (mentioned earlier). This includes most of the traumatic events occurring in the cervical column anel, as mentioned above, can lead to loss of rachis stability for osteo, disc, capsular, and ligament lesions, immediately or after the initial trauma. Instability, meaning the loss of the normal vertebral structure, needs more substantial treatment, such as more extreme immobilization with, e.g., the halo-vest for lesions in which the instability is exclusively or almost all osseous (thus temporaneous), with the possibility of treatment by consolidation of the fracture (pillar fracture without radicular lesion).

Surgical treatment is suggested for permanent instable forms (severe sprain, decomposition articular fractures, unilateral dislocations, pillar fracture with severe decomposition, and simultaneous reticular lesion), with protrusions and discal hernias with medullar radicular lesion.

The surgical options include intersomatic discectomy, arthrodesis performed anteriorly by Smith and Robinson's technique, possibly associated with a plaque screwed on to the upper and lower vertebral bodies, and posterior osteosynthesis by screwing together the articular mass, perhaps associated with arthrodesis (Figs. 5.8 and 5.9).

5.5 Prognosis

Prognosis of whiplash injury has been found to be related to a number of sociodemographic, treatment, and clinical factors. Dufton et al. (2012) [14] attempted to identify prognostic factors for delayed recovery using a validated and reliable

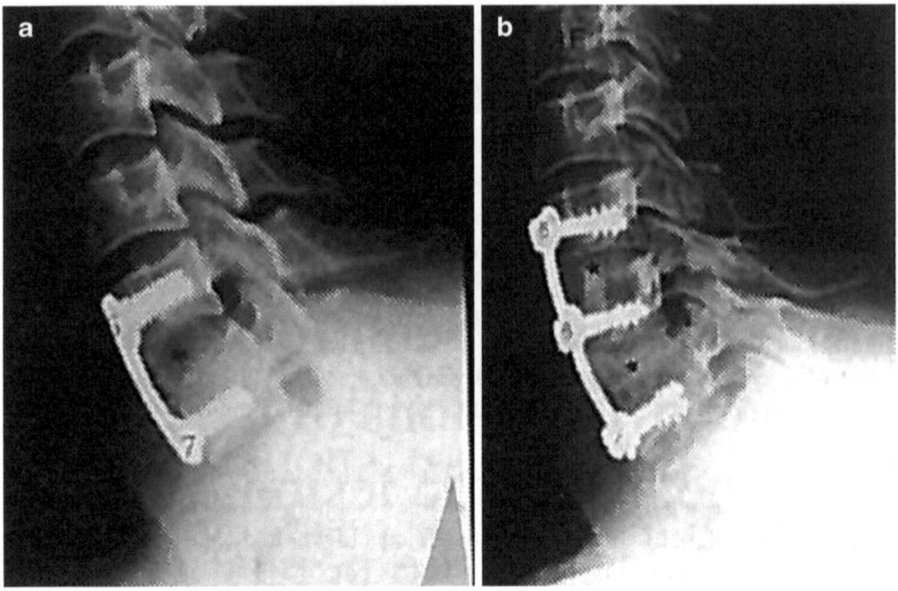

Fig. 5.8 Intersomatic arthrodesis performed by an anterior approach: at one level (**a**) or two levels (**b**) with different osteosynthesis devices. *Asterisks* indicate the autologous bone graft

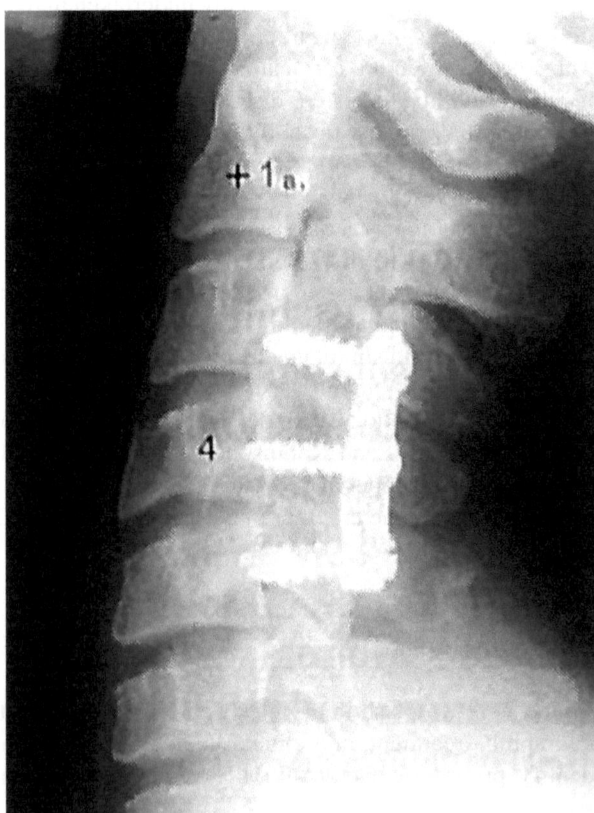

Fig. 5.9 Osteosynthesis with plate of the articular mass via a posterior approach

measure of recovery in a retrospective review of a large database from a national network of physiotherapy and rehabilitation service providers in Canada.

In a group of 5,581 individuals injured in motor vehicle collisions, they demonstrated positive outcomes to be proportionally fewer in the chronic cohort (52.1 %) relative to the early chronic (61.4 %), which was in turn lower than the acute cohort (72.3 %). Furthermore, individuals presenting with chronic pain were more likely to:

1. Be female
2. Be present with lower limb pain or nonorganic signs
3. Have returned to work
4. Have retained a lawyer or
5. have undergone previous spinal surgery

They were less likely to:

1. Be present with neck or mid-back pain
2. Live in Ontario or Nova Scotia
3. Have modified duties upon return to work

Generally speaking, recovery in whiplash-associated disorder appears to be multifactorial with both medical and noninjury-related factors influencing outcome.

References

1. Guo LY, Lee SY, Lin CF, Yang CH, Hou YY, Wu WL, Lin HT (2012) Three-dimensional characteristics of neck movements in subjects with mechanical neck disorder. J Back Musculoskelet Rehabil 25(1):47–53
2. Carroll LJ, Liu Y, Holm LW, Cassidy JD, Côté P (2011) Pain-related emotions in early stages of recovery in whiplash-associated disorders: their presence intensity, and association with pain recovery. Psychosom Med 73(8):708–715. Epub 2011 Sep 23
3. Lemming D, Graven-Nielsen T, Sörensen J, Arendt-Nielsen L, Gerdle B (2012) Widespread pain hypersensitivity and facilitated temporal summation of deep tissue pain in whiplash associated disorder: an explorative study of women. J Rehabil Med 44(8):648–657
4. White AA, Panjiabi MM (1990) Clinical biomechanics of the spine. Lippincott, Philadelphia
5. Elliott JM (2011) Are there implications for morphological changes in neck muscles after whiplash injury? Spine 36(25 Suppl):S205–S210
6. Clark CR, Igram CM, El-Khoury GY, Ehara S (1988) Radiographic evaluation of cervical spine injuries. Spine 13:742–747
7. Bohlman HH (1979) Acute fractures and dislocations of the cervical spine. J Bone Joint Surg Am 61A:1119–1141
8. Beyer CA, Cabanela ME, Berquist TH (1991) Unilateral facet dislocations and fracture-dislocations of the cervical spine. J Bone Joint Surg Br 73B:977–981
9. Davis SJ, Teresi LM, Bradley WG, Bloze AE, Ziemba MA (1991) Cervical spine hyperextension injuries: MR findings. Radiology 180:245
10. Walton DM, Macdermid JC, Nielson W, Teasell RW, Reese H, Levesque L (2011) Pressure pain threshold testing demonstrates predictive ability in people with acute whiplash. J Orthop Sports Phys Ther 41(9):658–665. doi:10.2519/jospt.2011.3668
11. Dvorak J, Froelich D, Penning L, Baumgartner H, Panjabi MM (1988) Functional radiographic diagnosis of the cervical spine: flexion/extension. Spine 13:748–755
12. Evans D (1976) Anterior cervical subluxation. J Bone Joint Surg Br 58B:318–321
13. Fuentes JM, Benezech J, Lussiez B, Vlahovitch B (1986) La fracture-separation du massif articulaire du rachis cervical inferieure. Ses rapports avec la fracture dislocation en hyperextension. Rev Chir Orthop Reparatrice Appar Mot 72:435–440

14. Dufton JA, Bruni SG, Kopec JA, Cassidy JD, Quon J (2012) Delayed recovery in patients with whiplash-associated disorders. Injury 43(7):1141–1147
15. Elliott J, Pedler A, Kenardy J, Galloway G, Jull G, Sterling M (2011) The temporal development of fatty infiltrates in the neck muscles following whiplash injury: an association with pain and posttraumatic stress. PLoS One 6(6):e21194. Epub 2011 June 16
16. Linnman C, Appel L, Fredrikson M, Gordh T, Söderlund A, Långström B, Engler H (2011) Elevated [11C]-D-deprenyl uptake in chronic Whiplash Associated Disorder suggests persistent musculoskeletal inflammation. PLoS One 6(4):e19182

Neurology of Whiplash

6

G. Meola, E. Bugiardini, and E. Scelzo

6.1 Introduction

Whiplash is an acceleration-deceleration mechanism of energy transfer to the neck which may result mainly from rear-end or side-impact motor vehicle collisions but also from diving or other mishaps [1]. Whiplash-associated disorder (WAD) is generally considered to be a soft tissue injury of the neck with symptoms such as neck pain and stiffness, headaches, cognitive and psychiatric disorders, dizziness, visual symptoms, paresthesias, and weakness. It is estimated that the incidence of whiplash injury is approximately 4 per 1,000 persons [2]. Although many persons involved in whiplash injuries recover quickly, between 4 and 42 % of patients report symptoms several years later [2, 3]. According to Quebec Task Force, late whiplash syndrome has been defined by the symptoms persistence for more than 6 months after the injury. Patients with neurological symptoms caused by whiplash syndrome are frequently referred to neurologists in everyday clinical practice.

The relevance of neurological signs in whiplash syndrome is highlighted by their role on determining the severity of the disease in Quebec Task Force classification of WAD (see Chap. 24).

6.2 Clinical Presentation

Clinical presentation of patients affected by whiplash syndrome may include different symptoms and signs involving both central and peripheral nervous system (see Table 6.1). Although it is one of the most relevant symptoms of whiplash syndrome,

G. Meola (✉) • E. Bugiardini • E. Scelzo
Department of Neurology,
University of Milan, IRCCS Policlinico San Donato Milanese,
Via Morandi 30, San Donato Milanese,
Milan 20097, Italy
e-mail: giovanni.meola@unimi.it

D.C. Alpini et al. (eds.), *Whiplash Injuries*,
DOI 10.1007/978-88-470-5486-8_6, © Springer-Verlag Italia 2014

Table 6.1 Neurological symptoms after whiplash injury

Headaches	Migraine-type headache Tension-type headache Cervicogenic-type headache Temporomandibular joint derangement Greater occipital neuralgia Third occipital headache
Cognitive and psychological symptoms	Memory, attention, or concentration impairment Sleep disturbance Psychiatric disorders: anxiety, depression, phobic travel, anxiety, and post-traumatic stress disorder
Dizziness	Vestibular dysfunction Cervical origin Brainstem dysfunction
Visual symptoms	Blurred vision Reduced visual field Photophobia Disordered fusion Reading and driving difficulties Reduced accommodation
Paresthesias	Trigger points Brachial plexopathy Cervical radiculopathy Spinal cord compression
Weakness	Brachial plexopathy Cervical radiculopathy Spinal cord compression
Rare symptoms	Torticollis Tremor Transient global amnesia Hypoglossal nerve palsy Superior laryngeal nerve paralysis Cervical epidural hematoma Brainstem infarct Internal carotid and vertebral artery dissection Symptomatic Chiari malformation

neck pain will not be discussed because in the majority of cases, it is thought to be due to a myofascial injury (of orthopedic pertinence).

6.3 Headaches

The incidence of headache in whiplash patients varies widely depending on methodologies utilized in the past studies. Unspecific headache in acute stage seems to be present in 50 % to more than 75 % of cases, while in 25–33 % of the cases, symptoms become chronic [4].

The origin of whiplash headache is probably multifactorial. In the second edition of the International Classification of Headache Disorders (2004) [5], whiplash headache has been classified in two categories: acute and chronic form. To fulfil the diagnostic criteria, headache, at the time accompanied by neck pain, must develop within 7 days after a whiplash injury. In the acute form, headache resolves within 3 months after whiplash injury, while in chronic form it persists longer. Diagnostic criteria do not specify typical characteristics of headache thus leading to question their application in clinical practice [6]. In previous studies, whiplash headache has been described as migraine-, tension-type headache, or cervicogenic headache [4]. A recent analysis showed that the headache after whiplash may represent a primary headache (mostly migraine- or tension-type headache) elicited by the stress of the situation [7].

Besides the unspecific headaches reported before, other factors as temporomandibular joint derangement [8], greater occipital neuralgia [9], and third occipital headache may contribute to the development of cephalalgia. Greater occipital neuralgia may be a consequence of whiplash injury especially in patients with anatomic entrapment of the nerve. Indeed in cases in which greater occipital nerve pass through the trapezius muscle, it may be damaged during neck flexion and extension typical of whiplash injury [9]. Third occipital headache was a condition investigated by Bogduk that consisted of referred headache caused by a C2–C3 zygapophyseal joint injury [10]. C2–C3 zygapophyseal joint is innervated by third occipital nerve whose afferent fibers converge with trigeminal afferents in spinal cord creating a neuroanatomical basis of referral pain to the head [10]. Using third occipital nerve block to diagnose this form of headache, Lord et al. [11] found a prevalence varying from 38 to 58 % in patients with headache post-whiplash.

6.4 Cognitive and Psychological Symptoms

Cognitive symptoms are a frequent complaint of patients with whiplash. In different studies, the prevalence of cognitive disturbances such as memory, attention, and concentration impairment was nearly 50 % [12, 13].

Previous neuropsychological examinations have found a deficit in attention tests [14] that was supposed to depend on the emotional dysfunction and the distracting effect of pain. Radanov [15] supports the concept that psychological and cognitive problems of patients with common whiplash are mainly related to somatic symptoms. Other works do not confirm the presence of deficit in neuropsychological test in patients with cognitive symptoms [13]. They suppose that cognitive problems appear to be indicators of heightened somatic vigilance rather than indicators of actual neuropsychological deficits. Additionally, somatization and inadequate coping may contribute to subjective complaints and poor performances in these patients [16]. Moreover, a recent study on MRI-based brain volumetry did not find any alteration in chronic whiplash patients [17]. Studies based on SPECT, PET, and functional MRI showed controversial results on the presence of specific brain alterations in whiplash [18, 19].

6.4.1 Sleep Disturbance

Sleep disturbances are common in patients after a whiplash injury ranging from 39 to 87 % of cases [20, 21]. Prevalence is higher immediately after the injury and patients' complaint falls significantly thereafter [21]. Sleep monitoring by actigraph failed to demonstrate significant alterations in sleep latency, sleep duration, number of arousals, or sleep efficiency. Otherwise, their subjective impression of sleep quality was significantly lower compared to controls [22].

Available data cannot exclude the presence of subtle, but clinically important, sleep disturbances demonstrable by polysomnography. Another recent work found an association between sleep disturbances and the intensity of pain [23] that is suggested to be one of the most relevant factors in determining sleep alteration.

6.4.2 Psychiatric Disorders

Mental symptoms after a whiplash injury are common. Psychological disorders have been found with a prevalence of 37 % at 3 months, 35 % at 1 year, and 35 % at 3 years after whiplash injury [24]. The alterations more frequently individuated are anxiety, depression, phobic travel anxiety, and post-traumatic stress disorder [24]. Reported psychiatric disorders are not specific of whiplash injury but are comparable to those following other types of injury (i.e., road traffic agents) [24]. The increased prevalence of anxiety disorders and depression is also supposed to be related to chronic pain suggesting that whiplash traumas should be considered in the same way as other chronic pain syndromes [25]. An interesting point of view is what emerges from the work of Mykletun et al. [26] which hypothesizes a reverse causality between whiplash and symptoms of anxiety and depression. Indeed, they found a higher incidence of chronic whiplash syndrome in patients already affected by anxiety and depression supporting that chronic whiplash may represent to some degree a functional disorder. The importance of psychological factors on the development of late whiplash syndrome is supported by recent evidences about the association between specific personality traits and the chronicization of symptoms [16].

6.5 Dizziness

Dizziness is a frequent complaint in patients with whiplash syndrome, reaching the 70 % of patients with chronic symptoms [27]. The dizziness may origin from an alteration of different systems that may be involved in whiplash-associated disorder. Direct dysfunction of the vestibular apparatus, such as benign paroxysmal positional vertigo (BPPV), may lead to true vertigo in whiplash patients. In a recent work of Dispenza et al. [28], it was found that 33.9 % of patients with whiplash injury present BPPV and it was underlined the importance of a correct individuation of these patients to perform a specific therapy. Dizziness of cervical origin is another frequent cause of dizziness in whiplash patients. Direct trauma on the neck may modify muscle spindle sensitivity leading to an alteration of cervical afferent input to the postural control system and a secondary impairment of the vestibular and visual system [29]. Vertebrobasilar artery insufficiency has been reported as a possible cause of dizziness, but more studies are needed to better define its role in whiplash syndrome [30]. Another cause of dizziness of cervical origin was that proposed by Barré and Lieou in 1928 [31] (posterior cervical sympathetic syndrome, Barré-Lieou syndrome). It was supposed that posterior circulation (including circulation of inner ear) was innervated by sympathetic nerve emerging from cervical roots. The cervical roots compression led to sympathetic irritation and consequently vasoconstriction and ischemia of inner ear. This theory is not widely accepted, and no recent papers supporting it have been published [32].

In conclusion, a brainstem dysfunction due to movement of brain within the skull may be a further cause of dizziness through an alteration of the inhibitory effect on the vestibular nuclei [33].

6.6 Visual Symptoms

Visual and ocular disturbances in whiplash syndrome have been widely reported in literature. They include not only disorders complained by patients as blurred vision, reduced visual field, photophobia, disordered fusion [29, 34], reading and driving difficulties [35], or reduced accommodation [29, 34] but also ocular alterations found in both symptomatic and asymptomatic patients (oculomotor system deficits, disturbances in smooth pursuit, eye movement with neck torsion, or saccadic eye movement) [29, 34, 36]. Most of the visual disturbances described in whiplash are thought to reflect an alteration in central connections between the eyes and the cervical afferents. Other visual symptoms may depend on injury to the brainstem or to higher centers in the central nervous system [37]. A significant reduction in the amplitude of accommodation was found in whiplash patients reporting visual disturbances [38]. Deficient accommodation has been attributed to an interruption or stimulation of the sympathetic pathway; to vascular disturbances of the vertebral, basilar, or internal carotid artery; or to lesions of the midbrain in the area of the third nerve nucleus [38]. Oculomotor system deficits have also been reported and seem to be mostly related to cervical afferent disturbances [39]; they are generally mild and are characterized by a good prognosis [40].

6.7 Paresthesias

Numerous clinical studies have documented paresthesias of neck, shoulders, upper back, and arms in whiplash patients. Norris and Watt found that the incidence of paresthesias acutely complained by patients ranged from 33 to 100 % depending on the presence of neurological abnormalities and the evidence of neurological loss. Symptoms tend to persist in a variable number of subjects after 6 months [41]. Paresthesias in the upper extremities can be caused by myofascial injuries with trigger points, by brachial plexopathy including thoracic outlet syndrome, and less often by cervical radiculopathy and spinal cord compression. Sometimes trigger points localized in several neck and trunk muscles can cause referred paresthesias in the upper extremities [42]. Whiplash injuries are a common cause of thoracic outlet syndrome (TOS) [43]. Whiplash injury would most likely affect a narrowing of the scalene triangle by spasm of the scalene muscles, but may also cause a reduction of the costoclavicular space by an elevation of the first rib, again secondary to continuous contraction of the scalene [44]. Some authors hypothesize that many patients with harm symptoms persisting more than some months after the injury might be affected by a neurogenic type of TOS caused directly by the trauma or by a secondary TOS related to cervical disc injury. The latter type of TOS is supposed to be caused by an alteration of anterior or posterior scalene muscles secondary to the involvement of the roots they are innervated by (C5–C7) [45]. Additionally, despite rarely, whiplash injuries can induce other brachial plexus lesions such as long thoracic and spinal accessory nerve injuries [46–48]. Paresthesias may also be associated with nerve root, ganglion, and spinal cord compression. During rear impact, the intervertebral levels of the lower cervical spine can undergo hyperextension, which may cause reduction in the cervical foraminal area and in canal diameter leading to nerve root, ganglion, and spinal cord damage [2, 49]. Several authors have found a strong association between radiculopathy and foraminal spondylosis preceding whiplash injury. Recent studies showed that rear impact may cause ganglion compression also in nonspondylotic foramen mainly at C5–C6 and C6–C7 levels but that the injury risk greatly increases in patients with spondylotic foramen involving also C3–C4 and C4–C5 levels [49, 50]. Repeated ganglion or nerve root compression caused by an increased joint laxity or instability induced by ligamentous injury has been supposed to be one of the most important risk factors for chronicization of radicular symptoms. This risk is exacerbated in individuals with foraminal spondylosis due to smaller bony foraminal dimensions [49]. Central cord injury without vertebral fractures is uncommon in whiplash syndrome. Although recent evidences have revealed that spinal cord injury is even possible in subjects with normal cervical canal, almost all cases are reported in patients with cervical stenosis and only after wide neck extension [51, 52].

6.8 Weakness

Complaints of upper extremity and neck weakness are common after whiplash injuries. Weakness may be caused by brachial plexopathy, cervical radiculopathy, and spinal cord compression with mechanisms similar to those described for paresthesias. Weakness is reported by patients even when there is no evidence of nervous system involvement. Some studies reported very low cervical strength scores in both acute and chronic whiplash patients [53, 54]. Prushansky et al. [54] found that cervical strength is reduced by about 80 and 90 % in women and men, respectively, compared to controls especially in extension patterns of movement. Although there is no consensus about it, recent studies have found no changes of cervical muscle volumes 6 months after whiplash injury and no consistent correlation of muscle volumes with clinical variables [55]. In the absence of severe atrophy or neurological dysfunctions, cervical muscles weakness has been suggested to be related to pain or to fear of pain [53]. A possible explanation of patients' sensation of weakness or heaviness is the reflex inhibition of muscle due to pain that can be contrasted only by central voluntary effort [56].

Conclusion

On the origin of the symptoms caused by whiplash, there is a wide debate especially regarding the late whiplash syndrome. Different nonorganic explanations have been proposed as the influence of psychological factors and the possibility of malingering. Indeed, the subjective nature of the majority of symptoms and the possibility of a financial compensation create the basis of the so-called compensation hypothesis. This theory is supported by the evidence that the incidence of whiplash syndrome varies between nations with different insurance systems and that the number of claims decreases after modification in financial compensation [57]. However, there are currently no sufficient data to accept this hypothesis [58]. The controversy between the organic and nonorganic etiology of whiplash has to be kept in mind to understand the conflicting data reported above.

In conclusion, irrespective of scientific debate, clinicians should carefully evaluate neurological symptoms to address patients to the correct diagnostic center and to choose the most appropriate treatment. Nevertheless, it is mandatory to consider the psychological aspects of this condition to achieve a correct "prise en charge" of the patients.

References

1. Spitzer WO, Skovron ML, Salmi LR, Cassidy JD, Duranceau J, Suissa S, Zeiss E (1995) Scientific monograph of Quebec Task Force on Whiplash-Associated Disorders: redefining "whiplash" and its management. Spine 20(8 Suppl):1–73
2. Eck JC, Hodges SD, Humphreys SC (2001) Whiplash: a review of a commonly misunderstood injury. Am J Med 110:651–656
3. Radanov BP, Sturzenegger M, DiStefano G (1995) Long-term outcome after whiplash injury. Medicine 74:281–297
4. Sjaastad O, Fredriksen T, Bakketeig L (2009) Headache subsequent to whiplash. Curr Pain Headache Rep 13(1):52–58
5. Headache Classification Subcommittee of the International Headache Society (2004) The International Classification of Headache Disorders: 2nd edition. Cephalalgia 24(1 Suppl): 9–160
6. Schrader H, Stovner LJ, Obelieniene D, Surkiene D, Mickeviciene D, Bovim G, Sand T (2006) Examination of the diagnostic validity of 'headache attributed to whiplash injury': a controlled, prospective study. Eur J Neurol 13(11):1226–1232
7. Stovner LJ, Obelieniene D (2008) Whiplash headache is transitory worsening of a pre-existing primary headache. Cephalalgia 28(Suppl 1):28–31
8. Epstein JB, Klasser GD (2011) Whiplash-associated disorders and temporomandibular symptoms following motor-vehicle collisions. Quintessence Int 42(1):e1–e14

9. Magnússon T, Ragnarsson T, Björnsson A (1996) Occipital nerve release in patients with whiplash trauma and occipital neuralgia. Headache 36(1):32–36
10. Bogduk N, Marsland A (1986) On the concept of third occipital headache. J Neurol Neurosurg Psychiatry 49(7):775–780
11. Lord SM, Barnsley L, Wallis BJ, Bogduk N (1994) Third occipital nerve headache: a prevalence study. J Neurol Neurosurg Psychiatry 57(10):1187–1190
12. Kischka U, Ettlin TH, Heim S (1991) Cerebral symptoms following whiplash injury. Eur Neurol 31:136–140
13. Robinson JP, Burwinkle T, Turk DC (2007) Perceived and actual memory, concentration, and attention problems after whiplash-associated disorders (grades I and II): prevalence and predictors. Arch Phys Med Rehabil 88(6):774–779
14. Di Stefano G, Radanov BP (1996) Quantitative and qualitative aspects of learning and memory in common whiplash patients: a 6-month follow-up study. Arch Clin Neuropsychol 11: 661–676
15. Radanov BP, Di Stefano G, Schnidrig A, Sturzenegger M (1994) Common whiplash: psychosomatic or somatopsychic? J Neurol Neurosurg Psychiatry 57:486–490
16. Guez M, Brannstrom R, Nyberg L, Toolanen G, Hildingsson C (2005) Neuropsychological functioning and MMPI-2 profiles in chronic neck pain: a comparison of whiplash and nontraumatic groups. J Clin Exp Neuropsychol 27:151–163
17. Sturzenegger M, Radanov BP, Winter P, Simko M, Farra AD, Di Stefano G (2008) MRI-based brain volumetry in chronic whiplash patients: no evidence for traumatic brain injury. Acta Neurol Scand 117(1):49–54
18. Otte A, Ettlin TM, Nitzsche EU, Wachter K, Hoegerle S, Simon GH, Fierz L, Moser E, Mueller-Brand J (1997) PET and SPECT in whiplash syndrome: a new approach to a forgotten brain? J Neurol Neurosurg Psychiatry 63(3):368–372
19. Bicik I, Radanov BP, Schäfer N, Dvorak J, Blum B, Weber B, Burger C, Von Schulthess GK, Buck A (1998) PET with 18fluorodeoxyglucose and hexamethylpropylene amine oxime. SPECT in late whiplash syndrome. Neurology 51(2):345–350
20. Radanov BP, Sturzenegger M, De Stefano G, Schnidrig A (1994) Relationship between early somatic, radiological, cognitive and psychosocial findings and outcome during a one-year follow-up in 117 patients suffering from common whiplash. Br J Rheumatol 33:442–448
21. Magnusson T (1994) Extracervical symptoms after whiplash trauma. Cephalalgia 14:223–227
22. Schlesinger I, Hering-Hanit R, Dagan Y (2001) Sleep disturbances after whiplash injury: objective and subjective findings. Headache 41(6):586–589
23. Valenza MC, Valenza G, González-Jiménez E, De-la-Llave-Rincón AI, Arroyo-Morales M, Fernández-de-Las-Peñas C (2012) Alteration in sleep quality in patients with mechanical insidious neck pain and whiplash-associated neck pain. Am J Phys Med Rehabil 91(7): 584–591
24. Mayou R, Bryant B (2002) Psychiatry of whiplash neck injury. Br J Psychiatry 180:441–448
25. Wenzel HG, Haug TT, Mykletun A, Dahl AA (2002) A population study of anxiety and depression among persons who report whiplash traumas. J Psychosom Res 53(3):831–835
26. Mykletun A, Glozier N, Wenzel HG, Overland S, Harvey SB, Wessely S, Hotopf M (2011) Reverse causality in the association between whiplash and symptoms of anxiety and depression: the HUNT study. Spine 36(17):1380–1386
27. Treleaven J, Jull G, Sterling M (2003) Dizziness and unsteadiness following whiplash injury: characteristic features and relationship with cervical joint position error. J Rehabil Med 35:36–43
28. Dispenza F, De Stefano A, Mathur N, Croce A, Gallina S (2011) Benign paroxysmal positional vertigo following whiplash injury: a myth or a reality? Am J Otolaryngol 32(5):376–380
29. Treleaven J (2011) Dizziness, unsteadiness, visual disturbances, and postural control: implications for the transition to chronic symptoms after a whiplash trauma. Spine 36(25 Suppl): 211–217

30. Endo K, Ichimaru K, Komagata M, Yamamoto K (2006) Cervical vertigo and dizziness after whiplash injury. Eur Spine J 15(6):886–890
31. Barré JA (1926) Sur un syndrome sympathique cervical postérieur et sa cause frequente, l'arthrite cervicale. Rev Neurol (Paris) 1:1246–1248
32. Yacovino DA (2012) Cervical vertigo: myths, facts, and scientific evidence. Neurología. doi:10.1016/j.nrl.2012.06.013
33. Chetana N, Claussen CF (2010) Vertigo in whiplash injury: a presentation of prevalent butterfly patterns of caloric tests. Indian J Otolaryngol Head Neck Surg 62(2):208–214
34. Treleaven J, Jull G, Grip H (2011) Head eye co-ordination and gaze stability in subjects with persistent whiplash associated disorders. Man Ther 16(3):252–257
35. Gimse R, Bjørgen IA, Straume A (1997) Driving skills after whiplash. Scand J Psychol 38(3):165–170
36. Mosimann UP, Muri RM, Felblinger J, Radanov PB (2000) Saccadic eye movement disturbances in whiplash patients with persistent complaints. Brain 123:828–835
37. Treleaven J, Jull G, LowChoy N (2005) Smooth pursuit neck torsion test in whiplash-associated disorders: relationship to self-reports of neck pain and disability, dizziness and anxiety. J Rehabil Med 37(4):219–223
38. Brown S (2003) Effect of whiplash injury on accommodation. Clin Experiment Ophthalmol 31(5):424–429
39. Heikkila HV, Wenngren BI (1998) Cervicocephalic kinesthetic sensibility, active range of cervical motion, and oculomotor function in patients with whiplash injury. Arch Phys Med Rehabil 79(9):1089–1094
40. Burke JP, Orton HP, West J, Strachan IM, Hockey MS, Ferguson DG (1992) Whiplash and its effect on the visual system. Graefes Arch Clin Exp Ophthalmol 230(4):335–339
41. Norris SH, Watt I (1983) The prognosis of neck injuries resulting from rear-end vehicle collisions. J Bone Joint Surg Br 65(5):608–611
42. Evans RW (2006) Whiplash injuries. In: Evans RW (ed) Neurology and trauma. WB Saunders, Philadelphia, pp 425–449
43. Roos DB, Owens JC (1966) Thoracic outlet syndrome. Arch Surg 93:71–74
44. Capistrant TD (1986) Thoracic outlet syndrome in cervical strain injury. Minn Med 69: 13–17
45. Kai Y, Oyama M, Kurose S, Inadome T, Oketani Y, Masuda Y (2001) Neurogenic thoracic outlet syndrome in whiplash injury. J Spinal Disord 14(6):487–493
46. Omar N, Alvi F, Srinivasan MS (2007) An unusual presentation of whiplash injury: long thoracic and spinal accessory nerve injury. Eur Spine J 16(3 Suppl):275–277
47. Bodack MP, Tunkel RS, Marini SG, Nagler W (1998) Spinal accessory nerve palsy as a cause of pain after whiplash injury: case report. J Pain Symptom Manage 15(5):321–328
48. Gupta V, Posner B (2004) Trauma to the long thoracic nerve and associated scapula winging in a low-velocity rear-end automobile collision: case report. J Trauma 57(2):402–403
49. Panjabi MM, Maak TG, Ivancic PC, Ito S (2006) Dynamic intervertebral foramen narrowing during simulated rear impact. Spine 31(5):E128–E134
50. Tominaga Y, Maak TG, Ivancic PC, Panjabi MM, Cunningham BW (2006) Head-turned rear impact causing dynamic cervical intervertebral foramen narrowing: implications for ganglion and nerve root injury. J Neurosurg Spine 4(5):380–387
51. Ito S, Panjabi MM, Ivancic PC, Pearson AM (2004) Spinal canal narrowing during simulated whiplash. Spine 29:1330–1339
52. Ivancic PC (2012) Cervical neural space narrowing during simulated rear crashes with anti-whiplash systems. Eur Spine J 21(5):879–886
53. Kasch H, Bach FW, Jensen TS (2001) Handicap after acute whiplash injury: a 1-year prospective study of risk factors. Neurology 56:1637–1643
54. Prushansky T, Gepstein R, Gordon C, Dvir Z (2005) Cervical muscles weakness in chronic whiplash patients. Clin Biomech (Bristol, Avon) 20(8):794–798

55. Ulbrich EJ, Aeberhard R, Wetli S, Busato A, Boesch C, Zimmermann H, Hodler J, Anderson SE, Sturzenegger M (2012) Cervical muscle area measurements in whiplash patients: acute, 3, and 6 months of follow-up. J Magn Reson Imaging 36(6):1413–1420
56. Aniss AM, Gandevia SC, Milne RJ (1988) Changes in perceived heaviness and motor commands produced by cutaneous reflexes in man. J Physiol 397:113–126
57. Cassidy JD, Carroll LJ, Côté P, Lemstra M, Berglund A, Nygren A (2000) Effect of eliminating compensation for pain and suffering on the outcome of insurance claims for whiplash injury. N Engl J Med 342(16):1179–1186
58. Spearing NM, Connelly LB (2011) Whiplash and the compensation hypothesis. Spine 36(25 Suppl):303–308

Radiological Evaluation

7

A. Bettinelli, M. Leonardi, E.P. Mangiagalli, and P. Cecconi

7.1 Introduction

The term "whiplash syndrome" was introduced by Crowe in 1928 [1], and it is normally used to describe a group of symptoms variously associated with unequal clinical importance. In most instances, the symptomatology is subjective, therefore the ensuring radiological evaluation may be elusive.

Generally speaking, patients complain about continuous pain to the posterior aspect of the occiput or the neck or both, sometimes bilaterally, with an area of reference to one or more muscles of the cervical paravertebral musculature; the trapezius is the muscle more frequently involved and, not uncommonly, there is a trigger zone lying outside the painful area [2]. The pain may irradiate to the axilla, to the arm, to the superolateral portion of the chest, and to the inferior tip of the shoulder blade. It is frequently associated with vertigo, tinnitus, diplopia, and dysphagia. In all such cases, the neurological exam is normal.

The pain worsens with movements of the cervical spine or with the strain involved in maintaining a posture.

Despite a large number of rear-end collisions on the road and a high frequency of whiplash injuries were reported, the mechanism of whiplash injuries is not

A. Bettinelli (✉) • E.P. Mangiagalli
Intermedica s.r.l., "Columbus" Private Hospital,
via Buonarroti 48, Milan, Italy
e-mail: intermedicarm@libero.it

M. Leonardi
Department of Neuroradiology, "Bellaria" Hospital,
via Altura 3, Bologna, Italy

P. Cecconi
Department of Neuroradiology, IRCCS "Don Carlo Gnocchi" Foundation,
via Capecelatro 66, Milan, Italy
e-mail: pcecconi@dongnocchi.it

D.C. Alpini et al. (eds.), *Whiplash Injuries*,
DOI 10.1007/978-88-470-5486-8_7, © Springer-Verlag Italia 2014

completely understood. One of the reasons is that the injury is not necessarily accompanied by obvious tissue damages detectable by X-ray or MRI.

Based on kinematical studies on cadavers and volunteers, there are three distinct periods that have the potential to cause injury to the neck. In the first stage, flexural deformation of the neck is observed along with a loss of cervical lordosis; in the second stage, the cervical spine takes an S-shaped curve as the lower vertebrae begin to extend and gradually cause the upper vertebrae to extend; during the final stage, the entire neck is extended due to the extension moments at both ends.

Experimental findings have examined strains across the facet joint as a mechanism of whiplash injury and suggested a capsular strain threshold or a vertebral distraction threshold for whiplash-related injury, potentially producing neck pain. Injuries to the facet capsule region of the neck are a major source of post-crash pain. There are several hypotheses on how whiplash-associated injury may occur and there are several possible injury criteria to correlate to the duration of symptoms during reconstructions of actual crashes. On a biomechanical basis, it has been hypothesized that the facet joint capsule is a source of neck pain and that the pain may arise from large strains in the joint capsule that will cause pain receptors to fire.

The aim of the chapter is to show the role of imaging in detecting and demonstrating spine and cervical soft tissues involvement due to whiplash.

7.2 Plain Standard X-Rays

Timely and accurate diagnosis of cervical spine injury is essential. A complete cervical spine series will diagnose almost 90 % of all cervical spine injuries and consists of a lateral roentgenogram from C1 to the top of T1, an AP roentgenogram, and an open mouth view (odontoid). In patients with large shoulders and/or short neck, it is often difficult to visualize the C7-T1 junction on the lateral film, and it may be necessary to apply traction to the arms to pull down the shoulders or obtain a swimmer's view [3]. Radiographs of the cervical spine after a whiplash injury are generally normal, except for the possible loss of physiological cervical lordosis [4].

The plain standard X-ray projections (anteroposterior, latero-lateral, oblique) obtained with the patient either in standing or sitting position may show a reversal of the physiological lordosis up to a hyperkyphotic appearance, sometimes coexisting with a lateral flexion of the cervical spine due to contraction of the lateral muscles of the neck. In this case, some authors [2] infer that the spasm of the neck muscle may be very disabling (i.e., in children it often reaches the features of a posttraumatic torticollis), especially if unilateral, and may interfere with the postural reflex of the neck ensuing a continuous and annoying vertigo which affects ambulation. Even a sprain to the longissimus colli may be associated with an injury of the cervical sympathetic plexus causing nausea and vertigo [2].

In the lateral projection, a widening of the vertebral interspace and perching of the facet joints can be noted due to a lesion of their facetal joint capsule. For this reason, lateral flexion and extension radiographs are useful to demonstrate the possible presence of an abnormal motion of one or more cervical vertebra disclosing injuries of the ligaments complex [5].

When an angular kyphosis is present, then an anterior or posterior subluxation may often be demonstrated, and the upper vertebral body is posteriorly or anteriorly displaced. Widening of the distance between the spinous processes (fanning) may be noted due to disruption of the interspinous and posterior ligament [29]. After a congruous period of time, discal and arthrosic modifications develop at the site of the kyphotic angulation.

Oblique radiographs in patients with flexion distraction injuries can be useful in the diagnosis of facet fractures. Obviously they should be obtained by angling the radiograph beam and not rotating the patient's head.

Pluridirectional tomography appears to be particularly advantageous in patients with injuries involving the facets. Computerized tomography appears to add the most additional information in patients with laminar and posterior element fractures and C1 fractures.

In unilateral dislocation on a lateral plain roentgenogram, the cephalad vertebra may appear translated up to 25 % of the width of the caudal vertebral body with splaying apart of the posterior spinous processes: The rotational deformity allows visualization of both facet joints on the lateral roentgenogram (normally superimposed), the so-called bow tie sign. On the AP roentgenogram, the spinous processes may be rotated with widening of the interspinous distance.

With bilateral dislocations, both inferior articular processes of the cephalad vertebra dislocate anterior to the superior processes of the caudal vertebra: This results in approximately 50 % anterior translation of the superior vertebral body on the inferior vertebral body. There is no rotational deformity (absent bow tie sign) on roentgenographic evaluation, and clinically the patient's head is held in the midline.

It is also very important not to neglect the first part of the thoracic spine, because it is not rare to see vertebral body fracture in T1 to T4. In fact, these vertebrae are functionally ascribed to the cervical spine by many authors.

Finally, the lower back must not be forgotten, because it is not rare that accident can involve this part of the body as well.

The role of dynamic lateral radiographs in an emergency setting remains controversial. These views are useful in alert, cooperative patients without neurological deficit and a normal spine series who continue to complain of neck pain. In this setting, a positive flexion-extension study has obvious clinical implications, but a negative roentgenogram does not rule out an acute flexion distraction injury. Patients with acute cervical spine subluxation may have muscle spasm which masks cervical instability for up to 2–3 weeks [5].

Static or dynamic flexion/extension lateral plain and AP roentgenogram can show subluxation of cervical vertebrae. Subluxation of the posterior cervical facet joints is caused by a partial disruption of the articular capsule and possibly the intervening intervertebral disk which allows anterior translation of the cephalad vertebra on the more caudal vertebra.

7.3 CT Scan

CT scan has no indication in the evaluation of patient with whiplash syndrome as we defined it here. Although CT allows good visualization of the bony structures, it does not yield a study of the ligamentous complex. CT with 3-D programs may demonstrate bony lesions not otherwise appreciated. It is true, CT permits imaging of the cervical disks and their lesions; however, an acute posttraumatic cervical disk herniation is very seldom without neurological deficits. Hence, within the framework of this chapter, CT evaluation is usually normal.

7.4 Magnetic Resonance Imaging

MRI clearly visualizes the anterior and posterior longitudinal ligaments and the interspinous ligament; hence, it is useful in defining their eventual tear. With the appropriate sequences, MRI permits evaluation of the soft tissues and the muscles. The presence of edema and/or hemorrhage in such spinal structures produces alteration in the magnetic signal [6].

MR imaging at 1.5 T reveals only limited evidence of specific changes to the cervical spine and the surrounding tissues in patients with acute symptomatic whiplash injury compared with healthy control subjects [7], but it is the choice imaging exam for cervical spine when radiographs show pathological findings or the clinical examination demonstrated signs suggestive of medullar involvement. The choice depends on the ability to show soft tissues and particularly nervous structures better than CT.

The principal disadvantage of MRI is the inability to show the cortical bone, making difficult the diagnosis of small fractures or the revelation of displaced bony fragments.

In the acute phase, plain radiographic films may only disclose, in lateral neutral position, a straightening or reversal of the physiological lordosis, or in lateral flexion-extension projection, an increased mobility of the cervical spine. In a selected number of patients, MRI may demonstrate the presence of paravertebral soft tissue edema or hematoma in the muscle of the neck.

Hypothesis that loss of integrity of the membranes in the craniocervical junction might be the cause of neck pain in patients with whiplash-associated disorders (WADs) has been proposed [8, 9]. In recent years, with the development of more detailed imaging techniques, morphologic changes of the ligaments and membranes in the craniocervical junction, especially alar and transverse ligaments, have been discussed. A meta-analysis was performed by Li et al. [10] to evaluate the relationship of MRI signal changes of alar and transverse ligaments and WADs. According to the authors, MRI signal changes of alar and transverse ligaments are not supposed to be caused from whiplash injury, and MRI examination of alar and transverse ligaments should not be used as the routine workflow of patients with WADs.

Schmidt et al. [11] demonstrate that high-field 3-T MRI provides better visualization of the alar ligaments compared with 1.5-T MRI. The higher signal-to-noise ratio allows detection of small signal changes. A great interindividual variety of the MRI morphology of the alar ligaments was found in participants with no history of neck trauma. Rupture of the alar and transverse ligaments due to whiplash injury can lead to upper cervical spine instability and subsequent neurological deterioration. The purpose of their study was to evaluate the normal anatomical variability of the alar ligaments in asymptomatic individuals with 3-T magnetic resonance imaging and to compare the findings with standard 1.5-T examinations. Magnetic resonance imaging findings were analyzed by classifying the alar ligaments with regard to the features detectability, signal intensity compared with muscle tissue, homogeneity, shape, spatial orientation, and symmetry. Delineation of the alar ligaments was significantly better on 3-T images, which were subjectively preferred for evaluation. The alar ligaments showed great variability. In the majority of participants, the alar ligaments were hypointense to muscle tissue, inhomogeneous, and different in shape and orientation.

Lummel et al. [12] showed an high variability of rotational mobility at the craniocervical junction and an attenuation of width of the subarachnoid space during head rotation also in an asymptomatic population. Their results indicate that the assessment of these parameters is of limited diagnostic value in patients with whiplash-associated disorders.

Cervical muscles involvement can be specifically investigated by mean of MRI. According to Elliot et al.'s [13] current evidence from structural MRI-based studies demonstrates the widespread presence of fatty infiltrates in neck muscles of patients with chronic whiplash. Such findings have not shown to feature in patients with chronic insidious-onset neck pain, suggesting traumatic factors play a role in their development. Recent studies have revealed that muscle fatty infiltrates manifest soon after whiplash but only in those with higher pain and disability and symptoms of posttraumatic stress disorder. The possibility that such muscle changes are associated with a more severe injury including poor functional recovery remains the focus of their research efforts. Authors hypothesized that cervical muscle hypotrophy would be evident after a 6-month follow-up and that cervical muscle hypotrophy would correlate with symptom persistence probably related to pain or inactivity. They performed in 90 symptomatic patients (48 females) MRI cross-sectional muscle area (CSA) measurements, bilaterally, of the cervical extensor and sternocleidomastoid muscles using transverse STIR (short tau inversion recovery) sequences at the C2 (deep and total dorsal cervical extensor muscles), C4 (sternocleidomastoid muscles), and C5 (deep and total dorsal cervical extensor muscles) levels. They found that women consistently had smaller CSAs than men. They found no significant changes of CSAs over time at any of the three levels. There were no consistent significant correlations of CSA values with the clinical scores at all time points, except with the body mass index. In conclusion, authors did not support a major role of cervical muscle volume in the genesis of symptoms after whiplash injury.

Long-term follow-up studies focusing on the posterior extensor muscles in patients suffering from whiplash injury are scarce. The purpose of Elliot et al. study [14] was to elucidate the changes in the posterior extensor muscles 10 years after whiplash injury. They performed MRI using a 1.5-T superconductive imager in 23 patients who had suffered from whiplash injury in 1994–1996 (13 males, 10 females, mean age 51.8 years, mean follow-up 11.5 years). In addition, 60 healthy volunteers who had undergone MRI in the same period were included as controls (36 males, 24 females, mean age 47.8 years, mean follow-up 11.1 years). All participants underwent follow-up MRI. The cross-sectional areas of the deep posterior muscles (CSA) including the multifidus, semispinalis cervicis, semispinalis capitis, and splenius capitis were digitally measured at C3–C4, C4–C5, and C5–C6 using NIH image. The long-term changes in the CSA were compared between the two groups. In addition, correlations between the CSA and cervical spine-related symptoms were evaluated. The mean total CSA per patient (the sum of the area from C3–C4 to C5–C6) was 4811.6 ± 878.4 mm2 in the whiplash patients and 4494.9 ± 1032.7 mm2 in the controls at the initial investigation ($p=0.20$) and 5173.4 ± 946.1 mm2 and 4713.0 ± 1065.3 mm2 at the follow-up ($p=0.07$). The mean change in CSA over time was 361.8 ± 804.9 mm2 in the whiplash patients and 218.1 ± 520.7 mm2 in the controls ($p=0.34$). Ten whiplash patients (43.5 %) had neck pain and 11 (47.8 %) had shoulder stiffness. However, there was no difference in the change in CSA over time between the symptomatic and asymptomatic patients. In conclusion, authors showed no significant difference in the change in CSA between whiplash patients and healthy volunteers after a 10-year follow-up period. In both groups, the cross-sectional area slightly increased at follow-up. In addition, there was no association between the change in CSA and clinical symptoms such as neck and shoulder pain. These results suggest that whiplash injury is not associated with symptomatic atrophy of the posterior cervical muscles over the long term [15–18].

Modic changes (MC) are a common phenomenon on magnetic resonance imaging (MRI) in spinal degenerative diseases and strongly linked with low back pain. They are due to signal intensity changes of vertebral endplates and subchondral bone. In 1988, Modic et al. [19] summarized these changes and classified them into three types, and then modic changes (MC), as a medical term, were used in the studies on spinal degenerative diseases.

There are few studies on MC of the cervical spine in patients suffering from whiplash. Matsumoto et al. [20] investigated relationships between modic changes and clinical symptoms or potentially related factors. They showed that while modic changes became more common in whiplash patients in the 10-year period after the accident, they occurred with a similar frequency in control subjects. We did not find any association between modic changes and the nature of the car accident in which the whiplash occurred. Modic changes found in whiplash patients may be a result of the physiological ageing process rather than pathological findings relating to the whiplash injury.

MRI can be used also to investigate extra-vertebral cervical involvement [21]. Elliot et al. through a [22] cross-sectional investigation has identified reductions in the size and shape of the oropharynx in subjects with chronic whiplash-related disability when compared to healthy controls. Repeated T1-weighted magnetic resonance imaging was used to measure and compare cross-sectional area (CSA) in square millimeters and shape ratio (SR) of the oropharynx in subjects with acute whiplash injury. MRI was performed at 4 weeks, 3 months, and 6 months post-injury. Subjects were classified at 6 months by their Neck Disability Index scores into the following categories: recovered (less than 8 %), mild disability (10–28 %), and moderate/severe disability (greater than 30 %). The effects of time and group and the interaction effect of group by time on oropharynx [23] morphometry (CSA, SR) were investigated using repeated-measure, linear, mixed-model analysis. Based on previous research findings, age, gender, and body mass index were entered into the analyses as covariates. Where significant main or interaction effects were detected, pairwise comparisons were performed to investigate specific differences in the dependent variable between groups and within groups over time. Authors found a significant interaction effect for group by time for both the CSA and SR values. Age significantly influenced SR, and body mass index significantly influenced CSA – there was no difference in CSA or SR across all groups at 4 weeks post-injury. However, at 6 months, CSA was significantly different between the recovered group and the moderate/severe group. The recovered group demonstrated a significant increase in CSA over time, whereas the moderate/severe group significantly decreased. At 6 months, the moderate/severe group had a reduced SR compared to the mild group. No differences in CSA or SR of the oropharynx were found between the mild and recovered groups throughout the study. In conclusion, authors showed temporal reductions in CSA of the oropharynx occur following whiplash, reductions that persist to a greater extent in those with moderate/severe symptoms at 6 months post-injury.

7.5 Echography and Duplex Sonography

Echography of the cervical soft tissue has to be considered as a second-level investigation. It can be used to depict the size of the cervical multifidus muscle in asymptomatic and symptomatic subjects [24]. The cross-sectional area (CSA) and the transverse versus the anterior-posterior dimensions (shape ratio) are measured at the C4 level. The size of the multifidus muscle may be significantly reduced in symptomatic subjects, which indicates loss of clarity of the fascial layer between the semispinalis cervicis muscle and the cervical multifidus muscle. In this way, echographic findings, in long-lasting symptomatic patients, may be a diagnostic sign of muscle atrophy [25].

Whiplash can induce lesion of deep oro-cervical soft tissues like retropharyngeal hematoma, resulting in airway obstruction and mortality due to bleeding amongst deep cervical fascias. Echography is the examination of choice when this situation is suspected [26].

Transcranial Doppler (TCD) sonography may be used for the assessment of vertebrobasilar circulation in patients with a whiplash injury of the cervical spine. Seric et al. [27] examined a group of WAD patients by TCD within a month and then 6 months following the accident. The obtained values were compared to normal blood flow velocities and correlated with the severity of clinical picture. During the first month after the injury, statistically significant disturbances in the vertebrobasilar circulation were recorded, such as the increase in mean blood flow velocities in

Table 7.1 Radiological strategy

Early trauma			
Plain standard X-rays			
Normal	Bone lesion?	Posture abnormalities	Facets abnormalities
Stop	**CT scan**	**Dynamic radiograms/echography**	**MRI**
Late trauma			
Plain standard X-rays			
Normal	Arthrosis ***Without*** neurological symptoms	Arthrosis ***With*** neurological symptoms	Posture abnormalities ***Without*** arthrosis
Stop	**Stop**	**MRI**	**Dynamic radiogram and/or echography**

AVL (68 %), AVR (62 %), and BA (51 %) (mostly as spasm). Six months later, normal findings were obtained in about 50 % of the vessels, whereas in the rest of the patients, vasospasm persisted in one, two, or all examined blood vessels.

TCD of the vertebrobasilar circulation is a very useful method in the diagnostics and follow-up of patients with a whiplash injury. Vertebral artery flow evaluation can be considered an effective supplementary method in a precise workup especially in polytrauma patient as well as in patients presenting with delayed onset of symptoms; in fact the V3 segment of the vertebral artery, especially where it courses through its groove behind the superior facet of the atlas, is particularly vulnerable to injury. Flow velocity is measured at the V3 segment from a point just below and roughly 2–3 cm dorsal to the mastoid process [28].

Conclusions

At a later date the neutral lateral view may reveal the evolution of a reversed lordosis in an angular kyphosis with the presence of a narrowed intervertebral space and an unco-arthrosis.

However, it can be very difficult to correlate patient's claim with X-ray findings, especially if the radiological evaluation is "normal or almost normal."

Posttraumatic disturbances may be present and, in some cases, disabling even with a normal radiological examination. Radiological strategy is presented in Table 7.1. Planning CT scan or MRI or echography is partially based on X-ray plain findings but mostly on clinical symptoms and signs.

References

1. Crowe HE (1928) Injuries to the cervical spine. Presented at the annual meeting of the Western Orthopedic Association, San Francisco
2. Macnab I (1973) The whiplash syndrome. Clin Neurosurg 20:232–241
3. Harris JH, Eideken-Monroe B (1987) The radiology of acute cervical spine trauma. Williams and Wilkins, Baltimore

4. Dosch JC (1985) Trauma: conventional radiological study in spine injury. Springer, Berlin/Heidelberg
5. Wimmer B, Hofmann E, Jacob A (1990) Trauma of the spine: CT and MRI. Springer, Berlin/New York
6. Grenier N, Halini PH, Frija G, Sigal R (1991) Traumatismes. In: Sigal R, Grenier N, Doyon D, Garcia-Torres E (eds) IRM de la Moelle et du Rachis. Masson, Paris/Milan
7. Anderson SE, Boesch C, Zimmermann H, Busato A, Hodler J, Bingisser R, Ulbrich EJ, Nidecker A, Buitrago-Téllez CH, Bonel HM, Heini P, Schaeren S, Sturzenegger M (2012) Are there cervical spine findings at MR imaging that are specific to acute symptomatic whiplash injury? A prospective controlled study with four experienced blinded readers. Radiology 262(2):567–575
8. Chen HB, Yang KH, Wang ZG (2009) Biomechanics of whiplash injury. Chin J Traumatol 12(5):305–314
9. Kongsted A, Sorensen JS, Andersen H, Keseler B, Jensen TS, Bendix T (2008) Are early MRI findings correlated with long-lasting symptoms following whiplash injury? A prospective trial with 1-year follow-up. Eur Spine J 17(8):996–1005
10. Li Q, Shen H, Li M (2013) Magnetic resonance imaging signal changes of alar and transverse ligaments not correlated with whiplash-associated disorders: a meta-analysis of case-control studies. Eur Spine J 22(1):14–20
11. Schmidt P, Mayer TE, Drescher R (2012) Delineation of alar ligament morphology: comparison of magnetic resonance imaging at 1.5 and 3 Tesla. Orthopedics 35(11):e1635–e1639
12. Lummel N, Bitterling H, Kloetzer A, Zeif C, Brückmann H, Linn J (2012) Value of "functional" magnetic resonance imaging in the diagnosis of ligamentous affection at the craniovertebral junction. Eur J Radiol 81(11):3435–3440
13. Elliott JM, Pedler AR, Theodoros D, Jull GA (2012) Magnetic resonance imaging changes in the size and shape of the oropharynx following acute whiplash injury. J Orthop Sports Phys Ther 42(11):912–918
14. Elliott JM (2011) Are there implications for morphological changes in neck muscles after whiplash injury? Spine 36(25 Suppl):S205–S210
15. Elliott J, Sterling M, Noteboom JT, Darnell R, Galloway G, Jull G (2008) Fatty infiltrate in the cervical extensor muscles is not a feature of chronic insidious-onset neck pain. Clin Radiol 63(6):681–687 [Epub 2008 Jan 31]
16. Cagnie B, Dolphens M, Peeters I, Achten E, Cambier D, Danneels L (2010) Use of muscle functional magnetic resonance imaging to compare cervical flexor activity between patients with whiplash-associated disorders and people who are healthy. Phys Ther 90(8):1157–1164
17. Matsumoto M, Ichihara D, Okada E, Chiba K, Toyama Y, Fujiwara H, Momoshima S, Nishiwaki Y, Takahata T (2012) Cross-sectional area of the posterior extensor muscles of the cervical spine in whiplash injury patients versus healthy volunteers – 10 year follow-up MR study. Injury 43(6):912–916
18. Elliott JM, O'Leary S, Sterling M, Hendrikz J, Pedler A, Jull G (2010) Magnetic resonance imaging findings of fatty infiltrate in the cervical flexors in chronic whiplash. Spine 35(9):948–954
19. Modic MT, Masaryk TJ, Ross JS, Carter JR (1988) Imaging of degenerative disk disease. Radiology 168:177–186
20. Matsumoto M, Ichihara D, Okada E, Toyama Y, Fujiwara H, Momoshima S, Nishiwaki Y, Takahata T (2013) Modic changes of the cervical spine in patients with whiplash injury: A prospective 11-year follow-up study. Injury 44(6):819–824
21. Ulbrich EJ, Eigenheer S, Boesch C, Hodler J, Busato A, Schraner C, Anderson SE, Bonel H, Zimmermann H, Sturzenegger M (2011) Alterations of the transverse ligament: an MRI study comparing patients with acute whiplash and matched control subjects. AJR Am J Roentgenol 197(4):961–967
22. Elliott JM, Pedler A, Beattie PF, McMahon K (2010) Diffusion weighted MRI for the healthy cervical multifidus: a potential method for studying neck muscle physiology following spinal trauma. J Orthop Sports Phys Ther 40(11):722–8

23. Elliott J, Cannata E, Christensen E, Demaris J, Kummrow J, Manning E, Nielsen E, Romero T, Barnes C, Jull G (2008) MRI analysis of the size and shape of the oropharynx in chronic whiplash. Otolaryngol Head Neck Surg 138(6):747–751
24. Churilov IK, Bagaudinov KG, Orel AM, Lapteva NV, Imenovskiĭ IE (2008) Clinical-neurological and radiological diagnostics of whiplash trauma and its consequences in flight crew. Voen Med Zh 329(6):22–26
25. Watson JD (2007) Whiplash injuries can be visible by functional magnetic resonance imaging. Pain Res Manag 12(1):49; Kristjansson E (2004) Reliability of ultrasonography for the cervical multifidus muscle in asymptomatic and symptomatic subjects. Man Ther 9(2):83–88
26. Nurata H, Yilmaz MB, Borcek AO, Oner AY, Baykaner MK (2012) Retropharyngeal hematoma secondary to whiplash injury in childhood: a case report. Turk Neurosurg 22(4): 521–523
27. Serić V, Blazić-Cop N, Demarin V (2000) Haemodynamic changes in patients with whiplash injury measured by transcranial Doppler sonography (TCD). Coll Antropol 24(1):197–204
28. Reddy M, Reddy B, Schöggl A, Saringer W, Matula C (2012) The complexity of trauma to the cranio-cervical junction: correlation of clinical presentation with Doppler flow velocities in the V3-segment of the vertebral arteries. Acta Neurochir (Wien) 144(6):575–580
29. Ducati A, Bettinelli A, Mangiagalli EP, Vaccari E (1979) Traumatic losions of the cervical spine: plain radiographic features of 140 cases. VRG CHIR Comment. 1979;2(3):321–325

Part II

Pathophysiology

The Vestibulo-vertebral Functional Unit

8

D.C. Alpini, G. Brugnoni, A. Cesarani, and P.M. Bavera

8.1 Introduction

The importance of the head as reference in dynamic control of balance is supported by evidence that the head itself supports three type of sensors: the vestibular system, which is sensitive both to gravity forces and head itself accelerations; vision, which is able to stabilise the head and the body with respect to the external space; and the neck muscle's proprioceptive input which conveys the position of the head with respect to the trunk providing an 'error signal' to central vestibular system in order to optimise vestibulo-spinal control.

The head stabilised in space serves as a reference frame for the postural organisation of the rest the body. In fact, while vertical alignment and centre of pressure displacement control during quiet standing are strictly important in postural control, head stability is important for balance in dynamic conditions like walking [1]. Static and dynamic head stabilisation is obtained through proper tonic and phasic contraction of the cervical muscles. Due to spine biomechanics, also dorsal and paravertebral muscles contribute to head stabilisation in space.

D.C. Alpini (✉) • P.M. Bavera
ENT-Otoneurology Service, IRCCS "Don Carlo Gnocchi" Foundation,
Milan, Italy
e-mail: dalpini@dongnocchi.it

G. Brugnoni
Italian Academy of Manual Medicine,
Italian Institute for Auxology, Milan, Italy
e-mail: guido.brugnoni@libero.it

A. Cesarani
Department of Clinical Sciences and Community Health,
University of Milan, Milan, Italy

Audiology Unit, IRCCS "Ca' Granda" Ospedale Maggiore Policlinico,
Milan, Italy
e-mail: antonio.cesarani@unimi.it

D.C. Alpini et al. (eds.), *Whiplash Injuries*,
DOI 10.1007/978-88-470-5486-8_8, © Springer-Verlag Italia 2014

For these reasons, it is possible to define the co-operation between vestibular cues and vertebral muscles activity as a functional unit, that is to say, the vestibulo-vertebral unit.

Because head stabilisation occurs during different tasks and conditions, some investigators speculate that motor system utilises a top-down control schema. The top-down schema corrects head displacements preventing upward transmission of movements from the trunk so that head remains stable in the space providing an inertial guidance system [2]. Stabilisation of head is thought to improve the interpretation of vestibular input for balance. In fact, head stabilisation reduces the inertial acceleration on otolithic membrane and semicircular canals, improving the estimation of gravitational acceleration and providing a stable gravitational reference. Head stabilisation also decreases the retinal slip of the image of the world on the retina and, in the specific, decreasing of retinal slip allows a more accurate visual control of the environment. Head control is not directly influenced by input from sensorial systems; rather, complex high order of sensory mechanisms combine inputs, forming frames of reference; so each sensory cue has a value of reference against which the changes of signal is interpreted. Finally, frames of reference of each cue are used to create body schema that is defined as 'a combined standard against which all subsequent changes of posture are measured'.

The internal representation of body schema allows CNS to represent body geometry, body kinetics and the attitude of the body with respect to gravity.

The importance of different body parts in the definitions of body schema relies on the specific characteristic of each segment itself. For example, the feet inform the position and attitude of support surface and the forces that are exerted by the support surface on the body; the importance of the trunk in the representation of body schema is justified by the fact that the trunk is the segment with bigger mass; a primary role of head in body schema is justified by the fact that visual and labyrinthine systems are located in the head and inform on the position of line of gravity and the horizontal; moreover, inputs from neck proprioceptors control the relationship between trunk and head.

This process leads to a better evaluation of the movement of the body segments with respect to the segment of reference and the position of the subjects with respect external world.

Vestibular function is dependent also by blood supply and venous drainage. Vascular inner ear system is regulated by sympathetic and parasympathetic cervical system. In this way, into the so-called vestibulo-vertebral functional unit, vascular and autonomic cervico-cephalic systems have to be taken in account.

8.2 Head Stabilisation Control

8.2.1 Vestibular Reflexes

During each movement of the head and/or body, it is necessary that the image of the perceived surrounding has to remain on the same place on the retina [3]. Thus, the image of the perceived part of the environment must be changed in a very quick way. During head movement, the eye has to make movements relative to the skull in such a way as to guarantee immobilisation of the image projection on the retina. If there is a 'retinal sip', the vision is blurred, and the surrounding is perceived as moving around. As a result, during head movement, that required eye movement has to be 'compensatory', in order to cancel the effect of the head movement. Such an eye movement is executed in a reflective manner, without conscious intervention, and it is called vestibulo-ocular reflex (VOR).

The achievement of correct erect standing position, both in static and in dynamic conditions, requires continuous adaptation of counterreaction of antigravity muscles to the gravity force, in order to stabilise head position and to maintain erect position itself. Maintaining of upright position of the body is acquired via a continual to and fro movement of the centre of gravity (CoG) around the point of mass equilibrium. This movement is called 'postural sway'. It is achieved in a reflective manner by the mean of the so-called vestibulo-spinal reflexes (VSR). The control of correct head position is possible through the activation of the neck muscles by the mean of a part of the VSR (the so-called vestibulo-collic reflex, VCR) and the cervical reflexes.

8.2.2 Cervical Proprioception

The receptors of the cervical region play a separate and particular role and constitute what can be considered as a 'secondary labyrinth' [3]. In a clinical context, attention has been devoted to the neck with respect to a possible origin of vertigo, the so-called cervical vertigo. Furthermore, its role in the posture of the head and the body seems undeniable. The cervical region with its structures intervenes in the elaboration of balance reflexes. Neck-body reflexes as well as cervical influences upon eye position have been described. It is the task of neck proprioceptors to inform the centres about movement or change of position of the head, so far as this concerns a differential movement between head and trunk. This is the fundamental difference from the vestibular system which is sensitive to head movements relative to space. Both sensory systems provide specific and proper information, thus complementing one another.

Peripheral proprioceptors of the muscles and the joints have a feedback control on the vestibular nuclei through spino-vestibular pathways. Neuromuscular spindles and Golgi receptors are dynamometers, and they are particularly sensitive to variations in muscle length and tension. Joint receptors, Ruffini corpuscles and Golgi bodies give information regarding the position of a joint and its movement. The portion of the neck including the first three vertebrae is particularly involved during the major part of everyday head movements. The paravertebral muscles of this region are very rich in proprioceptors. They are especially concentrated in the splenius capitis, the rectus capitis major, the longissimus capitis and the semispinalis capitis. These muscles compose the deep plane of the nuchal muscles. The splenius is just more superficial. They act in the extension homolateral bending and rotation of the head. During head movements they discharge to the vestibular nuclei.

Direct projection from the first three cervical roots to the inferior vestibular nucleus has been described as well as the convergence of cervical and labyrinth inputs on vestibular nuclei has been showed. Convergence regards especially inputs from horizontal semicircular canal: the electrical stimulation of the vestibular nerve induces action potentials in the contralateral abducens nerve. This response is increased when also neck roots are contemporary stimulated. Thus, facilitatory convergences of proprioceptive inputs from C2 to C3 receptors on the medial vestibular nucleus of the opposite side and an inhibition on the ipsilateral muscles have been demonstrated. The latency between electrical stimulation of the dorsal cervical roots and vestibular nucleus response is only 2 ms; thus, direct projections from neck to vestibular nuclei have been hypothesised. Proprioceptive nuchal afferences on the Schwalbe nucleus have been demonstrated as well as it has been shown that neurons in the dorso-caudal portion of the Deiters nucleus receive tonic cervical inputs, while the neurons in the rostro-ventralis portion receive especially otolithic inputs. Roller nucleus and the accessory group Y receive ipsilateral projections from the cervical muscles, and cerebellar projections on the nodulus and the flocculus have been demonstrated as well as projections on the cerebellar anterior lobus have been described.

Proprioceptive convergences in 80 % of the neurons in the suprasylvian parietal cortical vestibular area have been demonstrated and sensitive inputs run through IA and IIA fibres that raise along spinal cord and through the spino-reticular and spino-cerebellar fasciculus that seem to send direct projections to the vestibular nuclei.

From cervical proprioceptors arise the cervico-spinal reflexes (CSR): bending the neck and turning the head relative to the body evokes reflexes in the limb muscles either in decerebrate cats or in human beings.

These reflexes interact with the vestibulo-collic reflex (VCR) which is a part of the vestibulo-spinal reflexes (VSR).

Vestibulo-collic reflex moves the head and interferes with the VOR for stabilising the visual field. The VCR rotates the head in the plane of the canal. Natural canal stimulation results in contraction of neck muscles to counter the applied angular acceleration and thus results in stabilisation of the head. VCR augments the VOR for image stabilisation during head movement. Cervico-ocular reflex and cervico-collic reflex act to generate compensatory shifts of gaze which opposed those produced by rotation of the head. While the gain of COR is too small to make a significant contribution to gaze stability, the CCR is capable of generating large changes in neck muscles activity, which influences gaze and head position. In controlling gaze, the VCR and CCR damp oscillations of the head and produce counter-rotations that partially compensate for the rotation of the body, while the VOR compensates for residual rotation of the head with respect to space. In animals with vestibular lesions, COR and CCR increase to compensate partially. Head stabilisation contributes to gaze stabilisation [4].

8.3 Interaction Between Ocular Stabilisation Reflexes in Patients with Whiplash Injury

8.3.1 Autonomic Cervico-cephalic System

8.3.1.1 Sympathetic Supply to the Head and Neck

The preganglionic fibres, which supply the head and neck, arise from the spinal segments *T1 to T2*. They enter the sympathetic trunk and travel upward to synapse in one of the three ganglia in the neck:

1. The *superior cervical ganglion* (located anterior to vertebrae C1, C2)
2. The *middle cervical ganglion* (small, often absent, lying anterior to C6)
3. The *inferior cervical ganglion* which is usually fused with the first thoracic ganglion to form the *cervicothoracic* (or *stellate*) *ganglion* (located anterior to C7 and the neck of the first rib)

   Each of these ganglia gives rise to:

1. Cardiac branches.
2. Branches to blood vessels, sweat glands, and hair follicles in the neck and head. The superior ganglion sends branches to spinal nerves C1–C4, the middle ganglion to spinal nerves C5–C6 and the cervicothoracic ganglion to spinal nerves C7, 8–T1.
3. Vascular branches which pass to the vertebral, common, internal and external carotid arteries. Some of these branches 'hitchhike' along the arteries and their branches to reach their targets in the head and neck. The superior ganglion sends branches along the internal and external carotid arteries to reach structures in the orbit, face, nasal and oral cavities and pharynx. The middle ganglion sends branches along the inferior thyroid artery to reach the larynx, trachea and upper oesophagus. The inferior ganglion sends branches to the subclavian and vertebral arteries.

8.3.1.2 Parasympathetic Supply to the Head and Neck (See Also Chap. 10)

There are four ganglia in the head: ciliary, pterygopalataline, otic and submandibular.

The parasympathetic fibres of the oculomotor nerve enter the orbit with the inferior division of the nerve and synapse in the *ciliary ganglion*, which is located just lateral to the optic nerve. The postganglionic fibres with the short ciliary nerves enter the eye to supply the sphincter pupillae (that constricts the pupil) and ciliary muscles. Parasympathetic fibres also travel along the superior branch of the oculomotor nerve to supply the smooth muscle component of levator palpebrae superioris.

The parasympathetic fibres of the facial nerve supply the lacrimal gland, the mucous glands of the nose and palate and the submandibular and sublingual salivary glands. The fibres which supply the lacrimal, nasal and palatine glands leave the facial nerve (at its genu inside the petrous bone as the greater petrosal nerve), pass through the pterygoid canal (at the root of the pterygoid process as the nerve of the pterygoid canal) and terminate in the *pterygopalatine ganglion* (located in the pterygopalatine fossa). The postganglionic fibres travel in the branches of the ganglion or the maxillary nerve to reach the nasal and palatine glands. Other preganglionic fibres leave the facial nerve in its *chorda tympani* branch. This nerve passes over the internal surface of the tympanic membrane before emerging from the skull through a small fissure, the petrotympanic fissure, in the temporal bone. It joints the lingual nerve (a branch of the mandibular nerve) to travel to, and synapse in, the *submandibular ganglion*, which is suspended from the lingual nerve. The postganglionic fibres either pass into the submandibular gland or rejoin the lingual nerve to reach the sublingual gland.

The parasympathetic fibres of the glossopharyngeal nerve supply the parotid gland. The preganglionic fibres travel with the tympanic branch into the tympanic plexus in the middle ear. The fibres emerging from this plexus as the *lesser petrosal nerve*, which synapses in the *otic ganglion* (located medial to the mandibular nerve, just below the foramen ovale). The postganglionic fibres then hitchhike the auriculotemporal nerve (a branch of the mandibular nerve) to reach the parotid gland.

8.3.2 The Cervico-oto-ocular Interaction

Interspecies and human neuroanatomy provides the most important advances on the influence of some tracts and cortical areas on others and how they may be felt as secondary sensorineural otic symptoms.

The protagonism of constant deep pain, trigemino-vascular auditive control, somatosensorial-auditory multimodal integration, cortical and subcortical sound broadband interpretation, corticofugal modulation and limbic behavioural interferences as CNS phenomena has been demonstrated in referred otic symptom pathophysiology.

In 2005 and 2007 Franz et al. [5, 6] widely investigated the neurophysiological connections between inner ear and intrinsic ocular function, connections mediated via trigeminal nerve and cervical sympathetic system.

They focused their attention to Ménière's disease. Ménière's disease not only includes the symptom complex consisting of attacks of vertigo, low-frequency hearing loss and tinnitus but comprises symptoms related to the Eustachian tube, the upper cervical spine, the temporomandibular joints and the autonomic nervous system. Particularly these AA observed some patients presenting normal hearing levels, a mild Eustachian tube dysfunction, mydriasis on the side of the affected ear and a functional disorder of the upper cervical spine. These patients were given a diagnosis of cervicogenic oto-ocular (COO) syndrome.

Authors described hypothetical reflex (Fig. 8.1) pathway that links joint injury and the autonomic nervous system, where Eustachian tube function is under their influence and is the critical link. In this hypothetical reflex pathway, irritation of facet joints can first lead to an activated anterior cervical sympathetic system via an independent pathway in the mediolateral cell column; it can simultaneously lead to an axon reflex involving nociceptive neurons, resulting in neurogenic inflammation and the prospect of a Eustachian tube dysfunction. The Eustachian tube dysfunction is responsible for a disturbed middle ear-inner ear pressure relationship. This reflex

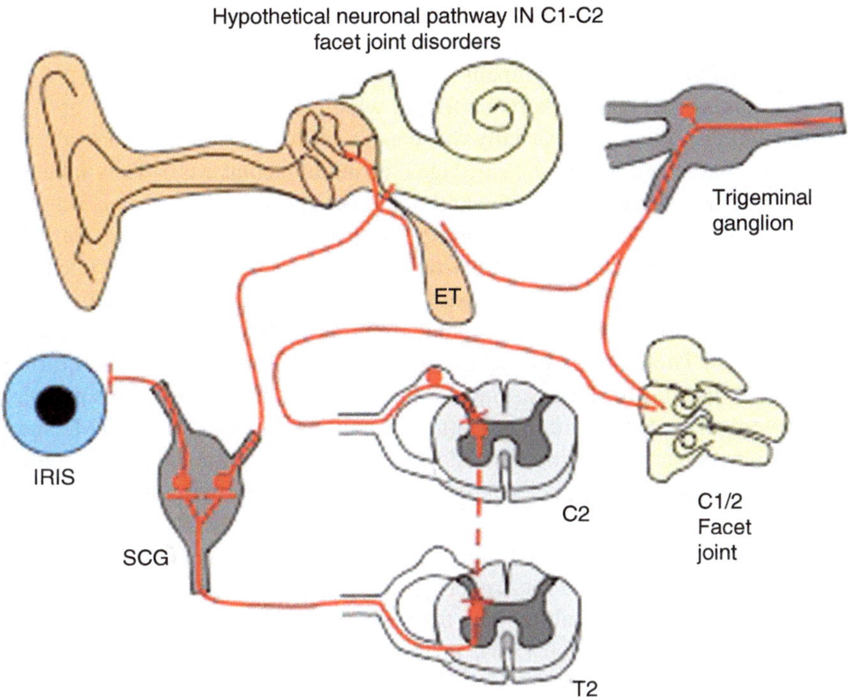

Fig. 8.1 The pathway that links first cervical joints and the autonomic nervous system, influencing Eustachian tube function. In this hypothetical reflex pathway, irritation of facet joints can first lead to an activated anterior cervical sympathetic system via an independent pathway in the mediolateral cell column. The trigeminal nerve, whose afferents come from temporomandibular joint (TMJ), contributes to modulate both middle (Eustachian tube) and inner ear function (blood flow regulation and thus endolymph production) and intrinsic oculomotricity (original figure by prof. Burkhard Franz, Melbourne, Australia, with permission of the Author)

pathway is supported by recent animal experiments [7]. These experiments highlight also the role of trigeminal nerve. Temporomandibular joint (TMJ) trigeminal afferents contribute to modulate both middle (Eustachian tube) and inner ear function (blood flow regulation and thus endolymph production) and intrinsic oculomotricity.

An integral model concerning neurological, anatomical and physiological perspectives offers a wider angle for the multiple auditory innervation patterns involving the *trigeminal* nerve. Vass et al. [8–10] found that trigeminal vascular system innervation in guinea pigs controls cochlear and vestibular labyrinth function. This plays an important role in regulating and balancing cochlear vascular tone and vestibular labyrinth channel and may be responsible for the symptomatic complexity of some cochlear diseases related to inner ear blood flow. Trigeminal ophthalmic fibre projection to the cochlea through the basilar and anterior inferior cerebellar arteries may play an important role in vascular tone in quick and vasodilatatory responses to intense noise. Inner ear diseases that produce otic symptoms such as sudden hearing loss, vertigo and tinnitus can originate from reduced cochlear blood flow due to the presence of abnormal activity in the trigeminal ganglion.

Link between TMJ, trigeminal nerve and middle ear has an embryological explanation. TMJ development and other neighbouring structures in humans (such as pharynx, Eustachian tube and tympanic cavity) are complex. The mandible is formed from the ventral part of Meckel's cartilage, which is the first branchial arch. The ossicles (malleus, incus and partially the stapes) are formed from the dorsal part of Meckel's cartilage and Reichert's cartilage (second branchial arch). The malleus has a double origin in these ossicles; the anterior process originates from mesenchymal cells (os goniale), through intramembranous ossification, and the rest form from Meckel's cartilage, through endochondral ossification. The malleus is related to the TMJ (condylar and temporal blastemas) by fibrous connections (lateral pterygoid muscle) passing through the petrotympanic fissure, which Rees named the discomalleolar ligament. These lateral pterygoid muscular fibrous connections then form the interarticular disc in Meckel's cartilage by mechanical stimulation of this muscle.

Neurological, vascular and ligamental communication between the TMJ and the middle ear is preserved during TMJ development and continues during adult life because of continuity of Meckel's cartilage through the petrotympanic fissure (causing an incomplete closing in adults). This fissure holds the chorda tympani nerve in its middle ear egress to the TMJ, amongst other ear-TMJ vestige structures. The medial pterygoid muscle and the tensor tympani muscle develop from the temporal blastema. These structures (along with the tensor veli palatini) are innervated by the trigeminal mandibular branch (V3), in turn innervating the masticatory muscles coming from the first branchial arch mesoderm.

The ossicular chain and middle ear muscles primarily belong to the chewing system (i.e. embryologically) but finally serve the auditory system.

8.4 From the Neck to the Inner Ear (Through Vertebro-basilar System)

The vertebral artery is a major artery in the neck. It branches from the subclavian artery, where it arises from the postero-superior portion of the subclavian artery. It ascends through the foramina of the transverse processes of the sixth cervical vertebrae. Then, it winds behind the superior articular process of the atlas. It enters the cranium through the foramen magnum where it unites with the opposite vertebral artery to form the basilar artery (at the lower border of the pons).

The vertebral artery can be divided into four divisions:

1. V1 – it runs postero-cranial between the longus colli and the m. scalenus anterior; it is also called 'pre-foraminal division'.
2. V2 – it runs cranial through the foramina in the cervical transverse processes of the cervical vertebrae C2; it is also called foraminal division.
3. V3 – it is the part that rises from C2, from the latter foramen on the medial side of the rectus capitis lateralis, curving behind the superior articular process of the atlas. Then, it lies in the groove on the upper surface of the posterior arch of the atlas and enters the vertebral canal by passing beneath the posterior atlanto-occipital membrane.

4. V4 – that pierces the dura mater and inclines medial to the front of the medulla oblongata.

At the junction between the medulla oblongata and the pons, two vertebral arteries joint into the *basilar artery*, forming the so-called the vertebro-basilar system, which supplies blood to the posterior part of circle of Willis and anastomoses with blood supplied to the anterior part of the circle of Willis from the internal carotid arteries.

The basilar artery ascends in the central gutter (sulcus basilaris) inferior to the pons and divides into the posterior cerebral arteries and the superior cerebellar artery just inferior to the pituitary stalk. From the basilar artery arises the anterior inferior cerebellar artery (supplying the superior and inferior aspects of the cerebellum), as well as smaller branches for the supply of the pons (the pontine branches). In under 15 % of people, the basilar artery gives rise to the labyrinthine artery while, generally, the *labyrinthine artery* (*auditory artery*, *internal auditory artery*), a long slender branch of the anterior inferior cerebellar artery (85–100 % cases) or basilar artery (<15 % cases), arises from near the middle of the artery; it accompanies the vestibulocochlear nerve through the internal acoustic meatus and is distributed to the internal ear.

CNS interaction between the somatosensory system and multilevel vestibular tracts cranial and cervical muscular dysfunction producing hypertonicity and muscular spasm can irritate nerves and blood vessels by muscular trapping.

The vascular relationship between the TMJ and the middle ear may explain otic symptoms in the presence of a vascular reflex from TMJ disorders. The most medial anterior tympanic *artery* posterior group branches (behind the TMJ) irrigate the tympanic cavity and the outflow of the inner ear, which is completely drained by the vein of the cochlear aqueduct.

8.5 From the Inner Ear to the Spine (Through Venous Drainage)

The veins of the vestibule and semicircular canals accompany the arteries and, receiving those of the cochlea at the base of the modiolus, unite to form the *internal auditory veins* (or *veins of labyrinth*) which end in the posterior part of the superior petrosal sinus or in the transverse sinus [11].

The common modiolar vein enters the bony channel immediately adjacent to the aqueduct to become the vein of the cochlear aqueduct which in turn drains via the inferior petrous sinus into the internal jugular veins (IJVs). Injury or occlusion of this vessel would be particularly significant since it is widely believed to provide virtually the entire venous drainage of the cochlea [12].

The cochlear aqueduct and the internal auditory canal communicate with the subarachnoidal space; in the guinea pig model, an occlusion of the veins of the cochlear aqueduct results in an increase of perilymphatic endolymphatic pressure, a decrease of cochlear blood flow and endolymphatic potential. Furthermore, since many of the venous vessels in the scala tympani have little or no bony covering and are essentially exposed to the perilymphatic space, the venous system is a route of entry for the cells participating in the inner ear inflammatory process.

Another interesting point is that the blood leaves the brain by using the back propulsion of the residual arterial pressure (vis a tergo), complemented by antero-grade respiratory mechanisms (vis a fronte). The latter consist of the thoracic pump increased venous outflow during inspiration: the increase of negative thoracic pressure improves the aspiration of blood toward the right atrium. In addition to vis a tergo and vis a fronte, postural mechanisms play a fundamental role in ensuring a correct cerebral venous return.

The pattern of cerebral venous drainage changes, even under physiological conditions, depending on the body position. In the prone or supine position, the outflow through the IJVs is favoured, whereas passing to the upright position transfers most of the encephalic drainage to the vertebral *veins*.

Corrosion cast study highlights the complexity of the venous network in the craniocervical junction.

Schematically, two descending cerebral venous outflow tracks can be distinguished: the internal jugular veins anteriorly and the vertebral venous system posteriorly. The latter is composed of the external and internal vertebral venous plexuses, which are anastomosed by way of the intervertebral and basivertebral veins.

In the cervical region, the vertebral venous system is mainly represented by the anterior internal vertebral venous plexus, the vertebral artery venous plexus and the deep cervical veins.

As far as this posterior outflow track is concerned, the anterior, posterior and lateral condylar veins and the *anterior condylar confluent* (ACC) represent the most important connections between the intracranial cerebral venous circulation and the vertebral venous systems.

The posterior and lateral condylar veins allow for connections with the external vertebral venous system, whereas the anterior condylar veins are predominantly related to the internal vertebral venous plexus. It is noteworthy that even though the diameters of the anterior and lateral condylar veins were important, they were connected to the internal jugular vein by only a small anastomosis between the jugular bulb or internal jugular vein and the ACC.

Venous flow from the jugular bulb through the anterior condylar vein and into the anterior internal vertebral venous plexus occurs efficaciously by way of the ACC regardless of how indirect this pathway might seem.

The ACC appeared as an anatomic constant whose major tributaries, size-wise, were the anterior and lateral condylar veins, inferior petrosal sinus and internal jugular vein. The ACC was also connected to the carotid artery venous plexus by the inferior petro-occipital vein and to the prevertebral venous plexus. The numerous anastomoses of the ACC make it a crossroad between the cavernous sinus, dural venous sinuses of the posterior fossa and posterior cervical outflow tracks. ACC is a 'common canal' of the inferior petrosal sinus and the anterior condylar vein of the junction of the inferior petrosal sinus and internal jugular vein sinus posteriorly.

From a physiological point of view, one should also consider that the same postural influences affecting cerebral venous drainage might redirect the circulation of the internal and external vertebral venous systems. For instance, the cranial (as opposed to caudal) connections of the anterior internal vertebral venous plexus with the anterior condylar vein could offer a cranial escape route for thoracic and abdominal venous return when thoracic pressure and abdominal pressure are increased concomitantly. One could even consider venous blood from the anterior internal vertebral venous plexus draining into the superior ophthalmic vein and cavernous sinus through the basilar plexus and inferior petrosal sinuses and thus terminally into the pterygoid plexus and facial veins.

In conclusion, cervico-cephalic drainage system is very complex: cerebral, neurocranial and cervical venous blood might take different common, but variable, outflow tracks depending on posture, pressure and anatomic variations. Anterior, lateral and posterior condylar veins and occipital and mastoid emissary veins provide connections between the posterior fossa dural sinuses and internal jugular vein system with the cervical vertebral venous system. These emissary veins allow for encephalic blood to drain into the cervical internal and external vertebral venous plexuses, which represent the major outflow tract for encephalic drainage in the upright position.

The ACC, a venous entity ignored since Trolard described it in 1868, represents a major venous crossroad of the base of the skull.

References

1. Nadeau S, Amblard B, Mesure S, Bourbonnais D (2003) Head and trunk stabilization strategies during forward and backward walking in healthy adults. Gait Posture 18(3):134–142
2. Gracovetsky S (2002) Le role des membres superieurs dans le control du pelvis et du cou durant la marche. Rev Med Vertebr 8:4–8
3. Cesarani A, Alpini D (1999) Vertigo and dizziness rehabilitation. Springer, Milan
4. Montfoort I, Kelders WPA, van der Geest JN, Schipper IB, Feenstra L, de Zeeuw CI, Frens MA (2006) Interaction between ocular stabilization reflexes in patients with whiplash injury. Invest Ophthalmol Vis Sci 47(7):2881–2884
5. Franz B, Altidis P, Altidis B, Collis-Brown G (1999) The cervicogenic otoocular syndrome: a suspected forerunner of Ménière's disease. Int Tinnitus J 5(2):125–130
6. Franz B, Anderson C (2007) The potential role of joint injury and Eustachian tube dysfunction in the genesis of secondary Ménière's disease. Int Tinnitus J 13(2):132–137
7. Franz B, Anderson CR (2007) The effect of the sympathetic and sensory nervous system on active Eustachian tube function in the rat. Acta Otolaryngol 127(3):265–272
8. Vass Z, Dai CF, Steyger PS, Jancsó G, Trune DR, Nuttall AL (2004) Co-localization of the vanilloid capsaicin receptor and substance P in sensory nerve fibers innervating cochlear and vertebro-basilar arteries. Neuroscience 124(4):919–927
9. Dai CF, Steyger PS, Wang ZM, Vass Z, Nuttall AL (2004) Expression of Trk A receptors in the mammalian inner ear. Hear Res 187(1–2):1–11
10. Zheng J, Dai C, Steyger PS, Kim Y, Vass Z, Ren T, Nuttall AL (2039) Vanilloid receptors in hearing: altered cochlear sensitivity by vanilloids and expression of TRPV1 in the organ of corti. J Neurophysiol 90(1):444–455
11. Raphael R, Ciuman MD (2009) Communication routes between intracranial spaces and inner ear: function, pathophysiologic importance and relations with inner ear diseases. Am J Otolaryngol 30:193–202
12. Ruız DSM, Gailloud P, Rufenacht DA, Delavelle J, Henry F, Fasel JHD (2002) The craniocervical venous system in relation to cerebral venous drainage. AJNR Am J Neuroradiol 23:1500–1508

Pathophysiology of Whiplash-Associated Disorders: Theories and Controversies

9

M. Magnusson, M. Karlberg, C. Mariconda, A. Bucalossi, and G. Dalmazzo

9.1 Introduction

The term "whiplash" already suggests difficulties in assessing this problem. Patients suffering from "whiplash" or "whiplash-associated disorders" (WAD) are defined as having been exposed to similar types of trauma or sometimes even similar mode of impact, rather than as having a certain type of lesion or set of symptoms [1, 2]. The origin of the term "whiplash" is attributed to H. Crowe [3, 4], who suggested a trauma to the cervico-cranial junction based on the mechanism of acceleration and deceleration of the head impact.

The Quebec task force (QTF) [5, 6] on whiplash-associated disorders (WAD) defined whiplash as "bony or softy tissue injuries" resulting "from rear-end or side impact, predominantly in motor vehicle accidents, and from other mishaps as a result of an acceleration-deceleration mechanism of energy transfer to the neck." Whiplash is associated with a wide variety of clinical manifestations including neck pain, neck stiffness, arm pain and paresthesias, problem with memory and concentration, and psychological distress [7, 8].

Below, some different theories of the organic causes of the complaints will be discussed, but it should be pointed out that it would not come as a complete surprise to us if in the future it becomes apparent that several mechanisms contribute to the complaints of the heterogeneous group of patients suffering from WAD [9].

M. Magnusson • M. Karlberg
Department of Otorhinolaryngology, Lund University Hospital,
Lund University, Lund, Sweden
e-mail: mans.magnusson@med.lu.se

C. Mariconda (✉) • A. Bucalossi • G. Dalmazzo
Department of Physical Medicine and Rehabilitation,
Gradenigo Hospital, Turin, Italy
e-mail: carlo.mariconda@gradenigo.it

D.C. Alpini et al. (eds.), *Whiplash Injuries*,
DOI 10.1007/978-88-470-5486-8_9, © Springer-Verlag Italia 2014

9.2 Pathophysiologic Mechanisms

There are several different theories to explain the traumatic mechanisms of whiplash injuries, as one has to assume that in such lesions there may be concomitant mild brain injury [10, 11]. The possible pathogeneses may include lesions to the soft tissue of the neck, cervical roots, peripheral and central nervous neuronal tissues, and the inner ear.

9.2.1 Lesions to Soft Tissues and Peripheral Nerves

On the one hand, it has been suggested that WAD should be distinguished from sprained necks, traumatic disk protrusions, and damage to cord and nerve roots. On the other hand, it is clear that, to associate the symptoms with the trauma, the patient should present with neck pain in close connection with the trauma [12]. If the finding that the pain from the neck emanates from the soft tissue and perhaps not from a possible CNS injury as suggested [13, 14], it becomes increasingly difficult to make the suggested separation, especially when considering that the definition of WAD is based on the trauma rather than the lesion [15, 16].

The proposed pathomechanics of whiplash injury have evolved from an injury model of rapid hyperextension of the cervical spine, creating large sagittal-plane angular displacements, to the current model of injury resulting from the body's inertial response, causing the head-neck complex to undergo large amounts of displacement without being exposed to any direct impact. For example, during a rear-end impact, the occupant's torso is rapidly carried forward as it is contacted by the forward-moving vehicle's seat. This movement is responsible for the development of an ephemeral "S-shaped" cervical curve, forcing the cervical spine into abnormal, nonphysiological motion of lower segmental extension and upper segmental flexion. As a result of this nonphysiological motion, energy is stored in the elastic components of the cervical spine, followed by an abrupt release of energy and subsequent forward thrust of the head and neck (acceleration/deceleration of the head/neck and torso). The consequences of this energy release could potentially impact and injure any number of anatomical tissues in the cervical spine (intervertebral disks, joint capsules, ligaments, facet joints, muscles, and nerve tissues). This abnormal motion has been shown to produce elongation and subfailure strain of the facet capsular ligaments at the C6–C7 level during the initial "S-shaped" phase (between 0 and 75 ms). Maximum head and neck displacement is observed during the second phase of this abnormal motion (100 ms), and all cervical segmental levels are extended. Furthermore, the occurrence of facet joint spearing of the superior articular facet onto the compromised inferior articular facet and stretching of the anterior ligamentous tissues contributes to the mechanism of injury and may explain the nature of painful symptoms following whiplash [17].

There are a variety of unique injuries involving the cervical facet joints, spinal dorsal ganglia (DRG), ligamentous tissues, and intervertebral disks. In cervical facet joint injuries, these include the occurrence of hemarthroses, capsular tears, articular cartilage damage, joint fractures, and capsular rupture. Moreover, the facet joints are abundantly innervated with A-delta and C-nerve fibers that operate at a high threshold and may become sensitized or excited by local pressure changes, capsular stretching, and naturally occurring proinflammatory agents (substance P, phospholipase A, and interleukin 1β). The anatomical locations of the dorsal root ganglion (DRG) and nerve roots render them vulnerable to excessive stretching and injury during rapid acceleration/deceleration ("S-shaped" curve) or lateral bending of the neck. Each segmental cervical DRG contains distinct nerve fibers responsible for relaying specific information to the spinal cord and brain (e.g., proprioception, pain, and temperature). DRG compression and soft tissue changes, which remain largely undetected with conventional radiography, may contribute to adaptation in the overall functioning of the cervical DRG and may predispose an individual to abnormal, centrally mediated pain processing [18, 19].

It should be also pointed out that peripheral nerve lesions have been demonstrated to occasionally produce motor disturbance and such adverse symptoms as Parkinsonism, tremor, and dystonia [20, 21].

It has been shown potentially injurious musculotendinous strains of the sternocleidomastoid muscle during whiplash injury and larger strains in the superficial posterior neck muscles (semispinalis and splenius capitis and upper trapezius) during rear-end impacts.

Therefore, while evidence exists to suggest the occurrence of muscle strain during the eccentric phase of a rear-impact whiplash, it is currently unknown if differential responses are noted in the deep versus superficial extensor muscles. Future research is warranted to investigate this question.

The lack of in vivo, gold-standard diagnostic tests aimed at specifically identifying these proposed lesions appears to be due to the poor sensitivity of current radiological imaging techniques. While evidence from in vitro studies indicates that the injury can damage any number of anatomical structures in the cervical spine at any segmental level, it is largely unknown if these lesions occur either in combination or are independent of one another.

9.2.2 Central Nervous System Lesions

Patients commonly report symptoms such as irritability, emotional lability, insomnia, and difficulties with concentration after cervical spine hyperextension injury. Cerebral symptoms after a neck sprain have been taken as an indication of neurotic personality; however, the acceleration forces could produce significant intracranial injury in the absence of direct head impact, and this is provided by neuropsychological tests which have consistently shown deficits in attention, concentration, and memory consistent with injury to frontobasal and upper brain stem structures. These deficits have been found both early and late after the injury. Structural lesions have, however, been more elusive. Examinations with MRI and brainstem auditory evoked potentials, sensitive investigations for brainstem lesions, have been normal.

Neuroimaging techniques have failed to report visible structural damage after whiplash injuries [cf Chap. 6]. This has been taken as evidence that whiplash trauma does not produce significant cerebral lesions. The same may be said for mild brain injuries [22]. The cervical trauma resulting from a whiplash injury often coincides with a significant acceleration-deceleration of or even direct impact to the head, which can be suspected to produce mild traumatic brain injuries. Furthermore, some of the symptoms of WAD are similar or identical to those of mild traumatic brain injuries and post-concussional syndromes. For example, attention deficits, concentration disturbances, fatigue, and sleep disturbances as well as depression, anxiety, and pain are common findings [23]. Diffuse axonal injury produced by shear forces generated during acceleration-deceleration of the nervous tissue is considered to constitute the primary pathophysiologic cause of traumatic brain injuries especially to the parasagittal white matter [24, 25].

Decreased attention is a major result of mild traumatic brain injuries and is also considered to cause concomitant cognitive deficits [26]. The decreased attentiveness may remain for a longer period depending upon the age of the patient and may not be completely restored even after years. Especially demanding work situations, fatigue, or other disorders may unveil the imperfect recovery. An alternative pathophysiologic mechanism causing central nervous lesions in whiplash injuries has been suggested by Portnoy [27] in the monkey and Svensson in the pig [28]. During the intense deceleration of the head, there is a fast and short rise of the intracranial and also intraspinal cerebrospinal fluid pressure, approaching values as high as 150 mmHg. The authors argue that such a pressure peak may cause damage to the neural tissue and be responsible for the concomitant symptoms. Again, the validity of the hypothesis remains to be tested further.

9.2.3 Vestibular Lesions

Several investigators report a high frequency of abnormal central vestibular signs in patients with whiplash injuries [29].

Complaints of dizziness and disorders of balance occur in as many as 23 % of patients after acceleration injuries to the cervical spine. As clinical examination is usually normal, the pathological basis for these symptoms is unclear and has variously been attributed to vertebral artery or inner ear or disturbance of the neck righting reflex induced by paraspinal muscle spasm. Objective evidence of vestibular involvement has been demonstrated by the correlation of symptoms with electronystagmograms: some patients with dizziness after neck injury show latent nystagmus, abnormal caloric tests, and abnormal rotatory tests.

The acceleration forces could cause significant damage to the delicate middle and inner ear structures, and faulty inner ear function leads to ineffective muscular control of balance and erect posture. Perilymph fistulae requiring surgery were found in few patients.

Conclusions

There is no consensus about the pathophysiological mechanisms of whiplash or WAD. There is no consensus about the pathophysiological mechanism of whiplash or WAD. It seems possible that the combination of CNS lesions and soft tissue or peripheral neural lesions might enhance each other or coincide to produce the diverse set of symptoms that one might encounter in these patients. Furthermore, a disturbed attention span may result in different sets of cognitive impairments, concentration deficits, and fatigue. Long standing pain may also trigger psychiatric conditions. WAD per se seems to evoke psychiatric conditions such as anxiety and depression. Although it is unclear to what extent this is due to the lesion itself or secondary to other symptoms, these psychiatric impairments may themselves contribute to the distress of the patient.

The possibilities of malingering ones' symptoms to receive medicolegal benefits have not been discussed here.

Improvements in medical imaging techniques may allow better definition of these specific injuries and the development of more appropriate treatment.

At the present we have to conclude that we do not have a specific unifying explanation of WAD.

References

1. Pearce JMS (1994) Polemics of chronic whiplash injury. Neurology 44:1993–1997
2. Alexander MP (1995) Mild traumatic brain injury: pathophysiology, natural history, and clinical management. Neurology 45:1253–1260
3. Crowe H (1928) Injuries to the cervical spine. Presentation to the annual meeting of the Western Orthopedic Association, San Francisco
4. Yadla S, Ratliff JK, Harrop JS (2008) Whiplash: diagnosis, treatment, an associated injuries. Curr Rev Musculoskelet Med 1(1):65–68
5. Sterling M, McLean SA, Sullivan MJ, Elliott JM (2011) Potential processes involved in the initiation and maintenance of whiplash-associated disorders. Spine 36:S322–S329
6. Spitzer WO, Skovron ML, Salmi LR, Cassidy ID, Duranceau J, Suissa S, Zeiss E (1995) Scientific monograph of the Quebec Task Force on whiplash-associated disorders. Spine 20 (8 Suppl):1S–73S
7. Johansson H, Bring G, Rauschning W, Sahlstedt B (1991) Hidden cervical spine injuries in traffic accident victims with skull fractures. J Spinal Disord 4:251–263
8. Elliot JM, Noteboom JT, Flynn TW (2009) Characterization of acute and chronic whiplash-associated disorders. J Orthop Sports Phys Ther 39(5):312–323
9. Jull GA, Sterling M, Curatolo M, Carroll L, Hodges P (2011) Toward lessening the rate of transition of acute whiplash to a chronic disorder. Spine 36(25 Suppl):S173–S174
10. Johansson H, Sojka P (1991) Pathophysiological mechanisms involved in genesis and spread of muscular tension in occupational muscle pain and in chronic musculoskeletal pain syndromes: a hypothesis. Med Hypotheses 35:196–203
11. Tencer AF, Huber P, Mirza SK (2003) A comparison of biomechanical mechanisms of whiplash injury from rear impacts. Annu Proc Assoc Adv Automot Med 47:383–98
12. Johnson G (1996) Hyperextension soft tissue injuries of the cervical spine-review. Emerg Med 13:3–8

13. Hai-bin C, Yang H, Zheng-guo W (2009) Biomechanics of whiplash injury. Chin J Traumatol 12(5):305–314
14. Karlberg M (1995) The neck and human balance. Thesis, Lund University Hospital, Lund, Sweden; Jankovic J (1994) Post traumatic movement disorders: central and peripheral mechanisms. Neurology 44:2006–2014
15. Rodriguez A, Barr KP, Burns SP (2004) Whiplash: pathophysiology, diagnosis, treatment and prognosis. Muscle Nerve 29:768–781
16. Schott GD (1986) Induction of involuntary movements by peripheral trauma. An analogy with causalgia. Lancet 2:712–716
17. Jankovic J, Van der Linden C (1988) Dystonia and tremor induced by peripheral trauma: predisposing factors. J Neurol Neurosurg Psychiatry 51:1512–1519
18. Cole ID, Illis LS, Sedgewick EM (1989) Unilateral essential tremor after wrist immobilization: a case report. J Neurol Neurosurg Psychiatry 52:286–287
19. Bhatia KK, Bhatt MH, Marsden CD (1993) The causalgia-dystonia syndrome. Brain 116:843–851
20. Yarnell PR, Rossie GV (1988) Minor whiplash head injury with major debilitation. Brain Inj 273:255–258
21. Cusick J, Pintar FA, Yoganandan N (2001) Whiplash syndrome: kinematic factors influencing pain patterns. Spine 26:1252–1258
22. Barnsley L, Lord S, Bogduk N (1998) The pathophysiology of whiplash. Spine 12:209–242
23. Ettlin TM, Kischka U, Reichmann S, Radii EW, Heim S, Wengen D, Benson F (1993) Cerebral symptoms after whiplash injury of the neck: a prospective clinical and neuropsychological study of whiplash injury. J Neurol Neurosurg Psychiatry 55:943–948
24. Povlishock JT, Becker DP, Cheng CLY et al (1986) Axonal change in minor head injury. J Neuropathol Exp Neurol 42:225–242
25. Gennarelli TA, Thibault LE, Adams JH et al (1982) Diffuse axonal injury and traumatic coma in the primate. Ann Neurol 12:564–574
26. Binder LM (1986) Persisting symptoms after mild head injury: a review of the postconcussive syndrome. J Clin Exp Neuropsychol 8:32
27. Portnoy HD, Benjamin D, Brian M, McCoy LE, Prince B, Edgerton R, Young J (1970) Intracranial pressure and head acceleration during whiplash. In: Proceedings of the 14th STAPP Car Crash conference, SAE paper no 700900, SAE Inc, USA, LC 67-22372 3-346
28. Svennson MY (1993) Neck injuries in rear-end car collisions. Thesis, Chalmers University of Technology, Gothenburg, Sweden
29. Chester JB Jr (1991) Whiplash, postural control, and the inner ear. Spine 16(7):716–720

The Contribution of Posturology in Whiplash Injuries

10

P.M. Gagey, D.C. Alpini, and E. Brunetta

Posturology studies disorders of the central nervous system (CNS), thanks to the categories of space and time. Indeed, at the end of the nineteenth century, Jean-Marie Charcot and the Salpetriêre's French school suggested to isolate the disorders of the CNS that were caused by a lesion—i.e., belonged to a spatial, anatomic category. That fertile suggestion led to the foundation of neurology.

Jean-Bernard Baron [1] was the first doctor, as far as we know, to observe the "butterfly effect" during his experiences (1955) on the regulation of the postural tonic activity. Butterfly effect has been described by Lorentz [2]: "A butterfly beats his wings in Brazil and a tornado is released to Texas" to say that the logic of the postural control systems make a minor modification of one of their parameters that could bring consequences without proportionality between causes and effects. Following and continuing those works, many doctors in southern Europe started to study disorders of the central nervous system whose logical structure is based not on an anatomical lesion but on the chaotic logic of chained temporal series. Such studies—particularly vigorous in the field of postural control—constitute posturology.

The fundamental concept of posturology is the "Fine Postural Control System" to say that postural control adapts itself to the various behaviors of man: if he is walking or quiet standing, mechanisms implied in his postural control are not the same [3, 4].

P.M. Gagey (✉)
Institut de Posturologie, Av. de Corbera 4, Paris, France
e-mail: pmgagey@club-internet.fr

D.C. Alpini
ENT-Otoneurology Service, IRCCS "Don Carlo Gnocchi" Foundation, Milan, Italy
e-mail: dalpini@dongnocchi.it

E. Brunetta
Private Dentist, Conegliano (TV), Italy
e-mail: elvio.brunetta@fastwebnet.it

D.C. Alpini et al. (eds.), *Whiplash Injuries*,
DOI 10.1007/978-88-470-5486-8_10, © Springer-Verlag Italia 2014

Human being, indeed, controls his position in his environment according to a fundamental operational scheme, common to all behaviors:

- He anticipates his posture according to what he decides to do.
- He controls it by the different inputs of his postural control system.
- He corrects it by muscle activity, either phasic or tonic.

This global scheme may be modulated. Adaptation of postural control to quiet standing, specified by this behavior, is characterized by:

- A predominance of tonic muscle activity
- A discontinuity of the functioning of some system inputs
- A predominance of feedback loops

Whiplash injuries impact strongly on the "Fine Postural Control System" both on tonic muscle activity and on sensorial feedbacks. Whiplash leads, in the great majority of patients, to the so-called disharmonious postural syndrome typically characterized by the absence of proportionality between the mechanical forces of the impact and the consequent effects on static and dynamic postural control.

10.1 Disharmonious Postural Syndrome

Clinical theory suggests that altered alignment of the shoulder girdle has the potential to create or sustain symptomatic mechanical dysfunction in the cervical and thoracic spine. The alignment of the shoulder girdle is described by two clavicle rotations, i.e., elevation and retraction, and by three scapular rotations, i.e., upward rotation, internal rotation, and anterior tilt. The search for an abnormal postural tonic asymmetry forms the basis of the clinical postural examination. This asymmetry at the level of the axial musculature obeys to the laws of spinal movement as stated by Lowett (1907) (cited by Fryette [5]):

> lateral inclination of the spine of the subject standing up is accompanied by a contralateral rotation of the lumbar and dorsal vertebrae. This finding is easily perceived by gently placing one's hands on the patient's iliac wings and scapulae, while he leans sidewards.

Distal musculature can be explored by means of Fukuda's stepping test [6] followed by measurement of neck reflex gains [7].

When the muscle tone is abnormally asymmetrical, we can speak of a "postural syndrome": it is said to be "harmonious" when the hypertonicity is crossed between the axial and distal musculatures; in the opposite case, the postural syndrome is said to be "disharmonious." Barré's "vertical" provides a visual summary of these postural syndrome analyses (Fig. 10.1).

The overwhelming majority of whiplash victims present a disharmonious postural syndrome; this surprisingly high incidence of disharmonious postural syndrome following whiplash is statistically significant.

Uemura and Cohen [8] showed that by localized destruction of the vestibular nuclei in the monkey, it was possible to induce harmonious or disharmonious postural syndromes depending upon the level of the lesion. However, it is difficult

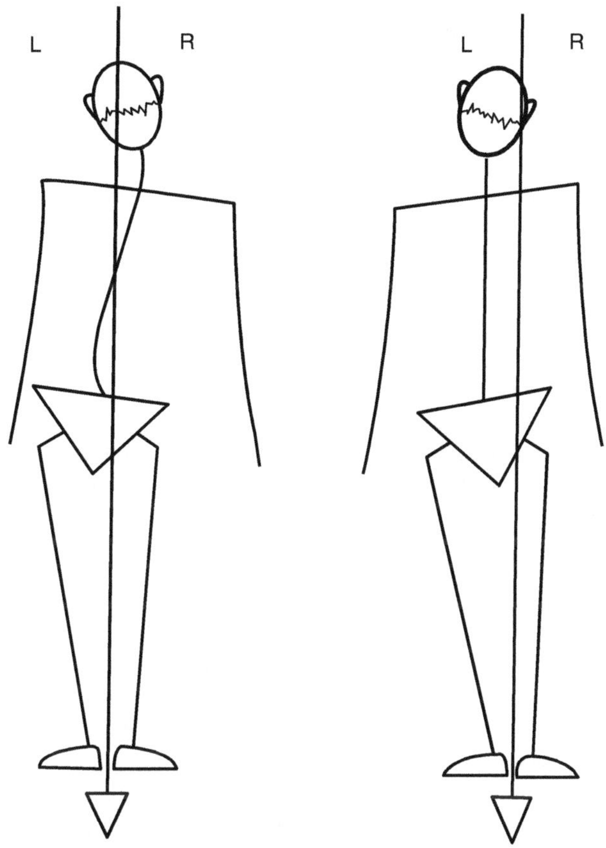

Fig. 10.1 Harmonious and disharmonious postural syndromes. *On the left,* in harmonious syndrome, the hypertonicity of the axial and distal muscles is crossed. *On the right,* in disharmonious postural syndrome, the hypertonicity of the axial and distal muscles is homolateral (From Ref. [7])

to imagine that whiplash systematically produces a lesion of the vestibular nuclei and even more difficult to think that such a lesion would always occur at the same site. Thus, the meaning of a disharmonious postural syndrome must be sought elsewhere. A clear-cut asymmetry of the electric activity of the neck muscles almost always exists following whiplash [9], and this does not seem strange when we remember the incidence of cervical articulation lesions caused by this type of trauma. The muscles contract to mitigate the consequences of rupturing ligaments. The postural importance of these cervical muscles could be showed by stabilometric recordings of these patients: significant asymmetry of the areas of the statokinesigrams appears between the recordings made with the head turned to the right and then to the left (Fig. 10.2).

Helgadottir et al. [10] confirmed the postural asymmetry in neck pain and WAD. Elevation and retraction have been assessed through a three-dimensional device measured clavicle and scapular orientation, and cervical and thoracic alignment in patients with insidious onset neck pain (IONP)and whiplash-associated disorder (WAD). An asymptomatic control group was selected for baseline measurements. The symptomatic groups revealed a significantly reduced clavicle retraction and

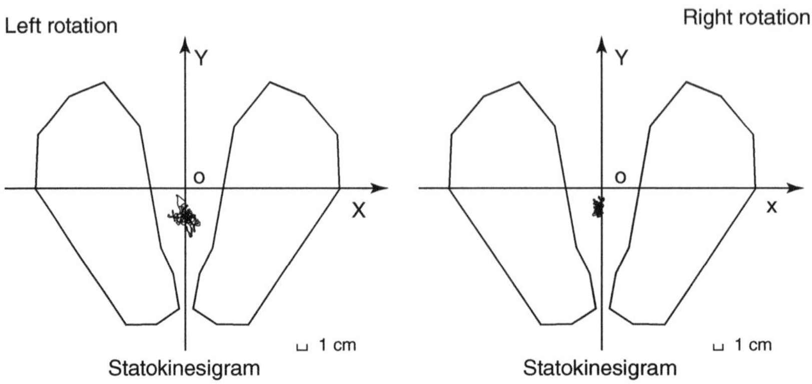

Fig. 10.2 Stabilometric recordings with the head turned to the left and the right. *On the left,* the subject's head was turned to the left during the recording session: the area of the statokinesigram is 2.092 mm^2. *On the right,* the subject's head was rotated to the right during the recording session: the area of the statokinesigram is 867 mm^2. The ration of the areas or the cervical quotient is statistically significant: 2.41 ($p<0.05$)

scapular upward rotation as well as decreased cranial angle. A difference was found between the symptomatic groups on the left side, whereas the WAD group revealed an increased scapular anterior tilt and the IONP group a decreased clavicle elevation. These changes may be an important mechanism for maintenance and recurrence or exacerbation of symptoms in patients with neck pain.

Furthermore, whiplash-associated posture modification in the sagittal plane has been studied by Johansson et al. [11] that investigated whether a kyphotic deformity of the cervical spine, as opposed to a straight or a lordotic spine, was associated with the symptoms at baseline and with the prognosis 1 year following a whiplash injury. MRI was performed in 171 subjects about 10 days after the accident, and 104 participated in the pain recording at 1-year follow-up. It was demonstrated that postures as seen on MRI can be reliably categorized and that a straight spine is the most frequent appearance of the cervical spine in supine MRI. In relation to symptoms, it was seen that a kyphotic deformity was associated with reporting the highest intensities of headache at baseline, but not with an increased risk of long-lasting neck pain or headache. According to the authors, a kyphotic deformity was not significantly associated with chronic whiplash-associated pain and that pain should not be ascribed to a straight spine on MRI.

10.2 The Fundamental Oscillation at 0.2 Hz

The ability to maintain balance is diminished in patients suffering from a whiplash injury. Stabilometry is a widely accepted method to document the impact of whiplash on static postural control.

Recently Madeleine et al. [12] investigated the variability of postural control in patients with chronic whiplash injury analyzing stabilometric recordings from 11

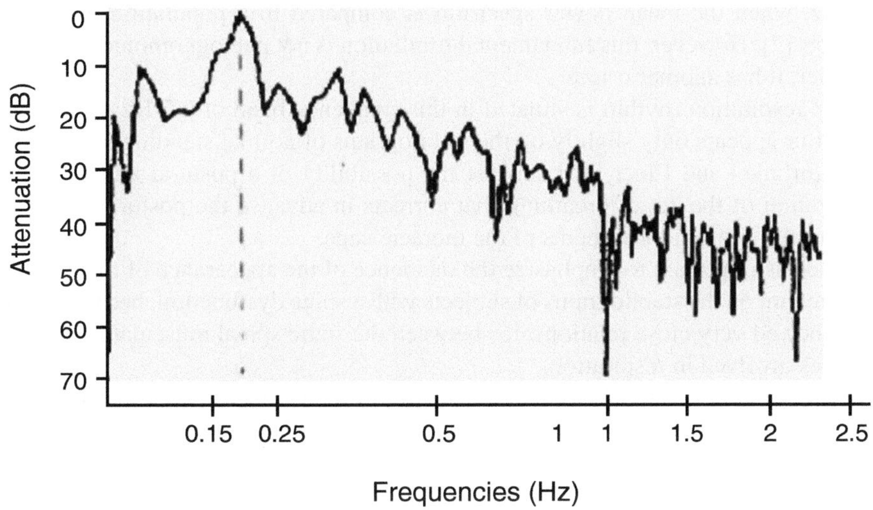

Fig. 10.3 Fourier's transform of the stabilometric signals of a whiplash victim. The fundamental oscillation GI is evident, clearly separated, at a frequency band of about 0.2 Hz (From Ref. [7])

whiplash patients and sex- and age-matched asymptomatic healthy volunteers. Spatial-temporal changes of the center of pressure displacement were analyzed to assess the amplitude and structure of postural variability by computing, respectively, the standard deviation/coefficient of variation and sample entropy/fractal dimension of the time series. The amplitude of variability of the center of pressure was larger among whiplash patients compared with controls ($P<0.001$), while fractal dimension was lower ($P<0.001$). They showed that sample entropy increased with both eyes closed and a simple dual task compared with eyes open ($P<0.05$). The analysis of postural control dynamics revealed increased amplitude of postural variability and decreased signal dimensionality related to the deficit in postural stability found in whiplash patients.

A specific contribution to comprehension of the complex phenomena that subserve postural control is the frequency analysis of the stabilometric signals. Using the Fourier transform in WAD patients, a fundamental oscillation around 0.2 Hz (Fig. 10.3) is frequently observed. This fundamental oscillation at 0.2 Hz appears equally on recordings made with the eyes open or closed.

This 0.2 Hz fundamental oscillation must not be confused with the fundamental oscillation at 0.3 Hz described by Taguchi [13]. The 0.3 Hz frequency corresponds to the resonance frequency of the inverted human pendulum that appears during dysregulations of the fine postural control system of which it is sometimes the only stabilometric witness. This fundamental oscillation simply demonstrates that the postural system is no longer able to damp out this resonance frequency of the human pendulum.

The 0.2 Hz fundamental oscillation has a completely different significance. Patients suffering from rachis pain is characterized by a peak at the frequency of

0.2 Hz, when the mean power spectrum is compared to a population of normal subjects [7]. However, this fundamental oscillation is not pathognomonic of a spine disorder; it has another origin.

The respiration rhythm is situated in this frequency band of 0.2 Hz; it does not appear or appears only slightly on the stabilograms of normal standing subjects [4, 14]. Gurfinkel and Elner [15] suggest the possibility of a postural adjustment in preparation of the act of breathing that corrects in advance the postural perturbations resulting from movements of the thoracic cage.

It seems important to emphasize the incidence of the appearance of this respiratory rhythm on the stabilograms of subjects with a spine dysfunction, because Tardy [16] showed very close relationships between the static spinal musculature and the muscles involved in respiration.

Postural control in WAD is disturbed even if subjects are seated as shown by Cote et al. [17] that investigated kinematic and electromyographic postural stabilization patterns in individuals with chronic WAD. Ten individuals with WAD and an age- and gender-matched group of healthy individuals were exposed to sudden forward and backward support surface translations while they were seated. Neck and trunk muscle activity and angular displacements as well as centers of mass (COMs) linear displacements at four levels of the head and trunk were computed. The displacement onset of the combined head, arms, and trunk COM was significantly delayed in persons with WAD. However, their peak trunk angles were smaller and were reached sooner. In the WAD group, the activation onset of the lumbar erector spinae was less affected by perturbation direction, and the sternocleidomastoid muscle, a neck flexor, showed a trend towards being activated later, compared to the healthy group. These results suggest that individuals with WAD may alter stretch reflex threshold and/or elicit a learned response for pain avoidance that may be direction specific. Such findings highlight the importance of assessing both spatial and temporal characteristics across different levels of the spinal musculoskeletal system to evaluate multidirectional postural responses in WAD individuals.

10.3 Asymmetry of the Activity of the Neck Muscles

Neck muscles are responsible for directing the head and for maintaining its posture. These functions are accomplished statically and dynamically, using various levels of contraction, by 22 muscle pairs that connect the head with the cervical spine and shoulder girdle. Optimal integration of this muscular complex is essential for normal functioning of the head-neck complex, whereas compromising it may result in associated pain and/or disability. Although assessing neck musculature may be conducted using imaging (ultrasound, computed tomography, magnetic resonance imaging) and electromyographic studies, from the functional point of view, the relevant parameter(s) refers to the mechanical expression of muscle function which is invariably reflected by the ability of neck muscles to develop force (strength) and to sustain it (endurance).

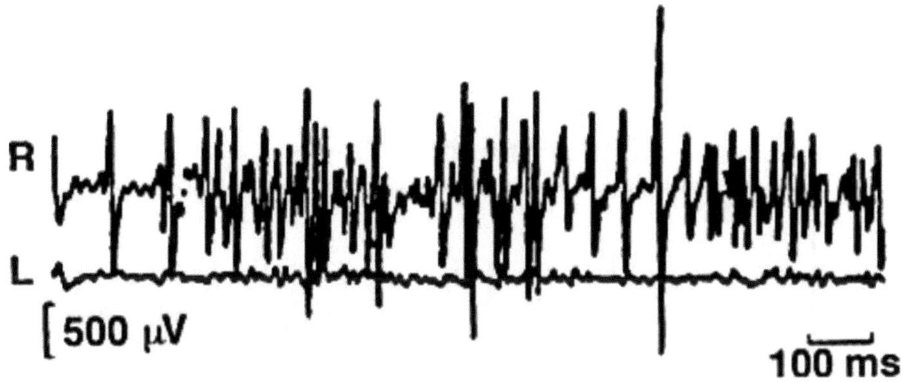

Fig. 10.4 Electromyograph (*EMG*) of neck muscles. EMG of the superior heads of the right and left trapezius muscles of a whiplash victim with his head in the normal position. The asymmetry of the tracings is obvious (From Ref. [7])

Manual muscle testing (MMT) [18] could be used for assessing sagittal and transverse plane strength. Testing is conducted with the patient at the prone (for extension) and supine (for flexion and rotation). Strength could be rated according to the MMT scale with grade 3 being equivalent to resisting gravity. Given the specific role of cervical muscles, preserving grade 3 would, in most cases, be sufficient for most functional activities since in these test positions the moment developed by the muscles is already in excess of the strength level required for normal activities. On the other hand, MMT is of a low validity when strength is to be rated as grade 4 or 5. Moreover, unlike the frontal plane, where the directional forces—lateral flexion to the right and to the left—are supposed to be symmetric and, hence, can serve reciprocally for comparison, such is not the case with flexion and extension as each depends largely on distinct muscle groups. Thus, MMT is not a recommended means for assessing cervical strength above grade 3.

Boquet and Boismare [19] studied comparatively the electromyograph (EMG) of the superior heads of the trapezius muscles, left and right. In whiplash victims, they almost always find marked asymmetry of these EMGs, with the patient's head in either the normal position (Fig. 10.4) or between positions with the head turned to the left and to the right (Fig. 10.5).

What is most remarkable on the EMG tracings of these patients is not only the asymmetry but also the amplitude of electrical activity.

Boquet noted signs of increased levels of vigilance, emotionalism, and basic anxiety in these patients. All whiplash victims do not necessarily have postural disorders. A supplementary factor is required which Boquet and Boismare link to this hypervigilance, that is, anxious individuals very often have neck pains and they blame it on early arthritis, but wrongly so, because one sees people with arthritis sufficiently severe to generate cracking sounds without any complain and contractures, but are calm individuals. This clinical contrast underlines the

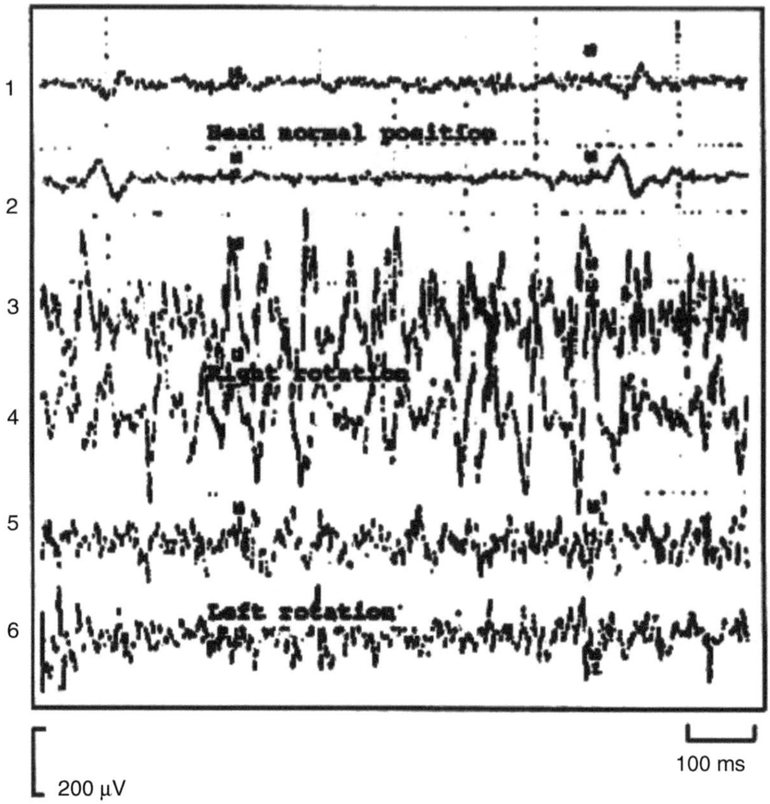

Fig. 10.5 Electromyograph (*EMG*) of neck muscles. EMG of the superior heads of the right (uneven numbers) and left (even numbers) trapezius muscles. 1–2: head in the normal position; 3–4: head turned to the right; 5–6: head turned to the left. The asymmetry appears when the head is rotated towards the right (From Ref. [7])

increased reactivity of neck neuromuscular spindles when the vigilance level is heightened [20]. This brings to mind the fundamental studies that demonstrated the noradrenergic innervation of the neuromuscular spindles and, more generally, the influence of the autonomous nervous system on the postural system. Ehrenborg and Archenholtz [21] showed that there is no support for the effectiveness of surface EMG biofeedback training as a supplement to an interdisciplinary rehabilitation program for people with long-lasting pain after whiplash.

10.4 Treatment

Treatment of post-traumatic cervical syndrome by strictly postural techniques (optical prisms, stimulation soles) has been a failure. But clinical posturology has taught us that, with every failure of postural treatments, a poorly understood lesion

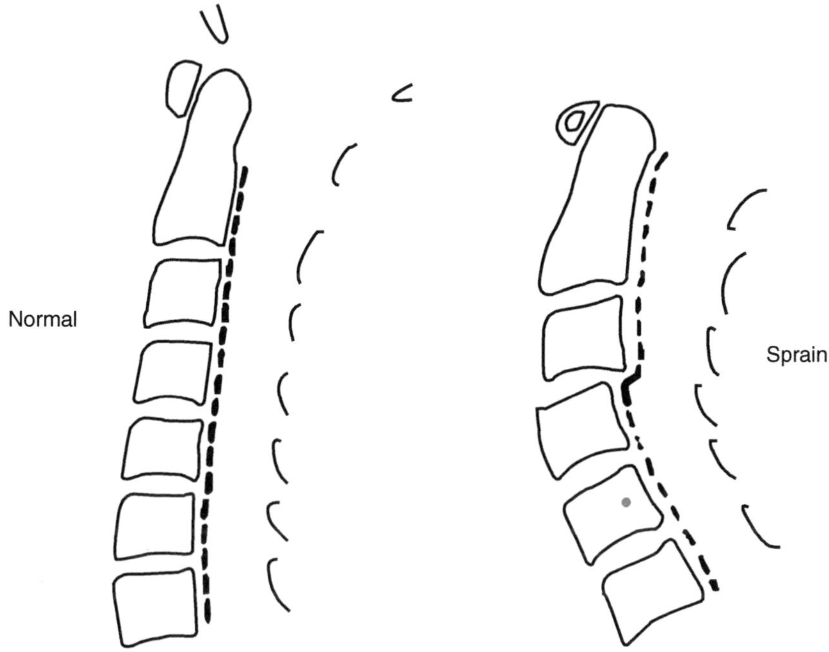

Fig. 10.6 Posterior walls, normal and after cervical sprain

must be sought. This is indeed the case, well established today, for mandibular lesions responsible for craniomandibular dysfunctions; we now know that the latter must be treated prior to initiating any postural therapy. This is also true for irritative lesions of plantar pressure points that are able to generate distant postural dysfunction; these lesions must be dealt with first. This hierarchy of treatments is easily explained: prisms and stimulation soles can only modify sensory integration. Addressing the lesion takes precedence over the subtleties of improving sensory integration.

Nowadays, lesions of the cervical spine after whiplash are far from always being poorly understood; medical imaging techniques have made enormous progress. Even before the era of computed tomography scanners and magnetic resonance imaging, Gentaz et al. [22], by multiplying the dynamic projections for radiography of the cervical spine, had detected obvious signs of cervical sprain, e.g., rupture of the continuity of the posterior wall of the vertebral bodies (Fig. 10.6) or overlapping of posterior articulations.

Normally, the posterior faces of the vertebral bodies remain perfectly aligned, even during hyperflexion and hyperextension of the neck. When a steplike shift appears in this posterior wall (between C3 and C4 in the drawing on the right of Fig. 10.6), a ligament has been torn, the neck sprained. These shifts usually only appear in dynamic positions, in this case, hyperextension.

Discovery of a cervical lesion subsequent to whiplash seems so important that we are tempted to say that no diagnosis of post-traumatic cervical syndrome can be made in its absence, especially when the whiplash is not recent. As long as the lesion is not found, it must be sought with perseverance.

If, despite the multiplication of tests, the lesion is not seen, the diagnosis should remain highly suspect. The neck is the privileged site of expression of all sorts of "distant" pathologies, such as oculomotor disorders, strabism, torticollis, occlusion pathologies, spinal, and even plantar disorders—that have nothing to do with whiplash. The cervical spine is a trap for the clinician.

It is useless to apply postural techniques to treat a whiplash victim with a cervical sprain. Therapy of the lesion takes precedence over attempts to manipulate sensory integration.

In contrast, Boquet and Boismare [19] insist upon the necessity to treat from the start the excessive anxiety, translated as permanent neurectasia, of these patients. The recommended therapeutic strategy is myoresolutive and sedative. The treatment starts pharmacologically with a diazepam (20 mg/ml) drip, in combination with 1-and f3-blockers that reduce the activity of the autonomous nervous system. The dosages are adjusted until the desired levels of vigilance and muscular tonus are obtained for each subject. Once the patient is "relaxed," work on the neck.

Conclusion

For more than 100 years, since the studies of Longet [23], we have known that the neck muscles are involved in postural control and we confirm this knowledge every day in whiplash victims. However, over the past few years, our attention has been drawn towards the overall level of vigilance of these patients that must be taken into account before starting therapy.

We are also better able to explore the traps posed by the cervical spine, where numerous postural tonic pathologies can express themselves without any local lesion. These observations lead us to insist upon searching signs of cervical sprain using all available means of medical imaging before settling on a diagnosis of whiplash.

The discovery of a cervical lesion is extremely important for determining the therapeutic strategy—it formally counter indicates the use of any postural techniques.

References

1. Baron JB (1955) Muscles moteurs oculaires, attitude et comportement locomoteur des vertébrés. Doctoral thesis in Science, Université de Paris
2. Lorenz EN (1993) The essence of chaos. UCL Press, London
3. Gagey PM, Martinerie J, Pezard L, Benaim C (1998) L'équilibre statique est contôlé par un système dynamique non-linéaire. Acta Otolaryngol 115:161–168
4. Gagey PM, Toupet M (1997) Le rythme ventilatoire apparaît sur les stabilogrammes en cas de pathologie du système vestibulaire ou proprioceptif. In: Lacour M, Gagey PM, Weber B (eds) Posture et Environnement. Sauramps, Montpellier, pp 11–28
5. Fryette HH (1978) Principes des techniques ostéopathiques. Maloine, Paris
6. Fukuda T (1959) The stepping test: two phases of the labyrinthine reflex. Acta Otolaryngol 50:95–108

7. Gagey PM, Weber B (1995) Posturologie; régulations et dérèglements de la station debout. Masson, Paris
8. Uemura T, Cohen B (1973) Effects of vestibular nuclei lesions on vestibulo-ocular reflexes and posture in monkeys. Acta Otolaryngol Suppl 315:1–71
9. Gagey PM (1986) Postural disorders among workers on building sites. In: Bles W, Brandt T (eds) Disorders of posture and gait. Elsevier, Amsterdam
10. Helgadottir H, Kristjansson E, Mottram S, Karduna A, Jonsson H Jr (2011) Altered alignment of the shoulder girdle and cervical spine in patients with insidious onset neck pain and whiplash-associated disorder. J Appl Biomech 27(3):181–191
11. Johansson MP, Baann Liane MS, Bendix T, Kasch H, Kongsted A (2011) Does cervical kyphosis relate to symptoms following whiplash injury? Man Ther 16(4):378–383. Epub 2011 Feb 3
12. Madeleine P, Nielsen M, Arendt-Nielsen L (2011) Characterization of postural control deficit in whiplash patients by means of linear and nonlinear analyses—a pilot study. J Electromyogr Kinesiol 21(2):291–297. Epub 2010 June 16
13. Taguchi K (1978) Spectral analysis of the movement of the center of gravity in vertiginous and ataxic patients. Agressologie 19B:69–70
14. Bouisset S, Duchene JL (1994) Is body balance more perturbed by respiration in seating thaò in standing posture? Neuroreport 5:957–960
15. Gurfinkel VS, Elner AM (1968) The relation of stability in a vertical posture to respiration in focal cerebral lesions of different etiology. Neuropathol Psychiatry 58:1014–1018 (in Russian)
16. Tardy D (1992) Systèmes moteurs posturaux du tronc, vieillissement, déclin. Crit Posturol 52:1–9
17. Côté JN, Patenaude I, St-Onge N, Fung J (2009) Whiplash-associated disorders affect postural reactions to antero-posterior support surface translations during sitting. Gait Posture 29(4):603–611. Epub 2009 Feb 7
18. Dvir Z, Prushansky T (2008) Cervical muscles strength testing methods and clinical implications. J Manipulative Physiol Ther 31(7):518–524
19. Boquet J, Boismare F (1982) Étude physiopathologique du syndrome cervical post-traumatique: ROie du tonus végétatif. Rev Fr Dommage Corpor 8:397–410; Hunt CC, Jame L, Laporte Y (1982) Effects of stimulating the lumbar sympathetic trunk on cat hindlimb muscle spindles. Arch Ital Biol 120:371–384
20. Grassi C, Perin F, Artusio E, Passatore M (1993) Modulation of the jaw jerk reflex by the sympathetic nervous system. Arch Ital Biol 131:213–226
21. Ehrenborg C, Archenholtz B (2010) Is surface EMG biofeedback an effective training method for persons with neck and shoulder complaints after whiplash-associated disorders concerning activities of daily living and pain -a randomized controlled trial. Clin Rehabil 24(8):715–726. Epub 2010 June 18
22. Gentaz R, Gagey PM, Goumot J, Rouquet Y, Baron JB (1975) La radiographie du rachis cervical au cours du syndrome post-commotionnei. Agressologie 16A:33–46
23. Longet FA (1845) Sur les troubles qui surviennent dans l'équilibration, la station et la locomotion des animaux après la section des parties molles de la nuque. Gaz Med Paris 13:565–567

11 Whiplash-Associated Autonomic Effects

R. Boniver, D.C. Alpini, and G. Brugnoni

11.1 Introduction

There is some evidence available indicating that autonomic disturbances are present in chronic WAD. Impaired peripheral vasoconstrictor responses have been demonstrated in both acute and chronic whiplash, but the relationship of these changes to the clinical presentation of whiplash or outcomes following injury is not clear. Gaab et al. [1] have shown reduced reactivity of the hypothalamic–pituitary–adrenal axis, a closely interacting system to the autonomic system, in a small sample of participants with chronic WAD. Autonomic nervous system dysfunction has been found to be present in other painful musculoskeletal conditions such as chronic low back pain, fibromyalgia, and cervicobrachialgia.

Individuals with posttraumatic stress disorder (PTSD) also show evidence of autonomic and hypothalamic–pituitary–adrenal dysfunction [2–5] which may have some relevance for WAD where recently it was shown that a significant proportion of injured people also have a probable diagnosis of PTSD.

There are obvious links between the cervical proprioceptors and the musculoskeletal system, but links to the autonomic nervous, vestibular, and visual systems and influence on pain modulation although important under a clinical point view are not yet well underlined.

R. Boniver (✉)
Department of Otolaryngology, Université de Liège, Rue de Bruxelles 21,
B-4800 Verviers, Belgium
e-mail: r.boniver@skynet.be

D.C. Alpini
ENT-Otoneurology Service, IRCCS "Don Carlo Gnocchi" Foundation,
Milan, Italy
e-mail: dalpini@dongnocchi.it

G. Brugnoni
Italian Academy of Manual Medicine, Italian Institute for Auxology, Milan, Italy
e-mail: guido.brugnoni@libero.it

D.C. Alpini et al. (eds.), *Whiplash Injuries*,
DOI 10.1007/978-88-470-5486-8_11, © Springer-Verlag Italia 2014

Dizziness is one of the most frequent complaints in those with persistent pain after a whiplash trauma, and it is often associated with postural control disturbances. Postural control may have potential to alter other systems and affect pain and should be considered as one of the processes that might influence the transition to chronicity after a whiplash trauma.

According to Trevalen [6, 7] transition from acute to chronic WAD is due to involvement of the autonomic system with special regard to cervical part of it. Besides its well-known action on muscle blood flow, the sympathetic nervous system (SNS) is able to affect the contractility of muscle fibers, to modulate the proprioceptive information arising from the muscle spindle receptors, and, under certain conditions, to modulate nociceptive information. Furthermore, the activity of the SNS itself is in turn affected by muscle conditions, such as its current state of activity, fatigue, and pain signals originating in the muscle.

The thesis of Trevalen et al. is sustained by the review of Passatore and Roatta [8] that focuses on the actions exerted by the sympathetic system at muscle level in WAD, with particular emphasis being devoted to sensorimotor symptoms.

The autonomic genesis of dizziness that could lead to postural disorders and then to chronic pain was sustained by Barrè [9] in 1924. He described the so-called *posterior cervical sympathetic syndrome* and proposed that cervical lesions might irritate the sympathetic vertebral plexus and result in a decreased blood flow to the labyrinth due to constriction of the internal auditory artery. Although numerous clinical reports of *Barré syndrome* have been published, few objective data exist to support an association between episodic vertigo and cervical sympathetic dysfunction. Since intracranial circulation is autoregulated independently of cervical sympathetic control, it is unlikely that lesions in the vertebro-sympathetic plexus could produce focal constriction of the vasculature to the inner ear.

Hinoki, first in 1971 [10] and in detail in 1985 [11], proposed a hypothesis in which the hypothalamus takes a fundamental place to explain vertigo due to whiplash injury.

11.2 The Autonomic Nervous System

The autonomic nervous system (ANS) is the part of the nervous system, both afferent and efferent, that innervates various body systems that are not under voluntary control. These include the constriction and dilation of blood vessels, the activity of the viscera, and the secretion of glands (secretomotor fibers), and assist the endocrine system to maintain a constant internal environment (homeostasis).

The *afferent* neurons have their peripheral receptors in the wall of viscera and blood vessels and their cell bodies in the dorsal root ganglia or cranial nerve ganglia. Their central processes end in the dorsal gray column of the spinal cord or the brain stem.

The *efferent* neurons supply the smooth muscles in the wall of hollow viscera and blood vessels. They can be either excitatory or inhibitory.

The efferent pathway is made up of two neurons:

1. A preganglionic neuron (myelinated), located in the spinal cord or brain stem, synapsing with
2. Postganglionic neuron(s) (unmyelinated) in an autonomic ganglion

Functionally, the ANS is divided into sympathetic and parasympathetic systems.

The *sympathetic nervous system* (SNS) prepares the body for "fright, fight, or flight." It increases the heart rate and ventricular contraction, dilates the blood vessels in skeletal muscles, constricts blood vessels in the skin and guts, increases blood sugar level, stimulates sweating, dilates the pupils, and inhibits activities of the guts and gastric secretion.

The sympathetic outflow from the central nervous system (CNS) is *thoracolumbar*, emerging from the spinal cord segments *T1–L3*. The sympathetic ganglia form a string of beads called the *sympathetic trunk*, lying on either side of the vertebral bodies. The two trunks extend from C1 to the level of the coccyx where they unite at the midline at the *ganglion impar*.

The preganglionic fibers leave the spinal cord with the ventral root of the corresponding spinal nerve and pass to the corresponding sympathetic ganglion via the *white ramus communicans* (white because the *fibers are myelinated*). In that ganglion, they may synapse with postganglionic fibers which leave the sympathetic trunk in the *gray ramus communicans*, rejoin the same ventral ramus, then are distributed to the target organs (smooth muscles of blood vessels, sweat glands…), travel up or down the trunk to synapse with postganglionic fibers in other ganglia (e.g., cervical, lumbar, sacral, which do not receive direct rami communicantes from the cervical, lower lumbar, or sacral segments), or pass through the ganglion without relay to synapse in *prevertebral ganglion* (e.g., celiac ganglion, known to lay people as "solar plexus").

The *parasympathetic nervous system* (PNS) is more active at rest, having in general anabolic effects. For example, it slows down the heart rate, constricts the pupils, and increases gastric secretion and intestinal motility.

The parasympathetic system outflow is *craniosacral*, emerging from the oculomotor, facial, glossopharyngeal, and vagus nerves and the spinal cord segments S2, S3, and S4. These fibers travel in the branches of sacral nerves S2–S4 (nervi erigentes) to the pelvic viscera.

The parasympathetic system supplies the heart, glands, and smooth muscles of the viscera, *not* the sweat glands, blood vessels, or erector pilorum muscles.

11.3 The Hypothalamus

The hypothalamus is unquestionably of great significance both phylogenetically and anthropologically. It plays striking roles in many aspects of mammalian physiology. It undoubtedly contains integrative mechanisms which, in addition to their effect on behavior patterns, also aid in regulating the basic life functions of the organism. However, this integration is apparently carried out through its relationship with other parts of the nervous system, including the so-called higher levels, as well as through the endocrine system.

It is in this field of interrelationship that some of the most pressing problems lie. It must be appreciated that while this interesting region of the brain is only part of a system of complex circuits, it is an extremely important link in these circuits and is so strategically placed that its derangement may have profound effects.

It is important that the hypothalamus be regarded as part of a series of complex neural circuits involving the brain stem, cerebral hemisphere, and other parts of the diencephalon. These circuits are poorly understood, but evidence for rich connections with septal, subcallosal, preoptic, and frontotemporal areas has been offered. The hypothalamus is considered to be the most rostral portion of the reticular formation and similarly is poorly differentiated with the exception of the magnocellular neurosecretory system. The hypothalamus is also the most caudal aspect of the limbic system and thus the brain region through which limbic system output comes to control autonomic and endocrine function.

The paraventricular nucleus of the hypothalamus (PVN) is one of the most vascularized areas of the brain. The PVN distinguishes itself from other hypothalamic nuclei in that it plays the dominant role in neuronally coupling autonomic, endocrine, and somatomotor responses to environmental stressors. It accomplishes this through a rich network of innervation from the forebrain, limbic system, other hypothalamic nuclei, and brain stem autonomic centers such as the nucleus of the solitary tract and the dorsal vagal complex. PVN innervates the median eminence, pituitary, brain stem nuclei, and spinal cord.

Concentrations in epinephrine (EPI) in the paraventricular nucleus in human hypothalamus are rather high [12]. If stressful motion were shown to lead to a significant rise in EPI and norepinephrine (NE), then this rise would be different from subject to subject and would therefore be more prominent in subjects more resistant to motion sickness. Strangely enough, in those cases, no correlations were found between measured levels of ACTH and EPI even though EPI exerts a stimulatory influence on the pituitary gland's release of ACTH. It is well known that ACTH and smaller peptides like ACTH 4–10 reduce latency in recovery of normal sensorimotor functions following unilateral labyrinthectomy.

Corticotropin-releasing factor (CRF), containing neurons, have been found in the medial vestibular nucleus and may contribute to CRF, containing climbing fibers shown to project from the inferior olive to the cerebellum.

11.4 Hinoki's Hypothesis

According to Hinoki, patients with whiplash injury present with a hypertonicity of the soft supporting tissues of the neck due to the overexcitation of the cervical proprioceptors, which is caused by an excitation of sympathical beta-receptors in the muscle spindles. He has demonstrated the development of granular vesicles at the end of unmyelinated nerve fibers near the motor nerve endings of these spindles.

Abnormal centripetal impulses arising from the injured cervical soft tissues may ascend along the spinoreticular tract to the brain stem. Among the ascending

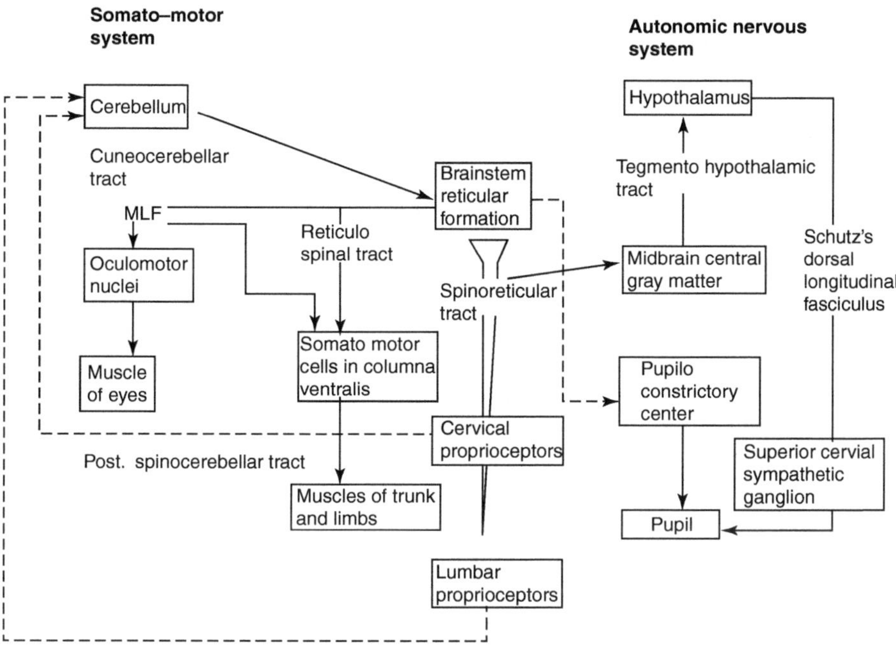

Fig. 11.1 Connections of lumbar and cervical proprioceptors within the somatomotor system

pathways from the cervical and lumbar proprioceptors to the brain stem, the spinoreticular tract seems to be the most important, since most of its fibers ascend along the lateral fasciculus and the anterior column and terminate in the reticular formation of both the medulla oblongata and the pons. However, some fibers of this tract ascend directly to the midbrain and are connected to Deiters' nucleus.

Furthermore, this tract changes neurons in the medulla oblongata, the pons, and the midbrain and terminates in the superior colliculus. It is generally accepted that the reticular formation of these parts of the brain, as well as Deiters' nucleus and the superior colliculus, is active in both ocular and spinal reflexes related to body equilibrium. Among the descending paths from the brain stem, the median longitudinal fasciculus (MLF) is important in cases of vertigo, because this tract originates in the brain stem and is connected to both the oculomotor nuclei and the somatomotor cells in the ventral column. The reticulospinal tract also originates in the brain stem reticular formation of both the medulla oblongata and the pons and is connected to the somatomotor cells in the ventral column. This tract is thought to have a close relationship with the spinoreticular tract mentioned above. Thus, the MLF and the reticulospinal tract seem especially important in the development of disequilibrium because of whiplash injury. The hypothalamus must also play an important role in producing vertigo due to whiplash injury, since most of Hinoki patients, with vertigo following whiplash injury, had various autonomic symptoms, such as lacrimation, abnormal sweating, and palpitation.

The cerebellum is, of course, involved in the development of this type of vertigo, since it is closely connected to the proprioceptors of the cervical and lumbar regions as well as to the brain stem (Fig. 11.1).

After several experiments, Hinoki further demonstrated that the abnormal autonomic reactions in patients with whiplash injury were not due to the irritation of the injured posterior cervical sympathetic nerves but to overstimulation of the proprioceptor of the neck.

On the basis of their report and the known fiber connections in the central nervous system, it may be assumed that in patients with whiplash injury, delayed pupil constriction in response to light is probably because of overstimulation of a sympathetic component in the hypothalamus-brain stem system brought about by centripetal impulses from the injured proprioceptors of the neck and waist. In addition, the spinoreticular tract is probably involved in the conduction of these impulses, since this tract ascends along the lateral fasciculus and the anterior column in the cervical and lumbar cords and terminates in both the reticular formation of the brain stern and the central gray matter of the midbrain [13].

The central gray matter of the midbrain is then connected to the hypothalamus both through the hypothalamotegmental tract and diffuse ascending neurons. There is evidence to support this assumption, since Hinoki found that, in patients with delayed pupil constriction in response to light, ataxia of the eyes and body tended to be aggravated by the subcutaneous injection of adrenaline.

Moreover, Kawamura and Oshurna [14] reported that adrenaline acts directly on the posterior hypothalamus, an important center of the sympathetic nervous system. Okada et al. [15] also reported that in cats the electrical activities of the short ciliary nerves, which are involved in pupil constriction, were significantly decreased by the injection of adrenaline. According to their explanation, overstimulation of the hypothalamus induced by adrenaline suppresses the activity of the pupillo-constrictory center of the midbrain, leading to pupil dilatation.

To summarize, the overexcitation of the arrival proprioceptors should be because of a hypersensitivity to sympathetic stimulation, inducing central disturbances by afferent nervous pathways at the level of brain stem, cerebellar, and hypothalamus, affecting the oculomotor system and gait control.

More recently Hinoki's hypothesis has been supported by Matsui et al. [16]. Authors found that abnormalities in the cervical muscles after whiplash cause autonomic dystonia, leading to headache, chronic fatigue syndrome, vertigo, and dizziness. They named this group of diseases cervical neuromuscular syndrome. In their experience treatment of the cervical muscle was effective for general whiplash-associated malaise.

Autonomic involvement after whiplash can provoke also short-lasting unilateral neuralgiform headache with conjunctival injection and tearing (SUNCT), a rare headache syndrome classified among the trigeminal autonomic cephalalgias. It is usually idiopathic, although infrequent posttraumatic forms have been described [17]. Recently the term short-lasting unilateral headache with cranial autonomic symptoms (SUNA) has been defined by the International Headache Society (ICHD-2) as similar to SUNCT with less prominent or absent conjunctival injection and lacrimation.

For this kind of posttraumatic neuralgiform headache, Choi et al. [18] proposed greater occipital nerve (GON) block as treatment.

11.5 Chronic Pain and Fatigue in Whiplash Patient

In spite of their clear traumatic origin, whiplash-associated disorders (WAD) appear to share many common features with other chronic pain syndromes affecting the musculoskeletal system. These features do not only include symptoms, like type of pain or sensory and motor dysfunctions, but possibly also some of the pathophysiological mechanisms that may concur to establish the chronic pain syndrome. Studies [19–22] show that injury produces plasticity changes of different neuronal structures that are responsible for amplification of nociception and exaggerated pain responses. There is consistent evidence for hypersensitivity of the central nervous system to sensory stimulation in chronic pain after whiplash injury.

Different mechanisms underlie and coexist in the chronic whiplash condition. Spinal cord hyperexcitability in patients with chronic pain after whiplash injury can cause exaggerated pain following low-intensity nociceptive or innocuous peripheral stimulation. Spinal hypersensitivity may explain pain in the absence of detectable tissue damage.

Whiplash is a heterogeneous condition with some individuals showing features suggestive of neuropathic pain. A predominantly neuropathic pain component is related to a higher pain/disability level [23, 24].

Chronic pain can lead to posttraumatic stress reaction (PTSR). On the other hand the sympathetic nervous system (SNS) could sustain a posttraumatic stress reaction (PTSR) at least in some whiplash-injured persons. Sterling and Kenardy [25] showed in fact that patients with persistent PTSR presented sensory hypersensitivity and impaired peripheral vasoconstriction compared to those whose PTSR resolved and those without PTSR. The early presence of sensory hypersensitivity was associated with PTSR at 6 months, but this relationship was mediated by pain and disability levels. Thus, authors showed the connections between chronic pain PTSR and SNS.

The correlation between chronicization of WAD and SNS has been investigated also by Kalezic et al. [26] that suggested a stronger autonomic reaction in WAD than in healthy subjects in response to dynamic loading of the jaw–neck motor system to explain impaired endurance during chewing as previously reported in WAD. Kalezic et al. correlated cardiovascular reactivity and EMG muscle fatigue indices, and perceptions of fatigue; exhaustion and pain were assessed during standardized chewing. More than half of the WAD subjects terminated the test prematurely due to exhaustion and pain. In line with their hypothesis, the chewing evoked an increased autonomic response in WAD exhibited as a higher increase in heart rate as compared to controls indicating pronounced vulnerability to dynamic loading of the jaw–neck motor system with increased autonomic reactivity to the test. Premature termination and autonomic involvement without EMG signs of muscle fatigue may indicate central mechanisms.

Conclusion

The correlation between ANS and whiplash injuries has been postulated until 1920s of the last century. In the following years more evidences have progressively sustained Barrè, before, and Hinoki's, after, hypothesis. Due to the complexity of the cervico-cephalic connections, the role of the ANS is not yet completely understood, but the role of central sensitization (both at the spinal cord and the brain level) is actually a matter of fact to explain chronicization of WADs [27].

References

1. Gaab J, Baumann S, Budnoik A, Gmunder H, Hottinger N, Ehlert U (2005) Reduced reactivity and enhanced negative feedback sensitivity of the hypothalamus-pituitary-adrenal axis in chronic whiplash associated disorders. Pain 119:219–224
2. Bogduk N (2006) Whiplash can have lesions. Pain Res Manag 11(3):155
3. Sterling M, Jull G, Kenardy J (2006) Physical and psychological predictors of outcome following whiplash injury maintain predictive capacity at long term follow-up. Pain 122:102–108
4. Sterling M (2010) Differential development of sensory hypersensitivity and a measure of spinal cord hyperexcitability following whiplash injury. Pain 150:501–506
5. Kamper S, Rebbeck T, Maher C, McAuley J, Sterling M (2008) Course and prognostic factors of whiplash: a systematic review and meta-analysis. Pain 138:617–629
6. Treleaven J (2011) Dizziness, unsteadiness, visual disturbances, and postural control: implications for the transition to chronic symptoms after a whiplash trauma. Spine 36(25 Suppl): S211–S217
7. Treleaven J, Jull G, LowChoy N (2005) Standing balance in persistent whiplash: a comparison between subjects with and without dizziness. J Rehabil Med 37:224–229
8. Passatore M, Roatta S (2006) Influence of sympathetic nervous system on sensorimotor function: whiplash associated disorders (WAD) as a model. Eur J Appl Physiol 98:423–449
9. Barré JA (1926) Sur un syndrome sympathique cervical postérieur et sa cause fréquente: l'arthrite cervicale. Rev Neurol (Paris) I33:1246–1294
10. Hinoki M (1985) Vertigo due to whiplash injury: a neuro-otological approach. Acta Otolaryngol Suppl 419:9–29
11. Hinoki M, Hine S, Tada Y (1971) Neurootological study on vertigo due to whiplash injury. Equilib Res (Suppl 1):5–29
12. Mefford IN, Oke A, Keller R, Adarns RM, Jonsson G (1978) Epinephrine distribution in human brain. Neurosci Lett 9:277–287
13. Stampacchia G, D'ascanio P, Hoin E, Pompeiano O (1988) Gain regulation of the vestibulospinal reflex following microinjection of a beta-adrenergic agonist or antagonist in to the locus coeruleus and the dorsal pontine reticular formation. Adv Otorhinolaryngol 41:134–141
14. Kawamura H, Oshima K (1962) Effect of adrenaline on the hypothalamic activating system. Jpn J Physiol I2:225–233
15. Okada H, Nakano O, Nishida I (1960) Effects of sciatic stimulation upon the efferent impulses in the long ciliary nerves of the cat. Jpn J Physiol 10:327–337
16. Matsui T, Ii K, Hojo S, Sano K (2012) Cervical neuro-muscular syndrome: discovery of a new disease group caused by abnormalities in the cervical muscles. Neurol Med Chir (Tokyo) 52(2):75–80
17. Jacob S, Saha A, Rajabally Y (2008) Post-traumatic short-lasting unilateral headache with cranial autonomic symptoms (SUNA). Cephalalgia 28(9):991–993. Epub 2008 May 30
18. Choi HJ, Choi SK, Lee SH, Lim YJ (2012) Whiplash injury-induced atypical short-lasting unilateral neuralgiform headache with conjunctival injection and tearing syndrome treated by greater occipital nerve block. Clin J Pain 28(4):342–343
19. Carroll LJ, Holm LW, Hogg-Johnson S, Côté P, Cassidy JD, Haldeman S (2008) Course and prognostic factors for neck pain in whiplash-associated disorders (WAD). Results of the bone and joint decade 2000–2010 task force on neck pain and its associated disorders. Eur Spine J 17(Suppl 1):83–92

20. Koelbaek-Johansen M, Graven-Nielsen T, Schou-Olesen A, Arendt-Nielsen L (1999) Muscular hyperalgesia and referred pain in chronic whiplash syndrome. Pain 83:229–234
21. Sterling M, Jull G, Vicenzino B, Kenardy J (2003) Sensory hypersensitivity occurs soon after whiplash injury and is associated with poor recovery. Pain 104:509–517
22. Lim E, Sterling M, Stone A, Vicenzino B (2011) Central hyperexcitability as measured with nociceptive flexor reflex threshold in chronic musculoskeletal pain: a systematic review. Pain 152:1811–1820
23. Davis CG (2013) Mechanisms of chronic pain from whiplash injury. J Forensic Leg Med 20(2):74–85
24. Van Oosterwijck J, Nijs J, Meeus M, Paul L (2013) Evidence for central sensitization in chronic whiplash: a systematic literature review. Eur J Pain 17(3):299–312
25. Sterling M, Kenardy J (2006) The relationship between sensory and sympathetic nervous system changes and posttraumatic stress reaction following whiplash injury – a prospective study. J Psychosom Res 60(4):387–393
26. Kalezic N, Noborisaka Y, Nakata M, Crenshaw AG, Karlsson S, Lyskov E, Eriksson PO (2010) Cardiovascular and muscle activity during chewing in whiplash-associated disorders (WAD). Arch Oral Biol 55(6):447–453. Epub 2010 Apr 21
27. Adeboye KA, Emerton DG, Hughes T (2000) Cervical sympathetic chain dysfunction after whiplash injury. J R Soc Med 93(7):378–379

Whiplash-Associated Temporomandibular Disorders (TMDs)

12

E. Brunetta

12.1 Introduction

Rear-end impacts account for more than one-third of vehicle accidents, and nearly 40 % of these accidents produce whiplash injuries. Whiplash injury to the neck has often been considered a significant risk factor for the development of temporomandibular disorders (TMDs) [1–4].

The state in which the stomatognathic musculoskeletal system is hyperfunctional, tender and exhausted is known as temporomandibular disorders (TMDs). TMDs can generate referred craniofacial symptomatology (where origin differed from its real location) that take influence in cervical and cranial diffuse discomfort. TMDs consist of musculoskeletal disorders, characterized by pain in the temporomandibular joint (TMJ) and/or mastication muscles, involving a wide range of craniofacial conditions with multiple origins that produces a large variety of nonobjective signs and symptoms. These could be primary, referred or combined from cervical muscles and associated cranial structures. The most frequent symptom is pain, usually localized in the muscles of mastication, the preauricular region and the temporomandibular joint (TMJ). Patients often complain of jaw ache, earache, headache and facial pain. In addition to pain, patients with these disorders frequently have limited or asymmetric jaw movement and joint sounds that are described as clicking or crepitus. The pathogenesis of TMDs remains unclear, and numerous factors have been implicated even when temporomandibular symptoms develop following motor-vehicle collisions (MVCs). Also in these cases TMDs are complex, representing a component of a symptom cluster of potentially regional and widespread pain impacted by psychosocial factors. Oral health-care providers must be aware of the complex relationship between temporomandibular symptoms and whiplash for appropriate diagnosis and management, because TMDs following

E. Brunetta
Private Dentist, Conegliano (TV), Italy
e-mail: elvio.brunetta@fastwebnet.it

D.C. Alpini et al. (eds.), *Whiplash Injuries*,
DOI 10.1007/978-88-470-5486-8_12, © Springer-Verlag Italia 2014

MVCs may result from both direct orofacial trauma and whiplash-associated disorder (WAD) without such trauma [5].

Furthermore, TMDs may not be identified at the time of first assessment, but may develop weeks or more after the MVC. TMDs in WAD appear to occur predominantly in females and can be associated with regional or widespread pain. TMDs following MVCs may respond poorly to independent therapy and may be best managed using multidisciplinary approaches [6].

According to Salè and Isberg [7, 8] the incidence of new symptoms of TMJ pain, dysfunction or both, between the inceptive examination and follow-up, was five times higher in WAD subjects (34 %) than in control subjects (7 %) and 20 % of all subjects reported that temporomandibular joint (TMJ) symptoms were their main complaint. Visscher et al. [9] showed that, irrespective of the classification system used, the chronic whiplash-associated disorder pain group more often suffered from temporomandibular disorder pain ($0.001 < P < 0.028$) and widespread pain ($0.001 < P < 0.003$) than the no neck pain group. Moreover, patients with whiplash-associated disorder showed more psychologic distress ($0.000 < P < 0.044$) than others. The higher prevalence of widespread pain and psychologic distress in patients with chronic whiplash-associated disorder suggests that the higher prevalence of temporomandibular disorder pain in these patients is part of a more widespread chronic pain disorder. There appears to be a risk of delayed onset of TMDs following an MVC. TMDs are reported as the primary complaint only by 5 % of the patients at the first visit and by 19 % at 1-year follow-up, with painful jaw clicking and/or locking, and they are higher in females than males.

The potential delay in onset of TMDs following an MVC raises concerns about diagnosis, prognosis, management and medico-legal issues.

12.2 Embryology

TMJ development and other neighbouring structures in humans (such as pharynx, Eustachian tube and tympanic cavity) is complex and continues to be investigated. The mandible is formed from the ventral part of Meckel's cartilage, which is the first branchial arch. The ossicles (malleus, incus and partially the stapes) are formed from the dorsal part of Meckel's cartilage and Reichert's cartilage (second branchial arch). The malleus has a double origin in these ossicles; the anterior process originates from mesenchymal cells (os goniale), through intramembranous ossification, and the rest form from Meckel's cartilage, through endochondral ossification. The malleus is related to the TMJ (condylar and temporal blastemas) by fibrous connections (lateral pterygoid muscle) passing through the petrotympanic fissure, named the discomalleolar ligament. These lateral pterygoid muscular fibrous connections then form the interarticular disc in Meckel's cartilage by mechanical stimulation of this muscle. The medial pterygoid muscle and the tensor tympani muscle develop from the temporal blastema. These structures (along with the tensor veli palatini) are innervated by the trigeminal mandibular branch (V3), in turn innervating the masticatory muscles coming from the first branchial arch mesoderm.

12.3 Anatomy

The temporomandibular joint (TMJ) consists of the glenoid cavity of the temporal bone, mandibular condyle, muscles and ligaments [10]. Between the two structures meniscus is interposed, a fibrocartilage disc connected to the joint capsule in front of the tendon of the lateral pterygoid muscle. The rear of the glenoid cavity, or temporal fossa, is very thin, and the rear tissue of the disc is sensitive to compression, as well as light traumas with great inflammatory reactivity. The upper side (temporomandibular meniscus) is used for the transfer of the jaw, and the lower side (meniscus-condyle) is for the rotation (first 2 cm of the opening of the mouth) [11].

TMJ moves by the masticatory muscles and the supra- and infrahyoid muscles. It is the only joint that is flat at birth and takes its shape with the masticatory function. It does this by determining its normal relationship with the temporal bone at 6 years of age, which is when the eruption of the permanent first molars determine the vertical dimension of dental occlusion.

The innervation consists primarily of the trigeminal nerve (V cranial pair) with three components: ophthalmic, maxillary and mandibular. Aside from the close connections with the other cranial nerves, anatomically, their motor nuclei intersect the brainstem reticular formation close to the basal ganglia, especially the locus coeruleus (noradrenergic nucleus).

Furthermore, the important correlation with the innervation at the level of the cervical vertebrae has been demonstrated (see vestibule-vertebral functional unit chapter).

12.4 Biomechanics of Whiplash-Associated TMDs

Several studies have investigated concomitant functional connections between TMDs and cervical spine disorders. The functionality of cervical and masticatory systems is complemented synergistically but pathologically too in a concomitant way. It has been reported [12, 13] that 45 % of TMD patients have headaches and 54 % have neck-shoulder pain confirming TMDs as a part of a more complex and widespread painful syndrome.

Lesions present in the classic whiplash at low speed are not normally seen through diagnostic imaging because the forces acting on the TMJ are most often offset by the strength of the assembly-muscle ligaments of the joint, added to the fact that the jaw weights little and has a little inertia.

WA TMD pathogenesis is still controversial. In the rear-end impact the inertia of the mandible caused it to move posteriorly slower than the head, and this resulted in downward and forward displacements of the disc-condyle complex relative to the cranial base. Consequently, a rapid and big mouth opening occurs. In contrast, during the frontal impact, the mouth hardly opened, because the superior maxilla pushed the mandible to move together. There was no differential movement between bony components of the joint, and therefore the soft tissues of the joint were not subjected to high loads. Neither a rear-end impact at low velocity nor a frontal impact would produce damage to the soft tissues of the joint.

In whiplash hyperextension phase of the neck, the jaw is pushed forward and down with disc displacement in the same direction, stretching the joint capsule with stabilizing contracture of the flexor muscles of the neck and of the supra- and infrahyoid muscles. At the time of the hyperflexion of the neck, the jaw is pushed upward in the posterior glenoid cavity with compression of the rear tissue of the disc and anterior medial displacement of the disc with contracture of the extensor muscles of the neck and jaw muscles. In this way, TMDs could be mainly due to traumatic retrusion of the condyle either directly, since the more sensitive anatomical part to compression is the posterior top of the glenoid cavity, as already mentioned, or indirectly, through the defensive muscle spasms, which tend to bring the jaw in retrusion, exacerbating the compression of the rear tissue of the disc.

Recent studies have determined that about one in three people who have suffered a whiplash injury develop TMD, even after a long time after the accident, with tenderness, abnormal joint kinematics, disturbances of jaw-head-neck coordination, possible dizziness and difficulty chewing, which happens to be the highest percentage in women, probably because of a weaker anatomical structure [13].

Hernandez et al. [4] investigated mandibular kinematics in low-impact rear-end impacts in 30 healthy adults. Subjects underwent three impacts (4.5 ms^{-2} expected, 10.0 ms^{-2}) unexpected and 10.0 ms^{-2} expected). Onset time and peak magnitude of angular head acceleration, angular mandibular acceleration and angular mandibular displacement were measured. Significant mandibular opening acceleration was not identified with rearward head rotation. The peak magnitude of mandibular closing angular acceleration approximately doubled with increased impact magnitude. No differences in peak angular mandibular acceleration regarding expectation were identified. Gender differences were detected in the fast unexpected impact. The peak time for the angular mandibular acceleration (mandibular closure) was approximately 84–120 ms later than peak rearward angular head acceleration for all impacts. Onset and peak times for angular mandibular acceleration (mandibular closure) were similar to the onset and peak times for forward head acceleration. There was also a positive correlation between the magnitude of the forward angular acceleration of the head and angular acceleration of the mandible for the slow (0.65, $P=0.015$) and fast expected (0.844, $P=0.001$) impacts. The average angular mandibular angular displacement (mandibular closure) was approximately 6°. The pure hyperextension hypothesis regarding mechanism of TMJ injury in low-impact rear-end collisions thus cannot be supported. Besides localized trauma to structural elements of the stomatognathic system (peripherally mediated and maintained pain), regional and widespread symptoms, may be due to dysfunction or dysregulation of central pain modulating systems and regional or widespread pain input, involving neuropsychological and cognitive changes (centrally mediated and maintained pain). Altered nociceptive input and central processing in WAD patients has also been reported in experimental pain studies.

We can conclude that the main aspect to be taken into account regarding WA TMDs in a specific patient is the threshold of "excitability" of the system jaw-cranium-neck, trigeminal controlled, as this buffer system is balanced and effective, for

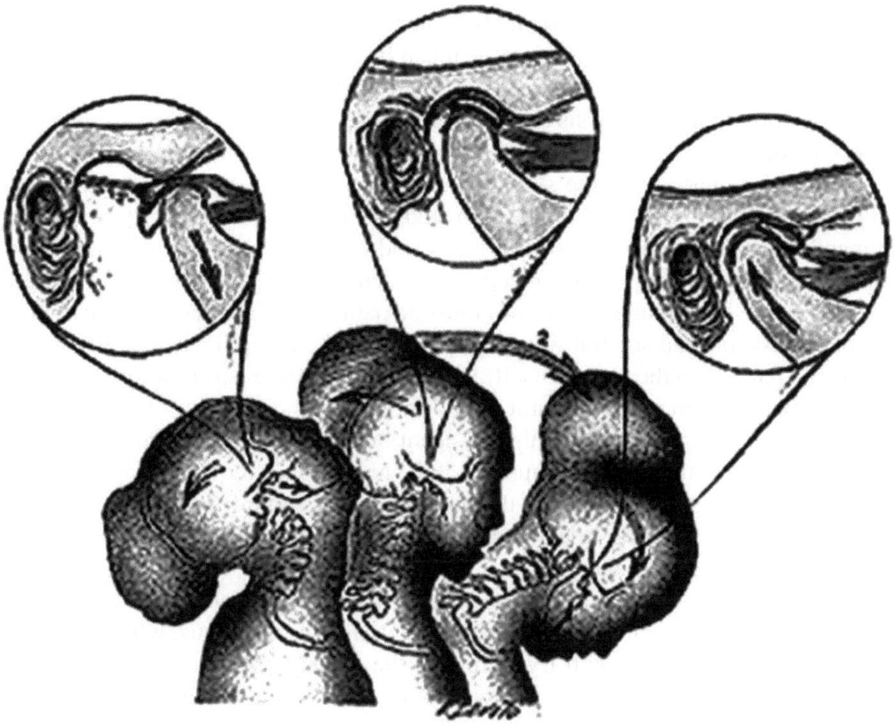

Fig. 12.1 Relative displacement of the condylus with respect to the skull (glenoid) in the hyperextension and hyperflexion phases of whiplash

the same energy absorbed, the greater the injury-dysfunction will be minor. The following sequence can be considered (Fig. 12.1):

1. Stretching and compression of the capsule-ligament-muscle complex of TMJ with or without meniscal dislocation, but with the reduction of the meniscus itself. Joint pain, myalgia, inefficient chewing, noises when opening and/or closing the mouth, sense of asymmetry in the chewing movements.
2. As above, but with dislocation and without reduction, the meniscus is blocked in the rear part, the painful symptom is higher and the mandible kinematic is altered, the dynamic asymmetry is evident, and the axiography reveals aspects, possible joint locking.
3. In regard to the above, it could add micro- or macro-ligamentous injuries to the rear tissue of the disc with possible inflammation and anatomical alteration of the joint.

12.5 TMJ and Posture

Eating requires mouth opening, biting, chewing and swallowing and should be performed without dysfunction or pain. Previous studies have shown that jaw opening-closing movements are the result of coordinated activation of both jaw and neck muscles, with simultaneous movements in the temporomandibular, atlanto-occipital and cervical spine joints. Consequently, it can be assumed that pain or dysfunction in any of the three joint systems involved could impair jaw activities. In fact, recent findings support this hypothesis by showing an association between neck injury and reduced amplitudes, speed and coordination of integrated jaw-neck movements.

The jaw is connected to the skull, which is connected to the spine and skeleton with a well-determined spatial position and is efficient for the vertical bipedal human being. The natural law of symmetry and orthogonality determines the neurogenic information of postural receptors; the cranio-cervical-mandibular posture obeys this rule. Upper and lower jaws must be parallel and aligned with each other in both transverse and sagittal ways and parallel to the bipupillary line, visual axis of human, parallel to the ground itself. We understand how a perturbation that could alter this balance can affect postural attitude.

The indirect mechanism of whiplash agent on TMJ, which determines a defensive contraction of the posterior muscles of the neck, brings the line of sight upward with a consequent hyperactivity of the muscles supra- and infrahyoid that, in order to restore such a line, brings the mandible in retrusion triggering a possible opposed mechanism starting from the TMJ.

The mandibular malpositioning, therefore, may cause an abnormal position of the skull that will determine a response of the vestibular apparatus, which, through the oculocephalic system, will try to restore the visual axis parallel to the ground with possible asymmetries of the various components of the skeleton.

Any sagittal-type mandibular alteration, as long as symmetric, will be compensated by the postural system in the opposite direction; there is, however, not the possibility of compensation in lateral direction, as whiplash, by its nature, always leads to asymmetric alterations which could lead to cross-like pathologies.

12.6 Diagnosis of Whiplash-Associated TMDs

WA TMD diagnosis presents considerable complexity reasons as follows:

1. The symptoms may be initially overwhelmed by the cervical one.
2. The dysfunction may develop months after the traumatic event.
3. The entity is sometimes very nuanced.
4. It is misunderstood, even by most insiders.
5. The patient may be unable to place a temporal connection with the symptoms. In fact, Salè et al. [7] demonstrated a high frequency of inaccurate recall of TMJ pain and dysfunction 1 year after whiplash trauma implies that clinicians and researchers should interpret with caution the results of previous studies that relied on retrospective data regarding whiplash-induced TMJ pain and dysfunction.
6. Pre-existing dysfunction cannot accurately determine the cause and effect of the trauma.
7. And, most importantly, it is very difficult to have a control group before the event. In reality, the percentage that a patient of a dental practice, followed at a

gnathological level, suffers a whiplash injury and is reviewed by the same doctor is very low.

To determine whether a patient who has been in a collision has a TMD, an appropriate history and examination of the head and neck should be undertaken, supplemented by diagnostic imaging, if necessary (e.g. pantomograph for screening bony abnormalities, cone beam computed tomography scanning for more detailed bony assessment, magnetic resonance imaging for soft tissue abnormalities). The history should include questions related to pain in the TMJ and masticatory muscle areas (and other areas of the head as well as the neck), TMJ sounds (e.g. clicking, crepitus) and catching or locking of the jaws with opening or closing.

Various TMD classification schemes are available to allow specific diagnoses based on the history and examination findings, but it would be desirable that every dentist at least compose a detailed history of any TMD to create a database for monitoring and that examination is performed according to criteria indicated in Helkimo index [14]. Generally speaking, it includes extraoral and intraoral palpation of masticatory muscles, evaluation of TMJ's symmetry; investigation of tenderness/pain, clicking or crepitus of TMJs during movements of the jaw; observation of any deviation of the mandible on opening or closing; and range of mandibular movements. Furthermore, cranial nerve function and the neck should be evaluated, including ranges of motion and sites of tenderness in the cervical musculature, according to the *Manual Medicine* procedure as described into the dedicated chapter.

Finally, on the basis of literature and personal experience, we propose to our patients a simplified questionnaire: Whiplash Impact on TMJ Questionnaire (WITQ) (Table 12.1).

Table 12.1 Whiplash Impact on TMJ Questionnaire (WITQ)

After your accident:	
1. Have you ever had a pain in your jaw?	Yes ( ) No ( )
2. Have you ever had difficulty chewing?	Yes ( ) No ( )
3. Has your sleep always been normal?	Yes ( ) No ( )
4. In the morning, have you ever had difficulty opening your mouth?	Yes ( ) No ( )
5. Have you ever had dizziness or feelings of instability standing?	Yes ( ) No ( )

It was tested on 20 patients already compensated by insurance in order to not be influenced by possible additional complaints. Patients were heterogeneous regarding age, sex, social position and the characteristics of the accident, but all of them had problems related to TMD (joint pain, difficulty chewing, unsatisfactory sleep, any equilibrium disturbances) followed at least 6 months after the collision. Seven patients (4 females and 3 males) answered affirmatively to all questions, four (2 females, 2 males) referred only TMJ pain, seven answered negatively, two patients did not answer. Despite the small sample, this simplified method agrees with the studies in the literature that lead to about 30 %, the percentage of referred TMDs after a MCV with whiplash.

12.7 Therapy

Multidisciplinary dental and medical management is necessary in many patients, and TMDs in these situations should not be interpreted as separate, independent conditions. Dentists should provide appropriate conservative, reversible forms of TMD management as part of a multidisciplinary team approach in order to eliminate or mitigate the pain as much as possible and restore a normal mandibular kinematic.

Apart from the use of pain medication and/or anti-inflammatory, benzodiazepines at low dosage for few days before sleeping is necessary, as this disease is more active especially at the end of the night, disturbing the normal rest.

Generally, we suggest that patients follow a programme of physical therapy, occupational therapy and pain management. At the start of their stay, they have to be examined both by a physician specialized in rehabilitation medicine and a dentist to perform a complete functional examination, both of the stomatognathic system, shoulder girdle and spine. This kind of programme is useful especially to increase maximum active mouth-opening capacity, but some authors [15] showed that therapeutic jaw exercises, in addition to the regular whiplash rehabilitation programme, did not reduce symptoms and signs of WA TMDs.

For this reason we combine physical therapy with low-level laser therapy (LLLT) directed on painful TMJ, main stomatognathic, cervico-dorsal trigger and tender points. This combination, from our experience, yielded the best results especially in cases without dislocation of the disc.

Other valid therapy is intraoral plates that are irreplaceable in cases with dislocation of the disc or joint locks.

The use of such devices must be well calibrated, especially in thickness, because when altering the vertical dimension (dimensional relationship between the dental arches), it is necessary to be sure that the system can tolerate the "new" jaw posture. It is also essential to check the correctness of the device with postural tests and possibly by the mean of stabilometry (see Chapter 17 on "Static posturography and whiplash" by P.L. Ghilardi, A. Casani, B. Fattori, R. Kohen-Raz and Dario C. Alpini).

12.8 Prognosis

Approximately 15–40 % of patients with acute WAD develop chronic symptoms [2]. Chronic WAD represents a physical, medical, economic and psychosocial problem. Severe neck pain, self-reporting of poor general health and stress in WA TMD patients are similar to that of nontrauma TMD patients, although the posttraumatic patients frequently require constant analgesic assumption, suggesting persistence of pain. In contrast, De Boever et al. [16] comparing two groups of TMD patients—one without a history of trauma to the head and neck (302 patients) and the other with a history of trauma that was linked to the onset of symptoms (98 patients)—showed that the trauma group's symptoms were more pronounced initially, but both groups responded equally well to conservative treatment after 1 year. Despite these findings, a minority of individuals develop a chronic condition that may reflect the more complex nature of regional and widespread pain, which may be the result of central hypersensitivity mechanisms or possible mild traumatic brain injury. Romanelli et al. [17] confirmed that post-MVC TMD patients do not respond to management and require more treatment compared to nontrauma cases. Other studies have demonstrated similar findings.

TMDs that develop post-MVC have a less favourable prognosis and affect quality of life. Anyway, most patients who develop TMDs following an MVC often improve with time or with standard therapy: active coping strategies (activity and exercise) is, in our experience, one of the most important aspects for recovery, while pessimism regarding return to usual activities may affect positive outcome.

References

1. Bucholtz MR (2007) TMJ and whiplash. J Am Dent Assoc 138(11):1422
2. Epstein JB, Klasser GD (2011) Whiplash-associated disorders and temporomandibular symptoms following motor-vehicle collisions. Quintessence Int 42(1):e1–e14
3. Grönqvist J, Häggman-Henrikson B, Eriksson PO (2008) Impaired jaw function and eating difficulties in whiplash-associated disorders. Swed Dent J 32(4):171–177
4. Hernández IA, Fyfe KR, Heo G, Major PW (2006) Mandibular kinematics associated with simulated low-velocity rear-end impacts. J Oral Rehabil 33(8):566–575
5. Eriksson PO, Häggman-Henrikson B, Zafar H (2007) Jaw-neck dysfunction in whiplash-associated disorders. Arch Oral Biol 52(4):404–408. Epub 2007 Feb 1
6. Epstein JB, Klasser GD, Kolbinson DA, Mehta SA (2010) Orofacial injuries due to trauma following motor vehicle collisions: part 2. Temporomandibular disorders. J Can Dent Assoc 76:a172
7. Salé H, Hedman L, Isberg A (2010) Accuracy of patients' recall of temporomandibular joint pain and dysfunction after experiencing whiplash trauma: a prospective study. J Am Dent Assoc 141(7):879–886
8. Salé H, Isberg A (2007) Delayed temporomandibular joint pain and dysfunction induced by whiplash trauma: a controlled prospective study. J Am Dent Assoc 138(8):1084–1091
9. Visscher C, Hofman N, Mes C, Lousberg R, Naeije M (2005) Is temporomandibular pain in chronic whiplash-associated disorders part of a more widespread pain syndrome? Clin J Pain 21(4):353–357
10. Kapandji AI (2001) Physiologie articulaire, 5th edn. Maloine, Paris
11. Norton NS (2011) Netter's head and neck anatomy, 2nd edn. Elsevier/Saunders, Philadelphia
12. Manfredini D, Bucci MB, Montagna F, Guarda-Nardini L (2011) Temporomandibular disorders assessment: medicolegal considerations in the evidence-based era. J Oral Rehabil 38(2):101–119
13. Pérez del Palomar A, Doblaré M (2008) Dynamic 3D FE modelling of the human temporomandibular joint during whiplash. Med Eng Phys 30(6):700–709. Epub 2007 Sep 5
14. Helkimo M (1974) Studies on function and dysfunction of the masticatory system. II Index for anamnestic and clinical dysfunction and occlusal state. Swed Dent J 67:101–121
15. Klobas L, Axelsson S, Tegelberg A (2006) Effect of therapeutic jaw exercise on temporomandibular disorders in individuals with chronic whiplash-associated disorders. Acta Odontol Scand 64(6):341–347
16. De Boever JA, Keersmaekers K (1996) Trauma in patients with temporomandibular disorders: frequency and treatment outcome. J Oral Rehabil 23(2):91–96
17. Romanelli GG, Mock D, Tenenbaum HC (1992) Characteristics and response to treatment of posttraumatic temporomandibular disorder: a retrospective study. Clin J Pain 8(1):6–17

13 Whiplash and Sport

M. Albano, D.C. Alpini, and G.V. Carbone

13.1 Introduction

Although sports-related injuries to the head and neck are much less common than injuries to the extremities, an estimated 70 % of mortality and 20 % of permanent disability result from injuries to the head and neck [1].

Whiplash is a term that refers to neck injuries that are incurred after the neck is forcibly bent forward, backward or both. Whiplash is a common injury associated with contact sports such as football, rugby and hockey. Symptoms of whiplash include neck pain and stiffness, pain in the back, arms and shoulders, dizziness, problems with concentration, blurred vision, ringing in the ears and irritability and patient needs an accurate diagnosis and appropriate treatment.

Head and neck injuries often occur simultaneously, and whiplash is often associated to concussion. Concussion is defined as a traumatically induced transient disturbance of brain function and involves a complex pathophysiological process. Concussion is a subset of mild traumatic brain injury (MTBI) which is generally self-limited and at the less-severe end of the brain injury spectrum [2]. Head and neck common injuries are frequent in American football, hockey and rugby that have the highest incidence of concussion, while soccer has the lowest. Male boxers and female taekwondo participants have the highest frequency of concussion

M. Albano (✉)
Sport Physiatrist "Galileo 18" Physiotherapy Centre, Juventus Football Club Medical Team, C.so Galileo Ferarris 18, Turin, Italy
e-mail: michele.albano4@virgilio.it

D.C. Alpini
ENT-Otoneurology Service, IRCCS "Don Carlo Gnocchi" Foundation, Milan, Italy
e-mail: dario.alpini@fastwebnet.it

G.V. Carbone
"Istituto Clinico Città Studi" City Hospital, Milano Hockey Medical Team, via Jommelli 17, Milan, Italy

D.C. Alpini et al. (eds.), *Whiplash Injuries*,
DOI 10.1007/978-88-470-5486-8_13, © Springer-Verlag Italia 2014

at the recreational level [3], and evidence indicates that female athletes may be at greater risk for concussion than their male counterparts. There also is some evidence that gender differences exist in outcomes of traumatic brain injury and concussions [4, 5].

Pure neck injuries in sports are less common, typically debilitating, and quite predictable in retrospect by mechanism of injury as to one of four natures – sprains/strains, fractures, brachial plexus pinches/stretches and spinal cord injury. Of these, the spinal cord injury, whether a concussion or contusion or physical disruption, is obviously the most severe (so-called Quebec Task Force WAD grade IV) and also, ironically, the best tracked because of its definition and notoriety when it is experienced [6–8].

The medical problem of neck injuries in sport is two-folded: diagnosis and treatment of acute lesion and adequate programming of athlete returning to sport practice. While most people can return to everyday activities a few days after sustaining a whiplash injury, athletes, in fact, need to achieve a full recovery before getting back on the field. Even if they feel ready, it's important to be completely free of whiplash symptoms and have medical clearance before returning to sports.

13.2 Neck Injuries in Sport Practice

Neck injury usually is secondary to high-velocity collisions between players, causing acceleration or deceleration of the head on the neck. Acceleration usually causes a whiplash type of extension force on the neck, while deceleration usually results in flexion forces. Serious injuries with neurological sequelae remain infrequent and most of these injuries are self-limited.

Regarding sport epidemiology, Tsoumpos et al. [9] recorded over 150 injuries between the years of 2008 and 2011, especially in contact sports, including indoor soccer, basketball, and wrestling but also in several noncontact sports, such as diving.

Whiplash spine injuries are estimated to occur in high percentage of indoor soccer players, and most commonly on defensive players.

According to the authors, there is no practical difference with healthy control group normalised with regard to sex, age, socioeconomic status and marital status after 6 months from initial trauma. They concluded that even if there is a significant risk of whiplash-type injuries in sports, serious injuries with neurological sequelae and chronic whiplash-associated disorders (QTF WAD grades III and IV) remain very infrequent.

Anyway, cervical spine injuries remain a serious concern in some games like American football, in which they have been estimated to occur in 10–15 % [10] of football players, most commonly in linemen, defensive ends and linebackers.

Also in ice hockey players, cervical injuries are frequently observed even if the overwhelming majority of such injuries are self-limited, and full recovery can be expected. However, the presenting symptoms of serious cervical spine injuries may closely resemble those of minor injuries. The orthopaedic surgeon frequently must make a judgment, on the field or later in the office, about the advisability of returning the athlete to the game. These decisions can have an enormous impact on the player, his team and his family. Most severe cervical spine injuries share the common mechanism of application of an axial load to the straightened spine. Advances in specific sport techniques, rules of the game and medical care of the athlete have been made throughout the past few decades to minimise the risk of cervical injury and improve the management of injuries that do occur.

Injuries have a wide spectrum of severity. The relatively common 'stinge' is a neuropraxia of a cervical nerve root(s) or brachial plexus and represents a reversible peripheral nerve injury. Less common and more serious an injury, cervical cord neuropraxia is the clinical manifestation of neuropraxia of the cervical spinal cord due to hyperextension, hyperflexion or axial loading.

Recent data [11] on American football suggest that approximately 0.2 per 100,000 participants at the high school level and 2 per 100,000 participants at the collegiate level are diagnosed with cervical cord neuropraxia. Characterised by temporary pain, paraesthesias and/or motor weakness in more than one extremity, there is a rapid and complete resolution of symptoms and a normal physical examination within 10 min to 48 h after the initial injury.

Stenosis of the spinal canal, whether congenital or acquired, is thought to predispose the athlete to cervical cord neuropraxia. Although quite rare, catastrophic neurological injury is a devastating entity referring to permanent neurological injury or death. The mechanism is most often a forced hyperflexion injury, as occurs when 'spear tackling'.

The mean incidence of catastrophic neurological injury over the past 30 years has been approximately 0.5 per 100,000 participants at high school level and 1.5 per 100,000 at the collegiate level. This incidence has decreased significantly when compared with the incidence in the early 1970s. This decrease in the incidence of catastrophic injury is felt to be the result of changes in the rules in the mid-1970s that prohibited the use of the head as the initial contact point when blocking and tackling [12].

In professional rugby union players, incidence, severity, nature, and causes of cervical, thoracic, and lumbar spine injuries sustained during competition and training have been studied by Fuller et al. [13]. They identified as risk factors player age, body mass, stature, playing position, use of headgear and activity and period of season. In their study the incidences of spinal injuries were 11 per 1,000 player match-hours and 0.37 per 1,000 player training hours. No player sustained a catastrophic spinal injury, but three players sustained career-ending injuries. Overall, players were more likely to sustain a cervical injury during matches and a lumbar injury during training. Forwards were significantly more likely to sustain a spinal injury than backs during both matches and training. During matches, injuries to the cervical and lumbar spine were more severe (calculated as days necessary to sport practice recovery) than injuries to the thoracic spine; during training, injuries to the lumbar spine were more severe than cerebral injuries.

Similar differences regarding injuries occurred during matches with respect to training have been observed also in professional soccer players. Nilson et al. [14], in a recent investigation, recorded a total of 136 head and neck injuries, that is to say 2.2 % of all injuries. The head and neck injury rate was 0.17 (0.06 concussions) per 1,000 h. There was a 20-fold higher rate of head and neck injury during match play compared with training and a 78-fold higher rate of concussions. Mean layoff for concussion was 10.5 days, but 27 % of the concussed players returned to play within 5 days. Defender was the playing position most at risk. Authors highlight that more than one-quarter of the concussed players returned to play before what is recommended in the consensus statements by the major sports governing bodies.

Kochar et al. investigated the risk of cervical injuries in mixed martial arts [15]. The kinematics of the athletic acts of these sports, from the point of impact, bears a considerable resemblance to the kinematics of a rear-end motor vehicle collision. With respect to car collisions, it has been shown that the biomechanics, kinetics and kinematics all contribute towards the outcome. It can be seen that the impact with the opponent on the ground can be directly correlated with the moment of impact in a rear-end collision. If one compares the force imparted on the driver from the seat with the reaction force of the ground on the opponent, one can see that they act at similar sites and in similar directions. There is also similar posterior translation of the head after impact in some martial arts manoeuvres (such as goshi and souplesse) and the car impact models. The action of the force causing pathological neck motion is of similar magnitude in the two scenarios (car and martial arts), and the gross pattern of motion seems to be comparable, including the mechanical obstruction from hyperextension of the cervical region by the floor and the car seat headrest, respectively.

13.3 The Role of Sideline Physician in the Management of Head and Neck Injuries

Head and cervical spine sports-related injuries are intimately associated. The on-field evaluation and management of the athlete with these injuries is of paramount importance to stabilise the athlete and prevent further injury.

The incidence of catastrophic cervical spine injury in sports is low compared with other sport injuries. However, cervical spine injuries necessitate delicate and precise management, often involving the combined efforts of a variety of health care providers. The outcome of a catastrophic cervical spine injury depends on the efficiency of this management process and timeliness of transfer to a controlled environment for diagnosis and treatment.

One of the most challenging roles of the team physician involves the intervention and decision-making processes regarding cervical spine injuries in contact sports. The team physician must be well versed in the prevention, evaluation, stabilisation and treatment of spine injuries. A high index of suspicion and an understanding of cervical alignment and architecture, as well as comprehension of the mechanics exerted during a sporting event, are imperative to diagnosing cervical injuries.

Sideline physicians must be attentive and prepared with an organised approach to detect and manage these injuries [16]. Evaluation of patients with suspected cervical spine injury includes a complete neurological examination while on the field or the sidelines. Immobilisation on a hard board may also be necessary. The decision to obtain radiographs can be made on the basis of the history and physical examination.

The goal in assessing neck injuries is to detect spinal cord injury and the potential for such injury resulting from instability of the cervical spine.

Cervical spine instability and the accompanying potential for neurological loss may be commonly underdiagnosed. The evaluation of neck injuries requires a regimented examination and a defined management protocol. A stepwise evaluation (Table 13.1), including a Spurling test that is to say a foraminal compression test, has to be used to evaluate cervical nerve root injury. In Spurling test, the examiner actively compresses the right and left foramina. Cervical radiculopathy is indicated if this position elicits radicular symptoms in the upper limb. Each step [17] in this examination presents a progressively greater risk to the spinal cord; therefore, if any part of the examination is abnormal, instability is presumed and testing is stopped. Furthermore, if an abnormality is found at any point of the examination, the neck should be immobilised and the patient prepared for transport to an emergency department. Any focal neurological symptom suggests a potential central nervous system injury. In particular, bilateral symptoms must be considered carefully [18].

Table 13.1 Combined Evaluation of Head and Neck Injuries (Whiteside [17])

1. Note the exact time of injury. Management decisions are based on duration of symptoms
2. Assess loss of consciousness. Management of unresponsive athletes should follow the ABCs of trauma care (i.e. check airway, breathing, and circulation)
3. Assess peripheral strength and sensation without moving the athlete's head or neck
4. Palpate the neck for asymmetric spasm or tenderness at the spine
5. Assess isometric neck strength without moving the athlete's head or neck
6. Assess active range of motion at the neck
7. Perform axial compression and Spurling test. If negative, athlete may be moved
8. Assess recent memory and postural instability
9. Inquire about symptoms such as headache, nausea, dizziness or blurred vision

This neck evaluation guideline cannot be used with unconscious athletes, and the detection of an unstable fracture is impossible. Instead, instability must be assumed, and care must be taken to avoid manipulation of the neck. In the absence of immediate danger, an unconscious injured athlete should remain at the site of the injury until the spine is fully immobilised. Three or four trained persons are required to safely 'log roll' the athlete into a supine position on a backboard. This procedure may require leaving the patient at the site until emergency medical personnel arrive. The physician should remind others involved in assisting the player that preventing further injury is the priority; the athlete should not be rushed from the field for the sake of continuing play [19].

Sideline physicians must protect the spinal cord from injury whenever instability is a consideration. A cervical collar alone never should be considered adequate protection for the spinal cord. Instead, full immobilisation on a backboard is required to stabilise the neck. When immobilising the neck, physicians should avoid movement and maintain proper alignment of the cervical vertebrae. This usually can be done with the helmet and other protective gear (e.g. shoulder pads) in place, and such equipment should not be removed. Studies using American football equipment on cadavers showed that removing the helmet and shoulder pads results in excessive movement of the cervical spine.

Symptoms of concussion are neurological in nature, occur immediately after a trauma and are transient. Concussion is common in sports; by conservative estimates, there are more than 300,000 sports-related concussions in the United States each year [20]. However, studies of relatively mild brain injuries, such as those typically sustained in sports, are limited.

Graded symptom checklists provide an objective tool for assessing a variety of symptoms related to concussions, while also tracking the severity of those symptoms over serial evaluations. Standardised assessment tools provide a helpful structure for the evaluation of concussion:

1. Assessment for loss of consciousness (LoC)
2. Inquiring about symptoms commonly associated with concussion
3. Evaluating recently acquired memory
4. Evaluating postural stability

Any athlete suspected of having a concussion should be stopped from playing and assessed by a licenced healthcare provider trained in the evaluation and management of concussions. Team physicians should restrict from play any athlete with persistent symptoms of concussion because these symptoms place them at risk of reinjury if they return prematurely. Recognition and initial assessment of a concussion should be guided by a symptoms checklist, cognitive evaluation (including orientation, past and immediate memory, new learning and concentration), balance tests and further neurological physical examination.

Concussion is defined by transient symptoms, and until those symptoms resolve, other diagnoses must be considered. Athletes with memory loss, imbalance or symptoms reported 15 min after the injury should be restricted from play for the rest of the day. Athletes with neurological symptoms persisting longer than 30 min, particularly those with prolonged LoC or any focal neurological sign, should be monitored closely and may require transport to an emergency department. Finally, athletes with seizures, persistent vomiting or suspected skull fracture should be urgently evaluated in an emergency department.

Balance disturbance is a specific indicator of a concussion, but not very sensitive. Balance testing on the sideline may be substantially different than baseline tests because of differences in shoe/cleat-type or surface, use of ankle tape or braces or the presence of other lower extremity injury.

Imaging is reserved for athletes where intracerebral bleeding is suspected. Athletes suspected or diagnosed with a concussion should be monitored for deteriorating physical or mental status with neuropsychological (NP) tests, as an objective measure of brain-behaviour relationships, more sensitive for subtle cognitive impairment than clinical exam. Anyway, it is unknown if use of NP testing in the management of sports concussion helps prevent recurrent concussion, catastrophic injury or long-term complications [2].

13.4 Recovering from Head and Neck Trauma

Treatment depends on the severity of diagnosed injury and can range from an individualised cervical spine rehabilitation programme for a 'stinger' (QTF WAD I grade) to cervical spine decompression and fusion for more serious bony or ligamentous injury (QTF WAD IV grade). Still under constant debate is the decision to return to play for the athlete.

After resting for a day or two, patients recovering from mild to moderate whiplash should resume normal physical activity so that they can work their muscles and maintain flexibility in their soft tissue. Patients suffering from more severe whiplash may require a longer period of rest and should resume activity based on the advice of a doctor. If whiplash patients remain inactive for too long, pain will actually become more severe and difficult to treat. This does not mean that whiplash sufferers should immediately return to contact sports. While a return to daily activity is recommended, anyone recovering from whiplash should avoid heavy lifting, severe neck strain, intensive stretching and risky behaviour including contact sports until they have fully recovered.

A history of concussion is associated with a higher risk of sustaining another concussion. A greater number, severity and duration of symptoms after a concussion are predictors of a prolonged recovery. In sports with similar playing rules, the reported incidence of concussion is higher in female athletes than in male athletes. Certain sports, positions and individual playing styles have a greater risk of concussion. Youth athletes may have a more prolonged recovery and are more susceptible to a concussion accompanied by a catastrophic injury. Preinjury mood disorders, learning disorders, attention deficit disorders (ADD/ADHD) and migraine headaches complicate the diagnosis and management of a concussion.

13.5 Criteria for Returning to Practice (RTP)

Serious injuries with neurological sequelae remain infrequent, and most of cervical injuries are self-limited. Injuries occur in all levels of play from the high school to the professional level. The decision of return to play following cervical spine injuries can be one of the most challenging with a wide variation in opinion as far as management.

In general, the literature [21–24] shows agreement for the basic necessities for return to collision sports to include normal strength, painless range of motion, a stable vertebral column and adequate space for the neurological elements. In addition, return to play in an unsafe environment is contraindicated.

Playing with defective equipment or with improper technique has been associated with catastrophic injuries and should be avoided. This particularly includes spear tackling, diving in unknown or shallow water, diving while intoxicated, checking from behind in hockey or using a trampoline without spotting equipment.

However, there is a lack of consensus on returning to play with the following: stenosis, spear tackler's spine, loss of normal lordosis or range of motion, surgically corrected instability, ligamentous instability, transient quadriparesis, healed disc herniation and congenital fusion.

Since contact sports can exacerbate a whiplash injury, patients should not return to sports like football, wrestling or hockey until given a clean bill of health by their doctors. Some doctors may recommend a return to practice or noncontact drills while recovery is still in progress, but a full-contact game is not advisable until pain and tenderness in the neck area has subsided completely.

Figure 13.1 is referred to two hockey players. They are homozygote twins, playing with the same role in the same hockey team. Head-to-neck stability has been calculated as mean head and trunk velocities while standing with eyes open or closed on firm or foam surface. Mean head and trunk velocities have been calculated by means of two accelerometers (Delos device, Turin, Italy) posed on the head and the sternum (for details, see chapter 19 and reference [25]). Both athletes were studied 12 h after the match. Player 2 reported a whiplash trauma during a strong contact. Posturography clearly shows how the head is unstable with respect to the trunk even simply standing.

Patients should experience a full range of motion in their necks, shoulders and arms, maintain proper pre-injury posture and pass a neurological assessment before engaging in any contact sport. If a player returns to sport prematurely, the risk of further injury to the neck is increased significantly. If the athlete experiences any long-term effects of whiplash, such as headache, chronic pain or problems with range of motion, he/she has to cease his/her participation in contact sports and consult a doctor as soon as possible.

The non-elite athlete may not have the same resources available as the elite athlete (such as the presence of trained medical staff during practise and competition, a concussion programme as part of sideline preparedness, the benefit of neuropsychological or postural testing, as well as consultants with expertise in concussion readily available) and as a result will generally be managed more conservatively.

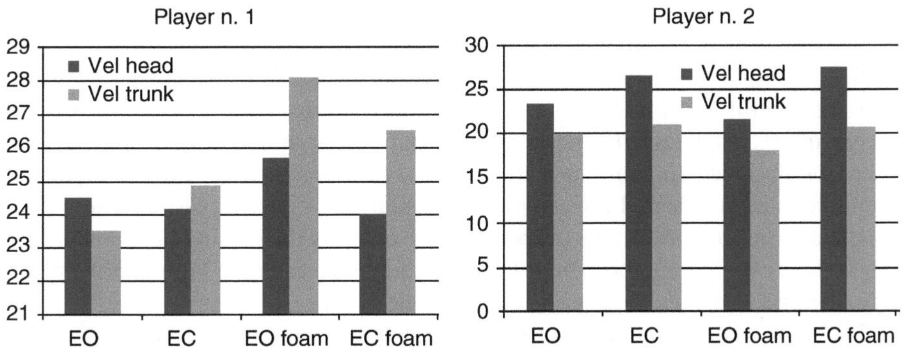

Fig. 13.1 Posturographic recording of head-to-trunk stability in stance after a hockey match. Mean head and trunk velocities have been calculated by means of two accelerometers (Delos device, Turin, Italy) posed on the head and the sternum. Players were required standing with eyes open or closed on firm or foam surfaces. Even both players show head velocity higher than trunk velocity when standing on firm surface with eyes open, only player 2 shows clear head instability in all four tests. Players are homozygote twins, playing with the same role in the same hockey team. Both athletes were studied 12 h after the match. Player 2 reported a whiplash trauma during a strong contact. Posturography clearly shows how the head is unstable with respect to the trunk even simply standing

Younger athletes often have a greater incidence of concussion with longer recovery time frames; however, they are often managed with less expertise and with limited resources.

Child athletes take longer to recover from concussions than adults. Concussion symptoms may resolve before cognitive function has completely recovered. Concussion assessment and management in children can be confounded by their growth and development, as well as the lack of trained medical personnel involved with youth sports. There are no child-specific assessment tools for concussion. RTP decisions in children should be made cautiously and should be individualised. No concussed child athlete should be allowed to RTP the same day. Physical and cognitive rest is very important to allow for the resolution of concussion symptoms. Child athletes should remain symptom free for several days before starting a medically supervised stepwise exertion protocol. Further research is needed to elucidate the effects of concussion in children and to determine the most appropriate RTP guidelines. Child-specific concussion assessment tools need to be developed to improve concussion assessment and management in children.

13.6 Preventing Future Injury

Primary prevention of some injuries may be possible with modification and enforcement of the rules and fair play. Helmets, both hard [25] (football, lacrosse and hockey) and soft (soccer, rugby), are best suited to prevent impact injuries (fracture, bleeding, laceration, etc.) but have not been shown to reduce the incidence and severity of concussions [26]. There is no current evidence that mouth guards can reduce the severity of or prevent concussions.

Secondary prevention may be possible by appropriate RTP management. Players must be careful when returning to contact sports so that they don't suffer from a repeat injury. Athletes who have experienced whiplash should perform specific exercises designed to strengthen their necks. A stronger neck with an expanded circumference of at least 1 cm can protect them from future whiplash injuries. They should also ensure to warm up properly before entering the playing field or working out at the gym. Playing football or hockey requires investing in high-quality, properly fitted neck and shoulder pads to protect the neck.

Ice hockey and American football are violent collision sport, and neck injuries are an unavoidable part of the game. What can be improved are the preventative measures, the treatment techniques and some standardisation of risk factors in playing after a neck injury. Prevention starts with decreasing the use of the head as an offensive weapon in American football and with proper shoulder pads in both sports.

Treatment begins with proper on-field evaluation and transportation techniques and is completed by good consultation services. Proper evaluation of risk demands requires open discussions with the patient of all factors involved. Clear advice has to be given to players and to the team through their medical staff [27].

References

1. Patterson D (1987) Legal aspects of athletic injuries to the head and cervical spine. Clin Sports Med 6:197–210
2. Harmon KG, Drezner JA, Gammons M, Guskiewicz KM, Halstead M, Herring SA, Kutcher JS, Pana A, Putukian M, Roberts WO (2013) American Medical Society for Sports Medicine position statement: concussion in sport. Br J Sports Med 47(1):15–26
3. Koh JO, Cassidy JD, Watkinson EJ (2003) Incidence of concussion in contact sports: a systematic review of the evidence. Brain Inj 17(10):901–917
4. Dick RW (2009) Is there a gender difference in concussion incidence and outcomes? Br J Sports Med 43(Suppl 1):i46–i50
5. Alla S, Sullivan SJ, McCrory P, Hale L (2011) Spreading the word on sports concussion: citation analysis of summary and agreement, position and consensus statements on sports concussion. Br J Sports Med 45(2):132–135
6. Clarke KS (1998) Epidemiology of athletic neck injury. Clin Sports Med 17(1):83–97
7. Cooper MT, McGee KM, Anderson DG (2003) Epidemiology of athletic head and neck injuries. Clin Sports Med 22(3):427–443
8. Maroon JC, Bailes JE (1996) Athletes with cervical spine injury. Spine 21:2294–2299
9. Tsoumpos P, Kafchitsas K, Wilke HJ, Evaνgelou K, Kallivokas A, Habermann B, Tsepis E, Bilis E, Matzaroglou C (2013) Whiplash injuries in sports activities. Clinical outcome and biomechanics. Br J Sports Med 47:e3
10. Thomas BE, McCullen GM, Yuan HA (1999) Cervical spine injuries in football players. J Am Acad Orthop Surg 7(5):338–347
11. Rihn JA, Anderson DT, Lamb K, Deluca PF, Bata A, Marchetto PA, Neves N, Vaccaro AR (2009) Cervical spine injuries in American football. Sports Med 39(9):697–708
12. Watkins RG (1986) Neck injuries in football players. Clin Sports Med 5(2):215–246

13. Fuller CW, Brooks JH, Kemp SP (2007) Spinal injuries in professional rugby union: a prospective cohort study. Clin J Sport Med 17(1):10–16
14. Nilsson M, Hägglund M, Ekstrand J, Waldén M (2013) Head and neck injuries in professional soccer. Clin J Sport Med 23(4):255–260. [Epub ahead of print]
15. Kochhar T, Back DL, Mann B, Skinner J (2005) Risk of cervical injuries in mixed martial arts. Br J Sports Med 39:444–447
16. Warren WL Jr, Bailes JE (1998) On the field evaluation of athletic neck injury. Clin Sports Med 17(1):99–110
17. Whiteside JW (2006) Management of head and neck injuries by the sideline physician. Am Fam Phys 74(8):1357–1362. www.aafp.org/afp
18. Swartz EE, Decoster LC, Norkus SA, Boden BP, Waninger KN, Courson RW, Horodyski M, Rehberg RS, National Athletic Trainers' Association (2009) Summary of the National Athletic Trainers' Association position statement on the acute management of the cervical spine-injured athlete. Phys Sportsmed 37(4):20–30
19. Ghiselli G, Schaadt G, McAllister DR (2003) On-the-field evaluation of an athlete with a head or neck injury. Clin Sports Med 22(3):445–465
20. Grindel SH, Lovell MR, Collins MW (2001) The assessment of sport-related concussion: the evidence behind neuropsychological testing and management. Clin J Sport Med 11:134–143
21. Morganti C (2003) Recommendations for return to sports following cervical spine injuries. Sports Med 33(8):563–573
22. Ellis JL, Gottlieb JE (2007) Return-to-play decisions after cervical spine injuries. Curr Sports Med Rep 6(1):56–61
23. Putukian M, Aubry M, McCrory P (2009) Return to play after sports concussion in elite and non-elite athletes? Br J Sports Med 43(Suppl 1):i28–i31. doi:10.1136/bjsm.2009.058230
24. Purcell L (2009) What are the most appropriate return-to-play guidelines for concussed child athletes? Br J Sports Med 43(Suppl 1):i51–i55. doi:10.1136/bjsm.2009.058214
25. Alpini D, Hahn A, Riva D (2008) Static and dynamic postural control adaptations induced by playing ice hockey. Sport Sci Health 2:85–92
26. Watkins RG (1986) Neck injuries in football players. Clin Sports Med 5(2):215–246
27. Bell K (2007) On-field issues of the C-spine-injured helmeted athlete. Curr Sports Med Rep 6(1):32–35

Whiplash Associated Somatic Tinnitus (WAST) 14

D.C. Alpini, A. Cesarani, and A. Hahn

14.1 Introduction

Approximately 10 % of patients who have suffered whiplash injury will develop otological symptoms such as tinnitus, deafness and vertigo [1]. Some of these are purely subjective symptoms. Tinnitus is a common and disturbing symptom; it is the perception of ringing, buzzing, hissing, or other noises in the ears or head in the absence of external sources for these sounds. These perceptions can be transient, intermittent, occasional, or constant. "Chronic" tinnitus is present all or most of the time during a person's waking hours.

Tinnitus is therefore also considered an auditory phantom percept similar to central neuropathic pain. Its pathophysiology remains unclear, but it is supposed to result from hyperactivity and neuroplastic pathological reorganization of cortical–subcortical auditory and nonauditory networks [2].

Chronic disabling tinnitus is due to emotional–affective involvement induced by a pathological shift of patient attention to his/her tinnitus. Coping with tinnitus thus requires a modification of the patient approach to one's self-perception through the modification of lifestyle, stressor removing and diverting pathological attention. The aim of the tinnitus cure, generally speaking, is to reach a golden point in which the patient is able to hear tinnitus but tinnitus is not disabling for the patient.

D.C. Alpini
ENT-Otoneurology Service, IRCCS "Don Carlo Gnocchi" Foundation, Milan, Italy
e-mail: dalpini@dongnocchi.it

A. Cesarani
Department of Clinical Sciences and Community Health,
University of Milan, Milan, Italy

Audiology Unit, IRCCS "Ca' Granda" Ospedale Maggiore Policlinico, Milan, Italy
e-mail: antonio.cesarani@unimi.it

A. Hahn (✉)
3ENT Clinic, 3rd Medical Faculty, Charles University Prague, Prague, Czech Republic
e-mail: hahn@fnkv.cz

D.C. Alpini et al. (eds.), *Whiplash Injuries*,
DOI 10.1007/978-88-470-5486-8_14, © Springer-Verlag Italia 2014

Whiplash associated tinnitus could be due to an auditory damage, as a consequence of inner ear damage with hearing loss due to labyrinth concussion or vertebral artery spasm. In these cases tinnitus has to be mainly treated into the context of inner ear damage treatment.

In some cases, tinnitus, even without any significant hearing loss, could be related to whiplash injuries of the temporomandibular joint (TMJ) and upper cervical spine through the interaction between the somatosensory and auditory systems. In these patients, neck and/or facial movements, movements of the upper extremities, tactile stimulation, changes in gaze, jaw opening or teeth clenching may induce or modulate tinnitus: the so-called somatic tinnitus.

Somatic tinnitus is a subgroup of tinnitus suffers. It was described by Pulec et al. in 1978 [3] as “cervical tinnitus”, considered as a consequence of degenerative changes in the cervical spine that could be, at least temporarily, reduced by injection of local anaesthetic into tender areas of the neck. This clinical entity was forgotten until Dehmel et al. [4] introduced the somatic tinnitus syndrome (STS) in which tinnitus is associated to a somatic disorder involving the head and neck. They presented the anatomical basis for the auditory–somatosensory interactions and showed how auditory neurons respond to somatosensory stimulation.

Particularly, whiplash associated muscle–skeletal disorders could become a chronic stress source that pathologically integrates with previous or whiplash-induced auditory disturbances, causing/increasing tinnitus. More specifically, somatic tinnitus suffers frequently present modulation of their spontaneous tinnitus through appropriate stimulation of trigger points in the cervical and shoulder muscles. Somatic tinnitus occurs when the patient feels the effect of head and neck muscle contractions, changing the intensity or quality of tinnitus, for instance, during clenching the teeth or head rotation. In these cases, tinnitus is modulated by stimulation of the somatosensory system as a result of muscle contractions. This is not surprising because the auditory system is part of the most complex sensory–motor system involved in the head position regulation, necessary to provide gravitation reference, prerequisite for a correct orientation of the human subject in the environment. The brainstem and cerebellum are the main sites of integration of multi-sensorial information from the inner ear, retina and proprioceptors regarding head position, body position, gravity, visual landmarks and movement of the jaw, the tongue and the pharynx.

Somatic tinnitus, generally, is a well-treatable condition by means of manipulations, physiotherapy and physical exercises, or at least, the removal of somatic component of patient’s tinnitus significantly decreases tinnitus annoyance and improves quality of life.

14.2 Diagnosis of Whiplash Associated Somatic Tinnitus (WAST)

The convergence between auditory and somatosensory inputs was shown by Levine et al. [5]: forceful manipulations or contractions of the muscles of the jaw, head or neck elicited the perception in 58 % of the subjects. Several studies have demonstrated the interactions between the somatosensory and auditory systems at the dorsal cochlear nucleus (DCN) [6], inferior colliculus and parietal association areas. In particular, auditory and somatosensory [7, 8] (proprioceptive and tactile) pathways converge into specialized multisensory brain areas, particularly the right inferior frontal gyrus and both right and left insulae, that work as multisensory operators for the processing of stimulus identity. In animals, it was shown that hyperactivity in the DCN, which is a second-order auditory structure [9], correlates with noise-induced tinnitus [10]. The DCN receives auditory input from the VIIIth nerve and somatosensory input, directly from the ipsilateral dorsal column and spinal trigeminal nuclei or indirectly via the dorsal raphe and locus coeruleus.

Diagnosis must combine investigation of auditory condition and somatic cervicocephalic condition. Diagnosis is threefold:

1. Identification of eventual auditory damage and main tinnitus characteristics.
2. Forceful manoeuvres of the neck and the mouth (so-called somatic tests) to identify somatic component of tinnitus: the more prevalent the somatic component, the higher the possibilities to cure tinnitus.
3. Identification of emotional and cognitive aspects of tinnitus-induced disturbances.

14.2.1 Identification of Eventual Auditory Damage and Main Tinnitus Characteristics

Pure tone audiometry and tympanometry are the basic steps to identify hearing loss. In this case it will be necessary to proceed as indicated in the specific chapter dedicated to inner ear WAD. The loudness of tinnitus can be estimated by asking the individual to adjust an external sound so as to match the loudness of the tinnitus. One method is for the listener to first select a sound that is similar to their tinnitus. For example, if the tinnitus is tonal, the listener might adjust the frequency of a pure tone until it matches the pitch of their tinnitus. Then, the external tone is adjusted in level so as to match the loudness of the tinnitus. For the scope of WAST assessment, Feldman test [11] and loudness discomfort level test [7] are enough to investigate auditory/somatic interaction under a therapeutic point of view.

14.2.2 Forceful Manoeuvres of the Neck and the Mouth (So-Called Somatic Tests) to Identify Somatic Component of Tinnitus: The More Prevalent the Somatic Component, the Higher the Possibilities to Cure Tinnitus

Levine et al. [5] proposed to identify somatic components of tinnitus through a series of forceful manoeuvres or pressures on some parts of the head or the neck, during which patients has to note modification of tinnitus loudness or pitch (Table 14.1)

Table 14.1 Somatic Testing According to Levine et al. [5]

All manoeuvres use maximal force applied by the examiner	
(a)	Jaw contractions
	Clench teeth together
	Open mouth with and without restorative pressure
	Protrude jaw with and without restorative pressure
	Slide jaw to the left and the right with and without restorative pressure
	Retrude jaw
(b)	Head and neck contractions
	With the head in the neutral position, contractions were made to resist pressure applied by the examiner to the:
	Forehead
	Occiput
	Vertex
	Left and right temple
	With the head turned to the left, before, and to the right, after, resist the torsional force on the ipsilateral zygoma
	With the head turned to the right and tilted to the left, before, and vice versa, after, resist force applied to the opposite temple (to test the sternocleidomastoid)
(c)	Pressure on muscle insertions
	Right and left mastoid attachment of the sternocleidomastoid
	Right and left suboccipital attachment of the splenius capitis
	Posterior pinna pressure
	Right and left pinna attachment of the posterior auricular
	Furthermore, examination protocol includes:
(d)	Estimation of neck range of movement in the three directions, in degrees
(e)	Palpation of the right and left trapezius, temporalis, masseter, medial pterygoid. For each muscle bulk tender and tension are subjectively quantified ranging from 0 to 5
	We have simplified the examination protocol as follows:
	1. Jendrassik manoeuvre
	2. Clench the teeth together – forced opening of the mouth – and protrude the jaw with and without restorative pressure
	3. With the head in the neutral position, contractions to resist pressure applied by the examiner to the forehead and occiput

On the basis of the results of these main manoeuvres, an accurate [12] evaluation/palpation of the TMJ and stomatognathic muscles and/or cervical and dorsal spine according the examination criteria of Manual Medicine as described elsewhere in the book (see Chap. 17 "Static Posturography and Whiplash" by P.L. Ghilardi, A. Casani, B. Fattori, R. Kohen-Raz, and Dario C. Alpini) is therefore performed. Generally speaking, Manual Medicine examination is mainly aimed to identify trigger and tender points of the facial and cervico-dorsal muscles. Trigger points are described as hyperirritable spots in the skeletal muscle that are associated with palpable nodules in taut bands of muscle fibres. Trigger points are small contraction knots and a common cause of pain. Compression of a trigger point may elicit local tenderness, referred pain or local twitch response. It is common to induce transient tinnitus when stimulating trigger points in the trapezius muscle. A tender point hurts to the touch and causes some degree of pain in that area, while a trigger point may not necessarily be painful to the touch but causes a degree of pain (or tinnitus in this specific field of investigation) to be felt in another area. Furthermore, Manual Medicine looks for the so-called painful minor intervertebral dysfunctions (PMID), in these cases, paying particular attention to the cervical and dorsal spine [13].

Particular attention is also paid to temporomandibular disorders (TMDs) very often underdiagnosed in whiplash patients (see dedicated chapter). TMDs are a group of related disorders of the masticatory system (the masticatory musculature and the temporomandibular joint). The most frequent symptom is pain, usually localized in the muscles of mastication, the preauricular region and the temporomandibular joint (TMJ). Patients often complain of jaw ache, earache, headache and facial pain. In addition to pain, patients with these disorders frequently have limited or asymmetric jaw movement and joint sounds that are described as clicking or crepitus.

The Jendrassik manoeuvre is useful to identify a specific activation of tinnitus, while Manual Medicine examination procedure provides the basis of the manipulative treatment. When TMDs are prevalent, manipulative and physical treatments have to be combined with adequate stomatognathic therapy.

14.2.3 Identification of Emotional and Cognitive Aspects of Tinnitus-Induced Disturbances

The Tinnitus Reaction Questionnaire (TRQ) [14] is useful to identify the tinnitus stress-induced phase of a specific patient. TRQ is a self-reported scale designed to assess perceived distress associated with tinnitus. It is composed of 26 items describing some of the potential effects of tinnitus on lifestyle, general well-being and emotional state. Respondents are asked to rate the extent to which each of the potential effects has applied to them over the last week on a 5-point scale (0, not at all; 4, almost all the time). Respondents are also asked to indicate how frequently tinnitus induces some reactions such as depression, anger and confusion (from not at all to always). The total score ranges from 0 to 104. A lower score represents slight reaction to tinnitus, while higher scores indicate deeply negative reaction.

To determine individual tinnitus-specific reaction besides TRQ, the Tinnitus Cognitive Questionnaire (TCQ) [15] was adopted. TCQ investigates patient approach to tinnitus with 13 negative (1–13) and 13 positive (14–26) thinking items, rated on a 0–4-point scale. For each item, respondents are asked to "indicate how often they have been aware of thinking a particular thought on occasions when they have noticed the tinnitus". The negative items are scored from 0 to 4, whereas the positive items are scored from 4 to 0. The total score is the sum of the scores of each item and ranges from 0 to 104. A high score represents a greater tendency to engage in negative cognitions in response to tinnitus and low engagement in positive cognitions.

Regarding general stressor identification, we adopted the CAPPE questionnaire [16] that investigates the presence of different kind of stressors: chemical (prolonged expositions to solvents, assumptions of ototoxic drugs), acoustic (noise exposure, acoustic neuroma, otosclerosis, hearing loss), pathologies (diabetes, thyroiditis, autoimmune diseases), physical (professional stress, worsening of tinnitus during physical exercises) and emotional (sleep disorders, job change, depression).

The general perceived stress (due both to WAST, general health and life conditions) is quantified through the Perceived Stress Questionnaire (PSQ) [17]. It is designed to represent the subjective perspective of the individual ("You feel…"). Because stress results from an overload of experienced unpredictability and uncontrollability of events, the existence of stress in a subject is partially inferred from information on the person's experience of lack of control. The presented stress experiences in PSQ were intended to be abstract enough, to be applicable to adults of any age, stage of life, sex or occupation, but at the same time interpretable as specific to a variety of real-life situations. For example, "you feel under pressure from deadlines" could refer to anything from a payment to an oncoming birthday party or to a grant proposal. This questionnaire asks the respondent how often certain experiences of stress occurred in the last month. The content of the items is not referred to tinnitus, but it focuses on a more cognitive appraisal of stress. PSQ is a 20-item questionnaire of 4 scales, each resulted with 5 items:

- Scale 1 (worries) covers worries, anxious concern for the future and feelings of desperation and frustration (e.g. "you have many worries").
- Scale 2 (tension) explores tense disquietude, exhaustion and the lack of relaxation (e.g. "you feel mentally exhausted").
- Scale 3 (joy) is concerned with positive feelings of challenge, joy, energy and security (e.g. "you are full of energy").
- Scale 4 (demands) covers perceived environmental demands, such as lack of time, pressure and overload (e.g. "you feel you are in a hurry").

Each positive (yes) answer to scales 1, 2 and 4 is scored 1 point. In joy scale the score is 1 point for each negative (no) answer because all items of this scale are positively worded. Thus, maximum possible score means that the most unbearable stress perception is 20: the higher the total score, the higher the perceived stress.

14.3 Identification of Treatable Patients

The inclusion criteria are:

1. Acute or chronic tinnitus with TRQ less than 80.
2. CAPPE's item "increasing with physical exercise" with a positive answer.
3. PSQ score at least 15 as total score OR 4–5 score in "tension" subscale.
4. Patient's tinnitus modulated by somatic manoeuvres as described above.
5. No tinnitus modulation by the Jendrassik manoeuvres. In our experience modulation by clenching, neck forceful flexion, etc. AND Jendrassik modulation mean a no-specific facilitation of tinnitus perception to be distinguished from specific, treatable, somatic involvement.
6. Trigger or tender point in the muscles, specifically activated during forceful somatic manoeuvres, e.g. the masseter or anterior temporal regarding clenching and sternocleidomastoid regarding neck flexion or rotation.

Feldman masking curve, LDL level, TRQ, PSQ and TCQ represent the outcome measures.

14.4 Treatment

WAST treatment is mainly based on the so-called Tinnitus School as described elsewhere [18–20]: Tinnitus School is a five-step programme as follows:

1. Amelioration of lifestyle through adequate counselling based on the case history and CAPPE questionnaire.
2. Removing cervico-cephalic sensory–motor disturbances, by means of Manual Medicine techniques (Maigne and Nieves [13]; see dedicated chapters) including also high-velocity low-amplitude vertebral manipulations directly performed by the physician.
3. Leading the patient to an awareness of own body and learning breath and neck tension control, through physical exercises performed with a physiotherapist in a gymnasium (Table 14.2). Tinnitus School physiotherapy programme is constituted by ten sessions subdivided into three sessions per week along 2 weeks followed by two sessions per week along two other weeks. The first step is to prepare the patient to cooperate in a complex programme involving movement, thinking and learning. Muscle–skeletal impairments are often provoked by or associated with tension and anxiety; that is why head and neck disorders have to be treated before training. Therefore, it is more necessary to begin treatment with simple relaxation exercises to manage patient's tension. Physical exercises are pointed to postural control because, in chronic somatic tinnitus as well in WAST, the abnormal alignment of body parts with respect to each other and to the base of support may be due to both muscle–skeletal cervico-cephalic impairments and changes in patient's internal perception of the own sensations induced by pathological attention to tinnitus. Simple exercises have to be planned, and they are generally pointed to mobilization of the pelvis, of the cervical rachis and of the thoracolumbar spine. In some cases massages can be useful either to relax the patient or to mobilize joints, including slow-velocity high-amplitude vertebral manipulations performed by the physiotherapist.
4. Shifting patient attention away from tinnitus, through home physical exercises (Table 14.3).
5. Bibliotherapy. Self-help books exist for a wide variety of psychological problems. Studies of their value indicate that they can help individuals to make substantial improvements [21], on average about as much as psychotherapy. We propose to our patients the Italian version (Springer, Milan, 2012) of *Tinnitus: A Self-Management Guide for the Ringing in Your Ears*. This self-help book by Henry and Wilson [22] is based on the cognitive–behavioural principles, including educational information on tinnitus, cognitive reappraisal and restructuring, relaxation and stress management techniques, attention control techniques, use of self-instruction, making lifestyle changes and maintaining gains.

Table 14.2 Tinnitus School Gymnasium Training Protocol

Supine (all the exercise are performed with patients' head comfortably lying on a pillow)

- Relaxation exercises with control of breathing, improving consciousness of abdominal or thorax breathing: deep inhaling followed, after few seconds, by a forced exhaling while pronouncing the word "one". This exercise is repeated 8–10 times
- Patients move the head first slowly and then faster in all directions, focusing on a target straight on the ceiling
- Patients take the right knee against the chest, then extend the leg and take the left knee against the chest. A gentle traction of the flexed leg is performed by the patient himself when the knee is taken against the chest
- Patients take both knees to the chest, simultaneously helping gently with the hands
- Patients lift the pelvis taking the arms extended over the head. Then patients retake the arms along the body lowering the pelvis
- Patients grasp a stick. Then they extend the arms over the head and then return in the primary position
- In the quadrupedal position, patients inhale and arch the back while taking the head between the arms. Then they exhale while retroflexing the head and rotating the pelvis in hyperlordosis
- In quadrupedal position, patients extend simultaneously the right arm and the left leg, repeating the same exercise with the left arm and the right leg
- In prone position, patients lift their left arm and the right leg, maintaining the forehead over the bed, repeating it with the right arm and the left leg

Sitting

- Patients move the head first slowly and then faster in all directions, focusing on a target straight in front
- Patients look for three targets sited, respectively, in front, at their left and at their right. Then patients focus on the front target, and then they move the head, focusing on the right-sited target. At last they rotate leftward the head, maintaining the focus on the right-sited target
- Patients focus on the frontal target. Then they move the head leftward and focus on the left-sited target. At last they rotate rightward the head, maintaining the focus on the left-sited target
- Patients turn the head rightward and focus on a target on the lateral wall. Then they are instructed to move the head straight, maintaining focus on the target, through eye counterrotation, and count until 10
- Patients turn the head leftward and focus on a target on the lateral wall. Then they move the head straight, maintaining focus on the target, through eye counterrotation, and count until 10
- Patients extend their right arm and lift their thumb. Thus, patients move slowly the arm to and fro before along a horizontal direction and then along a vertical direction. Patients pursuit the thumb with eyes only, first slowly and then increasing progressively the velocity of thumb displacement
- As above but moving simultaneously also the head, trying to maintain the eyes still
- Patients grasp a stick with both hands and take the stick behind the shoulder, positioning the stick at the level of cervico-dorsal junction. In this position they rotate to and fro the trunk, maintaining the head still also focusing on a target straight in front. Rotation of the trunk has to be harmonic with quiet breathing
- Patients put the stick forward on the sternum at the level of the sternoclavicular joint. Then they perform rhythmic backward displacements of the shoulders
- In this position they rotate to and fro the trunk, maintaining the head still also through fixation of a target straight in front. Rotation of the trunk has to be harmonic with quiet breathing

- Paying attention to quiet breathing, patients inhale. Then, exhaling, they bend forward, taking the head on the right knee. They wait for 10 s. Then, inhaling, they return in sitting position
- Paying attention to quiet breathing, patients inhale. Then, exhaling, they bend forward, taking the head on the left knee. They wait for 10 s. Then, inhaling, they return in sitting position
- Patients inhale. Exhaling, they bend forward to keep an object on the floor. Then they inhale and take it up over the head and then they fixate it for 10 s. Patients inhale. Exhaling, they bend forward and take the object on the floor

Standing

- Patients focus themselves on a mirror and align correctly their posture. Thus, they maintain quiet equilibrium for 1 min, paying attention to breathing, before they maintain their eyes open and successively they close their eyes, imagining the correct position in their mind. They remain in this position for at least 1 min, paying attention to breathing. Then they oscillate to and fro according to the breath rhythm, hearing the air that enters and then exits from the lungs
- Patients in quiet upright position fixate a target on a mirror. In this case they have two planes of fixation: the target and their image. Thus, they have to be able to extract the correct fixation information from visual inputs. Then they oscillate to and fro according to the breath rhythm, hearing the air that enters and then exits from the lungs
- Patients keep a little object and lift it over the head, fixating it. Then they deeply inhale. Exhaling, they bend forward, placing the object on the floor. They wait for 10 s and then, inhaling, they lift again the object over the head
- Patients take a little object over their head. Maintaining the object, they move it in small circles according to breath rhythm, hearing the air that enters and then exits from the lungs

Table 14.3 Tinnitus School Home Training Protocol

Supine

- Relaxation exercises with control of breathing, improving consciousness of abdominal or thorax breathing: deep inhaling followed, after few seconds, by a forced exhaling while pronouncing the word "one". This exercise is repeated 8–10 times
- Take your two knees to the chest, simultaneously, helping, gently, with the hands
- Lift your pelvis while taking simultaneously your arms extended over your head. Then retake your arms along the body while lowering your pelvis
- Grasp a stick. Take your extended arms over your head and then return in the primary position
- In prone position lift your left arm and your right leg, maintaining your forehead over the bed. Then repeat with the right arm and the left leg.

Sitting

- Move your head first slowly and then faster in all directions, focusing on a target straight in front of you
- Grasp a stick with both hands and take the stick behind the shoulder, positioning the stick at the level of the cervico-dorsal junction. In this position rotate to and fro the trunk, maintaining the head still also through fixation of a target straight in front. Rotation of the trunk has to be harmonic with quiet breathing
- Repeat the exercise, putting the stick forward on the sternum at the level of the sterno-clavear joint. Then perform rhythmic backward displacements of shoulders

Standing

- With your hands on a table, lift yourself on your tiptoes and maintain this position for 30 s. Pay attention to breathing!
- With your hands on a table, lift yourself on your heels and maintain this position for 30 s. Pay attention to breathing!
- Focus yourself on a mirror. Then oscillate to and fro, right and left, around your ankles while keeping your pelvis still, according to breath rhythm, hearing the air that enters and then exits from the lungs
- Repeat with your eyes closed
- Keep a little object and then lift it over your head and focus on it. With your extended arms move it over and over wide circles, maintaining focus on the object, according to the breath rhythm, hearing the air that enters and exits from the lungs
- Repeat with your eyes closed. Pay attention to breathing!
- Keep a little object and lift it over your head. Focus on it. Inhale. Then exhale and bend yourself forward, taking the object on the floor. Wait for 10 s and then, inhaling, lift again the object over your head. Pay attention to breathing!

14.5 Outcome

Decreasing TCQ, TRQ and PSQ scores represents a significant improvement in the quality of life of the patients; thus, generally speaking, WAST treatment results in a significant decrease of tinnitus disturbance (TRQ and TCQ) through a decreased perception of stress (PSQ). A strict selection of the subjects and patients strongly motivated "to feel better" is needed.

Tinnitus, in general, may represent a sort of auditory after-effect [23–25]: an interrupted sound can be perceived as continuous when noise masks the interruption, creating an illusion of continuity. It is reasonable to assume that WA somatic disturbances convey abnormal inputs on DCN, creating something like spinal segmental sensitization described by Fisher [26] to explain chronic myofascial pain. According to this idea, somatic inputs may represent the "sensorial noise" in the DCN that masks the interruption, creating an illusion of continuity, continuity that we know to be the prerequisite for inducing chronic tinnitus at both cortical and limbic level.

References

1. Tranter RM, Graham JR (2009) A review of the otological aspects of whiplash injury. J Forensic Leg Med 16(2):53–55
2. Axelsson A, Ringdahl A (1985) Tinnitus: a study of its prevalence and characteristics. Br J Audiol 23:53–62
3. Pulec JJL, Hodell SF, Antony DF (1978) Tinnitus – diagnosis and treatment. Ann Otol Rhinol Laryngol 87:821–833
4. Dehmel S, Cui YL, Shore SE (2008) Cross-modal interactions of auditory and somatic inputs in the brainstem and midbrain and their imbalance in tinnitus and deafness. Am J Audiol 17(2):193–209

5. Levine RA, Nam EC, Oron Y, Melcher JR (2007) Evidence for a tinnitus subgroup responsive to somatosensory based treatment modalities. Prog Brain Res 166:195–207
6. Zeng C, Yang Z, Shreve L, Bledsoe S, Shore S (2012). Somatosensory projections to cochlear nucleus are upregulated after unilateral deafness. J Neurosci 7;32(45):15791-801
7. Shulman A (1995) A final common pathway for tinnitus: the medial temporal lobe system. Int Tinnitus J 1:115–126
8. Jastreboff PJ, Hazell JWP (1993) A neurophysiological approach to tinnitus clinical implications. Br J Audiol 27(1):7–17
9. Norena AJ (2010) An integrative model of tinnitus based on a central gain controlling neural sensitivity. Neurosci Biobehav Rev 10:345–353
10. Kaltenbach JA (2010) Tinnitus: models and mechanisms. Hear Res 10(1):35–38
11. Feldman H (1971) Homolateral and contralateral masking of tinnitus by noise-bands and by pure tones. Audiology 10(3):138–144
12. Simmons R, Dambra C, Lobarinas E, Stocking C, Salvi R (2008) Head, neck, and eye movements that modulate tinnitus. Semin Hear 29(4):361–370
13. Maigne R, Nieves WL (2006) Diagnosis and treatment of pain of vertebral origin, 2nd ed. Pain management. CRC Press, Taylor & Francis Group: Boca Raton FL. ISBN 0-8493-3121_8
14. Wilson PH, Henry J, Bowen M, Haralambous G (1991) Tinnitus reaction questionnaire: psychometric properties of a measure of distress associated with tinnitus. J Speech Hear Res 34:197–201
15. Wilson PH, Henry J (1998) Tinnitus cognitions questionnaire: development and psychometric properties of a measure of dysfunctional cognitions associated with tinnitus. Int Tinnitus J 4(1):23–30
16. Nodar RH (1996) CAPPE – a strategy for counselling tinnitus patients. Int Tinnitus J 2(2):111–114
17. Fliege H, Rose M, Arck P, Walter OB, Kocalevent RD, Weber C, Klapp BF (2005) The Perceived Stress Questionnaire (PSQ) reconsidered: validation and reference values from different clinical and healthy adult samples. Psychosom Med 67(1):78–88
18. Alpini D, Cesarani A (2006) Tinnitus as an alarm bell: stress reaction tinnitus model. ORL J Otorhinolaryngol Relat Spec 68(1):31–36
19. Alpini D, Cesarani A, Hahn A (2007) Tinnitus school: an educational approach to tinnitus management based on a stress-reaction tinnitus model. Int Tinnitus J 13(1):63–68
20. Alpini D, Cesarani A, Hahn A (2011) Tinnitus School – An Integrated Management of Somatic Tinnitus, Up to Date on Tinnitus, Prof. Fayez Bahmad (Ed.), ISBN: 978-953-307-655-3, InTech, DOI: 10.5772/27354. Available from: http://www.intechopen.com/books/up-to-date-on-tinnitus/tinnitus-school-an-integrated-management-of-somatic-tinnitus
21. Malouff JJ, Noble W, Schutte NS, Bhullar N (2010) The effectiveness of bibliotherapy in alleviating tinnitus-related distress. J Psychosom Res 68(2):245–251
22. Henry JL, Wilson PH (2001) Tinnitus: a self-management guide for the ringing in your ears. Allyn & Bacon, Boston
23. Riecke L, Micheyl C, Vanbussel M, Schreiner CS, Mendelsohn D, Formisano E (2011) Recalibration of the auditory continuity illusion: sensory and decisional effects. Hear Res 27:765–771
24. Zenner HP, Zalaman IM (2004) Cognitive tinnitus sensitization: behavioural and neurophysiological aspects of tinnitus centralization. Acta Otolaryngol 124(4):436–439
25. Vanneste S, Plazier M, van der Loo E, Van de Heyning P, Congedo M, De Ridder D (2010) The neural correlates of tinnitus-related distress. Neuroimage 52:470–480
26. Fischer AA (ed) (1997) Myofascial pain – update in diagnosis and treatment, Physical medicine and rehabilitation clinics of North America. W.B. Saunders, Philadelphia, pp 153–169

Part III

Evaluation

Anamnesis and Clinical Evaluation of Whiplash-Associated Equilibrium Disturbances (WAED)

15

A. Cesarani, D.C. Alpini, D. Brambilla, and F. Di Berardino

15.1 Introduction

In all medical fields a good case history evaluation is the key of a correct diagnostic pathway. Patients' complaints have to be documented as completely as possible just from the beginning of the disease. Sometimes the examiner uses technical terms to question the patient, and this can lead to confusion and misunderstandings. The first diagnostic task is to differentiate between vertigo and dizziness or disequilibrium, ruling out the many varieties of indistinct dizziness such as faintness. *Vertigo* is linked with a spinning sensation around the head and frequently a vestibular disorder. Vertigo is the awareness of some dysfunction in the balance mechanisms, that is, a dysfunction in the balance mechanisms becomes a conscious experience. The sensation is characterized by feelings of "spatial disorientation", whereof the illusion of false movement is the most characteristic. "Rotatory sensation" is the most typical sensation, but it is not the sole feeling generated by balance dysfunction. The basic impression has to be the sensation of loss of stable subjective relationship with the environment. In this way less typical sensations must be included and are called "atypical" vertigo. On the other hand, syncopes, blackout, drop attacks, odd sensations in the head, etc., have to be denied as primary "vertigo" sensations, but

A. Cesarani • F. Di Berardino
Department of Clinical Sciences and Community Health, University of Milan, Milan, Italy

Audiology Unit, IRCCS "Ca' Granda" Ospedale Maggiore Policlinico, Milan, Italy
e-mail: antonio.cesarani@unimi.it

D.C. Alpini (✉)
ENT-Otoneurology Service, IRCCS "Don Carlo Gnocchi" Foundation, Milan, Italy
e-mail: dalpini@dongnocchi.it

D. Brambilla
Department of Otoneurology, IRCCS "E. Medea", "La Nostra Famiglia" Association, via Don Monza 20, Bosisio Parini, Italy
e-mail: daniele.brambilla@bp.lnf.it

D.C. Alpini et al. (eds.), *Whiplash Injuries*,
DOI 10.1007/978-88-470-5486-8_15, © Springer-Verlag Italia 2014

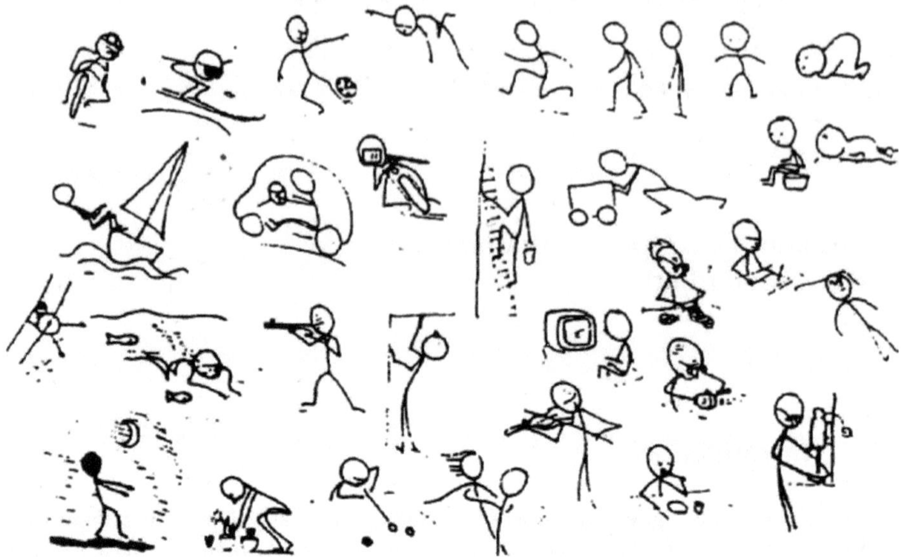

Fig. 15.1 Grateu's synoptic diagram for anamnesis

they can accompany true vertigo. *Dizziness* or a turning sensation inside the head may result from disturbances of integrating structures within the central nervous system. Atypical dizziness is usually confused with disequilibrium. The term "dizziness" is used popularly. It includes a multitude of symptoms related to the vestibular system or other aspects of the nervous system. Dizziness is applied to physical, emotional or intellectual disturbances, whose common denominator seems to be a loss of stability, a disruption of the pattern in which the individual is aware of his surroundings and their relation to him, whether these refer to his physical orientation in space, his emotional equilibrium or his intellectual clarity. It is important that the patient describes symptoms with his/her own words in the simplest way. In this sense Grateu [1] proposed a simplified chart to investigate vertigo and dizziness during common or less common daily activities (Fig. 15.1) every time the examiner has to lead the patient in order to identify the main elements of patient history.

In equilibrium disturbances particular attention has to be pointed on qualitative and quantitative aspects of symptoms.

15.2 WAED Anamnesis

The following aspects have to be investigated:

- Vertigo or dizziness. It is important to determine which symptom is prevalent or if both are present or if there is a particular and recurrent sequence between vertigo and dizziness. For example, after a whiplash injury, dizziness appears when the patient removes the collar, performing normal activities, while vertigo appears during rotation or flexo-extension of the head.

- Onset of the symptoms. Immediately after whiplash, or the day after, or when the collar was removed, or when physiotherapy began.
- Direction of vertigo rotation or the side of prevalent unsteadiness.
- Remission with particular position of the head/neck.
- Combination with spine pain and stiffness, with brachial paresthesias, with dysphagia or dysphasia, with neurovegetative symptoms such as nausea and vomiting, with cognitive symptoms such as amnesia and attention disturbances and with auditory symptoms such as hearing loss and tinnitus.
- Loss of conscious or combined with vertigo/dizziness.
- Headache and/or migraine immediately after vertigo attack or in the following days/weeks/months.
- Incidence of symptoms on daily life activities. These qualitative aspects of symptoms can be quantified using activities of daily living (ADL) questionnaires [2]. As with functional scales, there is a tendency to use different standards, depending on the type of lesion one aims to study. However, the usefulness of questionnaire and ADL estimations should not be underestimated. The clinician may well use this expertise to enhance the objective assessment of the patients. However, such estimations may be biased, and they cannot easily be quantified or documented for studies or evaluation of the effect of treatment. To get better objective estimations, several functional scales have been developed, generally designed for the study of a certain group of patients, thereby lacking the quality of general applicability. Well-known scales are the Tinetti [3] and the Berg Balance Scale [4, 5].
- Temporal distance between any first medical visit and whiplash.
- Temporal onset of each symptom and reciprocal combination.
- Frequence of spontaneous attacks.
- Intensity that can be quantified on a decimal scale.
- Duration: continuous, subcontinuous, transient, recurrent.
- Temporal correlation with hearing disturbances: no hearing disturbances, hearing symptoms before, during and after vertigo attacks, etc.
- Accident aspects
  - Whiplash of the driver or the passenger.
  - Anterior or posterior passenger.
  - Safety belts.
  - Rear-end or lateral or diagonal collision.
  - Collision with resting or moving car.
  - Position of the head during injury. For example, if the passenger, with safety belt, was speaking with the driver with the car stopped for a traffic light, then a pure rear-end collision would not induce a pure sagittal antero-retroflexion of the head but rather its torsional movement with the fulcrum on the first thoracic vertebra and with a torsion of the trunk with the fulcrum on the first lumbar vertebra. Such a complicated injuring mechanism usually induces stronger longer-lasting symptoms, sometimes with severe vertigo and dizziness.

The prognosis of WAED depends on concomitant diseases and/or previous vestibular disorders. Thus, it is important to investigate:

- Vertigo or unsteadiness months or years before whiplash
- Previous trauma
- Previous otoneurological visit/examinations either for symptoms or for working capability evaluation
- Previous auditory disorders
- Heart or brain or vascular diseases
- Hormonal disorders such as dysmenorrhoea or dysthyroidism
- Metabolic disorders such as diabetes
- Use of alcohol, drugs and tobacco products
- Exposure to solvents or other cerebro-toxic factors
- Epilepsy
- Previous treatment for scoliosis or orthodontic problems which could influence postural system compensation possibilities
- Kinetosis

During anamnesis the modality by which the patient tells his own history can suggest to the clinician some other characteristics, such as anxiety, restlessness or depression. Sometimes specific psychometric scales can be used, but they are generally noises and not well accepted to the subject. Computerized anamnestic systems, such as NODEC elaborated by Claussen [6], are very useful in order to standardize the series of questions, but it reduces the interpersonal interaction between clinician and patient. Generally speaking we can say that computerized anamnestic systems are particularly indicated for medicolegal expertise, while personal anamnesis is more useful in the treatment planning. The clinician has to identify psychological symptoms due to the stress and consequent symptoms. During anamnesis the examiner can, if necessary, simply evaluate attentional disturbances with easy temporal orientation (number of the present day), cultural (name of the Popes), memory (series of numbers) and logic reversal ability tasks.

A useful questionnaire is the Dizziness Handicap Inventory proposed by Jacobson and Newman [7] whose short form has been recently developed by Tesio et al. [8]. DHI investigates multiple aspects of activities of daily living and their correlation with evocation of equilibrium disturbances (Table 15.1). The short form is a simplified questionnaire which has been proved to be as reliable and accurate as the long form (Table 15.2). The questions are not restricted to the patient's problem (vertigo and dizziness), but they investigate the patient as an entire person. For example, it is possible that vertigo and dizziness don't cause difficulties in reading (answer "no" in DHI), but the patient may have a vision impaired for ophthalmological problems. In this way the correct answer in the DHIs will be "yes" because in every way reading is difficult and impaired vision, for any cause, may impair balance.

In elderly WAED the increased risk of falls may be quantified through the "Falling Risk Inventory" [9].

15.3 Clinical WAED Patient's Examination

As we said in the Introduction, whiplash is a true noncontact cerebral trauma. Thus, the otoneurological and equilibrium examinations have to evaluate some neurological, orthopaedic and psychiatric aspects.

Table 15.1 Dizziness Handicap Inventory

Instructions: The purpose of this scale is to identify difficulties that you may be experiencing *because of* your dizziness or unsteadiness. Please answer "yes", "no" or "sometimes" to each question. Answer each question as it pertains to your dizziness or unsteadiness problem only.
Does looking up increase your problem?
Because of your problem, do you feel frustrated?
Because of your problem, do you restrict your travel for business or recreation?
Does walking down the aisle of a supermarket increase your problem?
Because of your problem, do you have difficulty getting into or out of bed?
Does your problem significantly restrict your participation in social activities such as going out to dinner, going to movies, dancing or parties?
Because of your problem, do you have difficulties in reading?
Does performing more ambitious activities like sports, dancing and household chores such as sweeping or putting dishes away increase your problem?
Because of your problem, are you afraid to leave your home without having someone accompany you?
Because of your problem, have you been embarrassed in front of others?
Do quick movements of your head increase your problem?
Because of your problem, do you avoid heights?
Does turning over in bed increase your problem?
Because of your problem, is it difficult for you to do strenuous housework or yardwork?
Because of your problem, are you afraid people may think you are intoxicated?
Because of your problem, is it difficult for you to go for a walk by yourself?
Does walking down a sidewalk increase your problem?
Because of your problem, is it difficult to concentrate?
Because of your problem, is it difficult for you to walk around your house in the dark?
Because of your problem, are you afraid to stay at home alone?
Because of your problem, do you feel handicapped?
Has your problem placed stress on your relationships with members of your family or friends?
Because of your problem, are you depressed?
Does your problem interfere with your job or household responsibilities?
Does bending over increase your problem?

15.3.1 Cranial Nerves

Generally, the olfactory nerve is not investigated routinely also because it requires necessary instrumental equipments (olfactometry). The optic nerve is clinically investigated evaluating the fundus oculi by means of an ophthalmoscope. Extrinsic and intrinsic ocular motilities have to be always investigated. During oculomotricity, extrinsic evaluation smooth pursuit and saccadic eye movements have to be investigated using a pen or the examiner finger as target. Also the sensitivity of the face (trigeminus) and corneal reflexes has to be evaluated. Regarding the facial nerve, mimic aspects are sometimes evident, and dysesthesias of the auditory external meatus have to be searched. The Schirmer test can complete facial examination. The auditory function must be more correctly investigated with the different

Table 15.2 Dizziness Handicap Inventory Short Form

Instructions: The purpose of this scale is to identify difficulties that you may be experiencing that can cause your dizziness or unsteadiness. Please answer "yes" or "no" to each question *even if* disturbances are caused by problems different from vertigo, dizziness and unsteadiness.
Does looking up increase your symptoms?
Do you restrict your travel for business or recreation?
Do you have difficulty getting into or out of bed?
Do you have difficulties in reading?
Do quick movements of your head increase your problem?
Do you avoid heights?
Does turning over in bed increase your problem?
Is it difficult for you to go for a walk by yourself?
Does walking down a sidewalk increase your problem?
Is it difficult for you to walk around your house in the dark?
Are you afraid to stay at home alone?
Are you depressed?
Does bending over increase your problem?

audiometric tests, leaving the diapason tests to the history. Only the Weber test can be sometimes useful during clinical investigation. The inspective visit of the mouth and the larynx allows a complete evaluation of the IX, X and XII nerves, eventually completed with stimulation of the external auditory meatus and posterior pharyngeal wall to induce, respectively, cough and pharyngeal reflexes. The XI nerve is usually evaluated during postural examination, with palpation of the sternocleidomastoid and trapezius.

15.3.2 Posture

Several approaches may be used to estimate human postural control and they may be considered complementary. Clinical investigation can yield valuable information. The direct observation of patient behaviour, even during anamnesis, may contribute information otherwise overlooked. Several generally well-known examination procedures may be applied to help the examiner to evaluate the investigated subject. The use of standardized protocols also gives the examiner more experience in interpreting the outcome of the procedures. The active and passive movements of the head with respect to the neck, the trunk and the pelvis must be estimated. Pain and movement limitations have to be noted and in a certain way quantified. Palpations of the paravertebral extensor muscles, with special regard to those of the neck and the back, have to be performed in order to appreciate hypo- or hypertonus of the muscles. Simple muscular force test for the arm and leg extensors is useful. With the patient in supine position, a Babinski test is simple and useful to perform. General muscular tonus can be simply evaluated by asking to the patient to resist with his/her thumb and index contacting them in a circle during an opposite force of the examiner.

Tendon reflexes may be simply investigated. Trigger and tender points have to be routinely searched along all paravertebral muscles, and temporomandibular joints have to be inspected in static and dynamic (opening, protrusion, laterotrusion, etc.) positions of the jaw.

During postural evaluation some sensorial evaluation can be contemporarily performed especially if paresthesias are complained.

15.3.3 Eye Movements

Eye movements can be easily evaluated in a clinical manner and using instrumental devices. In clinical practice the investigator is in front of the patient. First the examiner lifts suddenly the right thumb in front of the patient (at about 50 cm from his eyes) asking him to fixate it without moving his head, then he lifts the left and so on the examiner continues lifting alternatively the right and left thumbs, and patient continues fixating them, producing saccadic eye movements. The most important features that can be noted are the latency of the eye movements and their conjugation. Also dysmetrias can be revealed because sometimes patients are not able to fixate the thumb with only one saccade but they require adjustments of the eye movements. Then the examiner asks to the patient to fixate his right thumb placed at 50 cm from patient's eyes, during a slow continuous to-and-fro movement. In this case a smooth pursuit can be elicited. The most important feature that can be noted is the regularity of the movement that must be continuous and harmonic.

15.3.4 Vestibulo-Ocular Reflex

Clinically, some information on vestibulo-ocular reflex (VOR) can be obtained by turning the patient's head while observing the optic disc during funduscopy. The patient must be instructed to maintain fixation on an object across the room. Normally, the disc remains steady in space, but if, say, the right labyrinth is hypoactive, the disc will seem to jerk during turning of the head to the right. When the vestibular loss is profound, this jerk eye movement in response to turns of the head can be seen by the naked eye. In this case it is best to instruct the patient to fixate on the examiner's nose (so-called Halmagyi sign, named also as the head impulse test or head thrust test) [10, 11].

Assessment of the otolith function clinically is even less easily done. Counterrolling of the eyes can be seen when the head is rotated to the ear down on to the shoulder; the eyes slowly deviate in the opposite sense and then there is a rotatory quick phase causing torsional nystagmus. This response is, however, mainly dependent on the vertical semicircular canals rather than the otoliths. Skew deviation of the eyes (vertical divergence of the eyes) without nystagmus is thought to reflect tonic otolith pathway imbalance. It can be seen with utricular nerve lesion or with lesions of the mesencephalon, especially those involving the interstitial nucleus of Cajal and medulla; this type of tonic rotation can be suspected from a head tilt or the eye covering test or seen from tilting of the optic disc.

Otolith-ocular reflexes may be investigated by means of a modified Halmagyi test using a brisk but small translational impulse of the head: head heave test [12].

One of the cardinal signs of abnormal vestibular function is nystagmus. *Nystagmus* (Ny) is a biphasic involuntary movement of both eyes (generally), and it is constituted by a slow displacement of the eyes in a direction (slow phase of nystagmus) followed by a rapid return of the eyes in the primary position of the gaze.

Nystagmus is classified according to the manoeuvres that are able to elicit it:

- Spontaneous nystagmus: it is present without any provocative manoeuvre.
  Vestibular nystagmus is caused by an imbalance between the paired vestibular structures. The nystagmus is called first degree if present only when gaze is directed towards the fast phase, second degree if present in the primary position or third degree if present when the eyes are deviated in the direction of the slow phase. Removal of fixation typically enhances the nystagmus if the lesion is peripheral and the eyes drift markedly towards the deranged side (fast phase towards the healthy side). This can be seen clinically with Frenzel's glasses that have high-dioptre convergence lenses which allow a magnified view of the eyes of the patient, without the patient being able to fixate due to the blur produced by the lenses.
- Gaze-evoked nystagmus.
  It is elicited by the eccentric position of the eyes that the patient has to maintain for at least 20 s. It is called also gaze-evoked nystagmus. When bilateral, it is usually a sign of central disorders due to a deficit of the central gaze neural integrator localized in the medial vestibular nucleus and in the prepositus hypoglossi nucleus.
- Positional nystagmus.
  Nystagmus may readily be induced or, if already present, modified by changes in position of the head. The conventional method is the Dix-Hallpike manoeuvre [13]. In this, the patient sits on a couch and the examiner firmly grasps the head which is turned 60° towards one shoulder. The patient is instructed to keep the eyes open and to fixate the examiner's forehead. The patient's head is rapidly lowered to below the level of couch and the eyes observed for any nystagmus. After an interval of 30 s, if nystagmus is not found, or after the nystagmus ceases, the patient is returned to the sitting position. Again, any nystagmus is normally noted. The test is repeated if nystagmus is found to see if there is any adaptation. After this, the test is performed with the opposite ear dependent. The variables noted are latency to onset of nystagmus, its duration and adaptation, its direction and, finally, associated symptoms. If any nystagmus is found after the Dix-Hallpike manoeuvre, nystagmus has to be investigated in supine position, in head hanging position and with briskly turning of the head to one side while the patient is in the supine position. Typical benign positional nystagmus indicates a peripheral dysfunction, it presents a latency, and it is generally horizontal rotatory, usually geotropic, fatiguable and adaptable. Although it is generally unilateral, occasionally what seems to be bilateral benign positional nystagmus occurs.

Typical central positional nystagmus occurs in a wide variety of lesions, especially those involving vestibulocerebellum. Spontaneous vertical nystagmus, either upwards or downwards, can often be modified by positional testing using the conventional Dix-Hallpike manoeuvre or by placing the subject supine or prone. If the nystagmus is increased in prone position, it is usually decreased lying supine. Nystagmus induced by canal stimulation can also be profoundly modified by alteration of position of the head, due to otolith/semicircular canal interaction.

- Vibration nystagmus.
  Mastoid or suboccipital stimulation by means of a 100 Hz vibration delivered by a specific vibration apparatus [14] evoked a nystagmus when canals or maculae are unbalanced. In whiplash patient is very frequent to observe nystagmus induced only by paravertebral cervical stimulation of one side, generally by the same side of more pronounced cervical muscle tension and pain, probably due to overstimulation of the cervical muscle spindles.
- Cervical nystagmus.
  It is due to the activation of the cervico-ocular reflex. It is elicited by the rotation of the subject with the head still. This provokes a stimulation of the neck muscles (stretching reflex), a stimulation of the vestibular nuclei and the elicitation of a nystagmus directed towards the opposite side of body rotation. In normal subjects nystagmus usually does not appear, thus the gain of the COR has been calculated to be very low (about 0.1). In patients cervical nystagmus can be more easily observed especially when the labyrinth is hypofunctional.
- Head-shaking nystagmus.
  In some patients vigorous head shaking may generate a nystagmus that is not clinically apparent. The head-shaking test (HST) (20–30 full cycles at around 2 Hz followed by Frenzel's glasses observation) is a useful addition to the clinical vestibular examination.
- Optokinetic nystagmus.
  Optokinetic nystagmus (OKN) is a nystagmus elicited by the rotation of the environment with respect to the patient. It is a compensatory movement of the eyes to pursue a target displacement more width than the visual field. It can be assessed at the bedside with a small stripped drum rotated in front of the patient. This is basically a pursuit task and not surprisingly correlates well with other pursuit measures.

15.3.5 Otolith Function

Some patients attending WAE disturbances clinics report symptoms of unsteadiness which suggest involvement of otolith rather than semicircular canal function. This may include a sense of bobbing up and down, being carried upwards and downwards in a lift, or lateral and sagittal pulsions. Certain disorders of head and eye coordination – for instance, the ocular tilt reaction combining head tilt and ocular skew deviation – are thought to be due to interruption of central graviceptive otoliths pathways.

15.3.6 Stance

Most common human activities require the ability to stabilize the human body in upright stance, to counteract perturbations and to allow voluntary movements, according to gravitational forces. The standing human is an unstable physical structure. To counteract the effects of gravity and comply with the requirements to stabilize the body during voluntary movements, there is a continuous modulation of motor activity, especially in the so-called antigravity muscles, based on the also continuously changing afferent sensory information. The postural control of the standing human can therefore be considered in part a dynamic feedback control. Furthermore, based on experience and visual information, the standing human may foresee perturbations or changing requirements in advance, thus adding a substantial degree of anticipatory or feedforward control. To evaluate the significance on postural control of observations or test results, it is necessary to bear in mind the physiological background and ability to maintain upright stance.

Regarding the clinical evaluation of stance, the classical Romberg test is easily applied even in the office and may yield some information. A patient unable to perform a Romberg test will probably have prominent difficulties in everyday life. During this test particular attention has to be paid to direction of the slow falling rather than the fast compensation. The Romberg test with feet in tandem position seems less appropriate as it requires a better than ordinary postural control and will yield a high degree of false-positive results. A Romberg test with the neck extended, however, may contribute further information. In this position the lateral semicircular canal is brought into line with the gravity vector. A patient with a vestibular lesion causing ataxia and nystagmus falls in the direction of the slow phase of nystagmus, while a patient with a cerebellar cause may fall towards the fast phase or the slow phase depending on the site of the lesion. According to Magnusson [15] a combination with the clinical headshake test and Romberg test may be performed. Nystagmus induced by a headshake test cannot differentiate between a CNS lesion and a peripheral vestibular lesion. One may, however, increase the sensitivity in tests of stance by combining the headshake test with a Romberg or a stepping test. The patient does headshakes for 10 s, standing with his back against a wall and then rapidly taking four steps forwards. If there is an evident deviation or fall towards the side of the fast phase of nystagmus induced by a previous headshake test, this may be taken as suggesting a posterior fossa lesion. Patients with compensated peripheral vestibular lesions seem to deviate only slightly.

15.3.7 Gait

Gait is certainly one of the most complex functions in which the equilibrium system must interconnect with inself and outself in order to provide a harmonious and coordinate progression of the body into the environment.

Gait can be evaluated either under a clinical point of view or by means of sophisticated equipments.

In order to investigate in clinical practice equilibrium control of gait, the patient has to walk quietly in a large room to-and-fro before with eyes open and then with eyes closed. Gait with eyes open provides generic informations regarding neurological aspects of gait.

Gait with eyes closed provides specific informations regarding the equilibrium system. Not only the direction of body deviation has to be noted but also the qualitative characteristic of gait: the width of the base of support, the position of the arms during gait, the presence of pendular synkinesias and the stability of the head.

A simple way to evaluate equilibrium control of gait is the investigation, with eyes closed, of *stepping*, a simplified gait on place. Generally the patient is asked to step for about one minute that it is equal to about 60–80 steps. During this time, with eyes closed, a certain forward progression of the patient is observed. The same characteristic of the gait can be revealed also during stepping: rotation of the stepping, body sway, coordination of the movement, width of base support, etc.

Conclusions

At the end of a complete anamnesis and a complete clinical otoneurological examination, the clinician has all the elements to plan the required instrumental tests. These cannot substitute for the clinical sensitivity of the examiner but have to confirm, specify and document alterations of the equilibrium system. On the basis of anamnesis and clinical examination, treatment planning can be generally completely performed even if instrumental tests are often indispensable to monitoring the results of therapy.

References

1. Grateau P (1992) Critique de l' objectivité? Neuromédia, Bull Club Neurosciences, 1986, DEA, Marseille
2. Cook CE, Richardson JK, Pietrobon R, Braga L, Silva HM, Turner D (2006) Validation of the NHANES ADL scale in a sample of patients with report of cervical pain: factor analysis, item response theory analysis, and line item validity. Disabil Rehabil 28(15):929–935
3. Panella L, Tinelli C, Buizza A, Lombardi R, Gandolfi R (2008) Towards objective evaluation of balance in the elderly: validity and reliability of a measurement instrument applied to the Tinetti test. Int J Rehabil Res 31(1):65–72
4. Berg KO, Maki BE, Williams N, Holliday PI, Wood-Dauphinee SL (1992) Clinical and laboratory measures of postural balance in an elderly population. Arch Phys Med Rehabil 73:1073–1080
5. Downs S, Marquez J, Chiarelli P (2013) The Berg Balance Scale has high intra- and inter-rater reliability but absolute reliability varies across the scale: a systematic review. J Physiother 59(2):93–99
6. Claussen CF (1992) Equilibriometric topodiagnosis as a basis of modern therapy of vertigo and dizziness. Neurootol Newsl 1(1):7–24
7. Jacobson GP, Newman CW (1990) The development of the Dizziness Handicap Inventory. Arch Otolaryngol Head Neck Surg 116(4):424–427
8. Tesio L, Alpini D, Cesarani A, Perucca L (1999) Short form of the Dizziness Handicap Inventory: construction and validation through Rasch analysis. Am J Phys Med Rehabil 78(3):233–241

9. Alpini D, Kohen-Ratz R, Braun R, Burstin A, Tesio L, Pugnetti L, Mendozzi L, Sambataro G, Cesarani A, Giuliano DA (2001) Falls in the elderly: the development of a risk questionnaire and posturographic findings. Int Tinnitus J 7(2):105–108
10. Halmagyi GM (2005) Diagnosis and management of vertigo. Clin Med 5(2):159–165
11. Ulmer E, Chays A (2005) Curthoys and Halmagyi Head Impulse test: an analytical device. Ann Otolaryngol Chir Cervicofac 122(2):84–90
12. Ramat S, Zee DS, Minor LB (2001) Translational vestibulo-ocular reflex evoked by a "head heave" stimulus. Ann N Y Acad Sci 942:95–113
13. Syed I, Ahmed W, Selvadurai D (2012) Dix-Hallpike and Epley manoeuvres. Br J Hosp Med (Lond) 73(10):C149–C151
14. Ulmer E, Chays A, Brémond G (2004) Vibration-induced nystagmus: mechanism and clinical interest. Ann Otolaryngol Chir Cervicofac 121(2):95–103
15. Magnusson M (1994) Evaluation of brainstem-cerebellar posture control. In: Cesarani A, Alpini D (eds) Equilibrium disorders: brainstem and cerebellar pathology. Springer, Milan, pp 52–59

Whiplash Effects on Postural Control 16

M. Magnusson and A. Hahn

The human ability to maintain upright stance in the presence of external disturbances such as gravity or body-support surface motion has intrigued researchers over the last century.

Interest arose from basic neuroscience [1] and from clinicians who diagnose and treat balancing problems [2].

Furthermore, most common human activities require the ability to stabilize the human body in upright stance, to counteract perturbations, and to allow voluntary movements, according to gravitational forces. The standing human is an unstable physical structure. To counteract the effects of gravity and comply with the requirements to stabilize the body during voluntary movements, there is a continuous modulation of motor activity, especially in the so-called antigravity muscles, based on the also continuously changing afferent sensory information (Fig. 16.1).

The postural control of the standing human can therefore be considered in part a dynamic feedback control [3]. Furthermore, based on experience and visual information, the standing human may foresee perturbations or changing requirements in advance, thus adding a substantial degree of anticipatory or feedforward control [4]. To evaluate the significance on postural control of observations or test results, it is necessary to bear in mind the physiological background and ability to maintain upright stance. Postural control cannot be considered a strictly hierarchical system but rather is characterized by decentralized or local decisions in a way which allows comparisons with the popular algorithms of neural networks. There is a substantial amount of redundancy. The complementary relationships between the afferent orientational information, i.e. the visual vestibular and somatosensory information, in

M. Magnusson (✉)
Department of Otorhinolaryngology, Lund University Hospital,
Lund University, 221 85 Lund, Sweden
e-mail: mans.magnusson@med.lu.se

A. Hahn
3ENT Clinic, 3rd Medical Faculty, Charles University Prague, Prague, Czech Republic
e-mail: hahn@fnkv.cz

D.C. Alpini et al. (eds.), *Whiplash Injuries*,
DOI 10.1007/978-88-470-5486-8_16, © Springer-Verlag Italia 2014

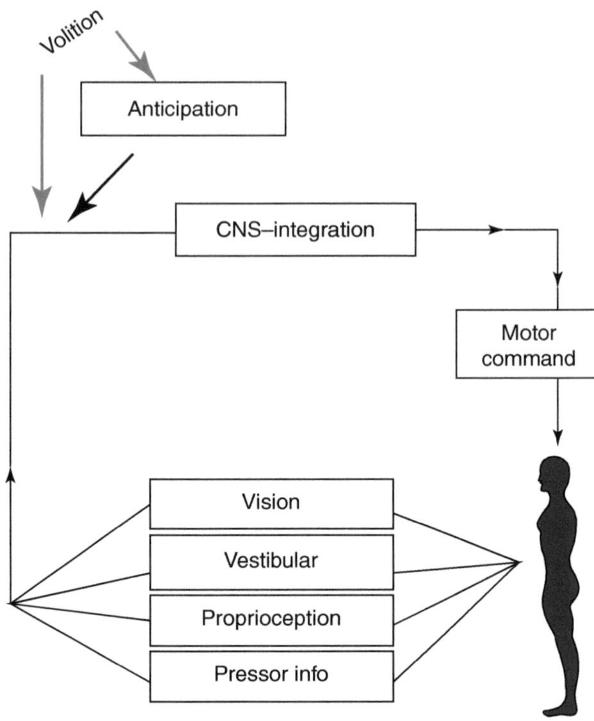

Fig. 16.1 A schematic representation of human postural control in quiet stance. To maintain upright position and stabilize the body, there are continuously changing visual, vestibular, proprioceptive and mechanoreceptive sensory inputs. As the standing human is an unstable physical structure, there can be stable static position. Stance is therefore maintained by dynamic feedback control with contribution of anticipatory or feedforward information

postural control have been well known since the observations of Romberg in the nineteenth century. However, the redundancies of the sensory systems or the central nervous pathways should not be interpreted as the information from the different sensory systems or neural pathways being equivalent and interchangeable.

Postural control is reactive and its task is body stabilization in the sense that the body is prevented from falling over. This may apply to different desired body-support (body on support) or body-space (body in space) orientations. Often, the task is to maintain a desired body-space orientation for stabilizing a given eye or hand work space. The balancing represents then the platform onto which volitional ('proactive') self-movements are superimposed. The balancing is relatively simple when it is restricted to the anterior–posterior, a–p, plane and when the body sway angles are small. Then, the head, arms, trunk, and legs essentially form a rigid segment, or link, that tends to sway about an axis through the ankle joints: this situation allows treating body biomechanics as a single 'inverted pendulum' [5]. This balancing is called the 'ankle strategy'.

In some situations, the balancing involves the hips to various degrees, depending on a number of factors such as disturbance magnitudes or restrictions of foot support or motor or sensory conditions ('hip strategy' [5]; then, in addition, the knees may get involved. Very large disturbance magnitudes may even evoke 'rescue reactions' such as steps, hopping, or holding with the hand. These reactions are then usually superimposed on the ankle joint stabilization.

There is evidence emerging which suggests that in cases of lesions or loss of information from one receptor or control system, another set of commands or strategy may be used to regain a sufficient postural control [6]. If so, there should be possibilities to evaluate the effects and differences of various lesions and the applied therapies.

The measuring and analysis of spontaneous or stimulus evoked sway is called posturography.

16.1 Posturography Without Perturbations

Quiet stance is called unperturbed stance. However, the standing body as an inverted pendulum is inherently unstable. Gravitational torque arising with its angular excursions away from the ideal gravitational vertical tends to tip it over. Therefore, gravity will here be considered an external stimulus.

Measurement of body movements to quantitatively and objectively evaluate postural control and responses led to the development of different sets of posturography. The basic concept depends on measurement of the forces actuated by the feet against the ground, measured with a forceplate. The forceplate consists of force transducers placed to pick up the distribution of forces which are vertical or horizontal to the ground. The simultaneous recordings from several transducers allow calculation of the moment produced by the standing human in different directions and shear (or transitional) forces to normalize effects of weight of different subjects.

The data may then be used to calculate the projection of forces against the ground. Although body sway is generally characterized in terms of kinematic and kinetic variables such as centre of mass (COM) rotation about the ankle joint and centre of pressure (COP) shifts on the support surface, respectively, it is of utmost importance to the understanding of posturography to realize that the recorded projection of all forces against the ground is not the same as a projection of the subject centre of mass (or gravity) but just the centre of forces. The trace that is recorded is thus not equivalent to movements, especially fast ones, but rather to the stabilizing forces.

Different variables may be derived from the force measurements. The sway amplitude, sway variance, of sway in either anteroposterior or lateral planes or sway path, sway velocity, and sway area describing two-dimensional movements are commonly used variables to evaluate postural competence [7].

The passive ankle joint stiffness is too weak to maintain the body upright during quiet stance. Instead, quiet stance is controlled actively, which is reflected in a continuously changing ‘spontaneous’ sway. Power density plots of the sway exhibit a clear preponderance at low frequencies [8]. The sway is not fully explained by internal motions due to heartbeat, breathing, etc., but appears to reflect mainly fluctuations of the active torque. Possible sources are sensor noise, central processing noise, and irregularities in actuator performance. Complete sway suppression appears not to be a goal of stance control. As a result of the sway, the COM excursion and the gravitational torque it evokes vary over time. This represents a sensory stimulus that in turn evokes changes in active torque. The active torque stands out in the COP as rapid variations [9]. Comparing experimental findings of such COM and COP changes with corresponding simulations using a COM angle control model.

Although measurements of quiet stance may contribute to separation of groups of subjects with different lesions, the normal variations are so wide that classification of individual responses and, hence, clinical usefulness becomes ambiguous. To master such shortcomings, different techniques to increase the demands on the postural control are applied. The idea is that if there is a deficit in the postural control system that is not evident because of the redundancy and adaptability of the systems, the deficit will become evident if further sensory information is lost or distorted. The classical Romberg test uses evasion of visual clues to load the postural system. Likewise, posturography can be performed and results compared with open and closed eyes. This is a standard procedure used in most test set-ups [10]. If the increase of sway compared to normals is greater with open eyes than with closed eyes, this might be taken as suggesting less effective use of visual clues and may be, but not unequivocally, interpreted as a sign of decreased CNS function. A foam rubber pad can be positioned between the feet of the subject and the forceplate to reduce mechanoreceptor sensation from the soles of the feet and increase the difficulties in stabilizing the body. The patient can be asked to place his head in different positions to increase difficulties with vestibular cervical interaction.

The role of static posturography in body sway assessment still has a limited clinical use because of its intrinsic high variability which does not permit a reliable diagnosis. There are no reports concerning the intersubject coefficients of variation (CV) of static posturography parameters in healthy subjects. In order to make static posturography a reliable clinical tool, it is necessary to use parameters with a CV lower than 15 %. It is possible using 'sensory ratio' formulas, like sensory integration tests of the EquiTest equipment, which is probably the most widespread commercially available equipment that utilizes six sets of disturbed sensory information to estimate a sensory integration set.

It is possible to calculate similar 'sensory ratio' with standard static posturographic equipments including values from the unstable condition on foam pads. According to Di Berardino et al. [11], the most reliable parameters in static posturography were given by the use of bilayer rubber foam pads. The CV of the visual and vestibular percentages were about 10 %. Therefore, the lowest variability suggests that these percentages derived from the 'sensory ratios' using bilayer foam pads, together with somatosensory one that was about 14.4 %, are the most acceptable parameters for clinical use. Furthermore, the role of 'sway-related' tests with foam pads, proposed by Allum et al. [12], is fundamental in order to make static posturography more useful.

16.2 Posturography with Induced Perturbations

Balancing is often investigated in response to three external mechanical stimuli, which are body-support surface tilt, surface translation, and contact force (e.g. a push or pull having impact on the body).

To further load human postural control with the purpose of revealing deficits, the standing subject may be exposed to different perturbations, and the responses to recover quiet stance are evaluated.

In the T-Post system from Toennies, the subjects stand, leaning somewhat backwards, and the platform then tilts and induces a further backward movement of the body. The subjects have to move forward to avoid falling; latencies and amplitudes of this movement can be combined with EMG recordings to estimate response latencies. The method can detect movement and probe synergistic muscle activity if combined with EMG. In the motor coordination test of the EquiTest, the platform is either tilted or translated with different velocities, and the postural reactions of the subject are measured.

Vibration toward the antigravity muscles induces a sensation of movement and involuntary body movements [12]. This has been used to perturb the standing human for diagnostic purposes, calculating vibration-induced body sway (VBS). Patients with posterior fossa lesions are reported to have larger responses when vibrated toward the neck muscles than the calf muscles, compared to subjects with vestibular lesions. Vibration toward the calf muscles according to a pseudorandom binary stimulus (PRBS) induces an on- and off-going perturbation which can be used to estimate an input–output relation and model postural control, which allows estimation of the so-called characteristic parameters of postural control. Comparing these parameters, one can get an estimation of the postural control of the subject. The use of these parameters can distinguish, for example, between an acoustic neuroma and an acute vestibular lesion and also distinguish subjects with cervical disorders. Patients who recover from hemispheric stroke demonstrate remaining differences in postural control when evaluated with those parameters [13].

A vestibular spinal perturbation may evoke both lateral and anteroposterior body sway by galvanic stimulation of the vestibular nerves. Evaluation of these responses may give further information in posterior fossa lesions, but so far clinical studies are lacking. Visual stimulation inducing a sensation of small amplitude translatory movements of the surroundings may induce perturbations in the anteroposterior plane, which, not surprisingly, differs in subjects with cerebellar lesions [14]. The effect of visual stimulation, however, may be dependent on attention and state of mind, and different patterns of response may be assumed in normal subjects. So far visually induced perturbations, with the exception of the so-called stabilized visual frame in EquiTest measurements, have not been used in clinical routine to the knowledge of the author [15].

References

1. Baloh RW, Honrubia V (2001) Clinical neurophysiology of the vestibular system, 3rd ed. Oxford University Press, New York; Trauma, pp 322–332
2. Brandt T, Krapczyk S, Malbenden L (1981) Postural imbalance with head extension. Improvement by training as a model for ataxia therapy. Ann N Y Acad Sci 374:636–649

3. Forth KE, Metter JE, Paloski WH (2007) Age associated differences in postural equilibrium control: a comparison between EQscore and minimum time to contact (TTCmin). Gait Posture 25:56–62
4. Clark S, Riley MA (2007) Multisensory information for postural control: sway-referencing gain shapes center of pressure variability and temporal dynamics. Exp Brain Res 310: 176–299
5. Nashner LM, Black FO, Wall C 3rd (1982) Adaptation to altered support and visual conditions during stance: patients with vestibular deficits. J Neurosci 2:536–544
6. Riley MA, Baker AA, Schmit JM, Weaver EE (2005) Effects of visual and auditory short term memory tasks on the spatio-temporal dynamics and variability of postural sway. J Mot Behav 37:311–324
7. Baloh RW, Jacobson KM, Beykirch K (1998) Static and dynamic posturography in patients with vestibular and cerebellar lesions. Arch Neurol 55:649–654
8. Contarino D, Bertora GO, Bergmann JM (2003) Balance platform: mathematical modeling for clinical evaluation. Int Tinnitus J 9:23–25
9. Di Fabio RP (1996) Meta-analysis of the sensitivity and specificity of platform posturography. Arch Otolaryngol Head Neck Surg 122:150–156
10. Shumway-Cook A, Horak FB (1986) Assessing the influence of sensory interaction of balance: suggestion from the field. Phys Ther 66:1548–1550
11. Di Berardino F, Filipponi E, Barozzi S, Giordano G, Alpini D, Cesarani A (2009) The use of rubber foam pads and "sensory ratios" to reduce variability in static posturography assessment. Gait Posture 29(1):158–160
12. Allum JHJ, Zamani F, Adkin AL (2002) Differences between trunk sway characteristics on a foam support surface and on the Equitest1 ankle-sway-referenced support surface. Gait Posture 16:264–270
13. Horak FB, Henry SM, Shumway-Cook A (1997) Postural perturbations: new insights for treatment of balance disorders. Phys Ther 77:517–533
14. Dehail P, Petit H, Joseph PA (2007) Assessment of postural instability in patients with traumatic brain injury upon enrolment in a vocational adjustment programme. J Rehabil Med 39:531–536
15. Magnusson T (1994) Extracervical symptoms after whiplash trauma. Cephalalgia 14: 223–227

Static Posturography and Whiplash

17

P.L. Ghilardi, A. Casani, B. Fattori, R. Kohen-Raz, and D.C. Alpini

17.1 Static Posturography

The quiet upright position (Stance) is controlled by three distinct sensorial cues organs: visual, somatosensorial (from skin and pressure sensors in the feet) and vestibular (mainly from otolithic maculae).

Posture is more stable when all the sensory systems operate. However, the weightening of each cue is adjusted in the vestibular nuclei and cerebellum [xxx] according to the surface, the environment and the task. SOT test (see part I) is designed to investigate the specific weightening of different cues in stance control. The sequence of posturographic test adopted is aimed to investigate postural interactions between sensorial cues, ranging from complete sensorial control (eyes open standing on a solid surface) to quite exclusively pure vestibular control (eyes closed standing on foam). Inputs from the vestibular canals and somatosensory system stabilize posture more effectively at higher frequencies of body sway, while visual and otolith-organ signals are more effective at lower frequencies. The amplitude threshold for detection of body sway differs between senses: the somatesthesic senses have the lowest threshold, vision the next and the vestibular system has the highest threshold.

Whiplash can affect the balance system through an involvement of one or more of these structures:

1. The neck proprioceptors
2. The peripheral vestibular system
3. The central vestibular system

P.L. Ghilardi • A. Casani • B. Fattori
Institute of Otorhinolaryngology, University of Pisa, 56100 Pisa, Italy

R. Kohen-Raz
The School of Education, The Hebrew University of Jerusalem, Har ha-Tsofim, Jerusalem, Israel

D.C. Alpini (✉)
ENT-Otoneurology Service, IRCCS "Don Carlo Gnocchi" Foundation, Milan, Italy
e-mail: dalpini@dongnocchi.it

D.C. Alpini et al. (eds.), *Whiplash Injuries*,
DOI 10.1007/978-88-470-5486-8_17, © Springer-Verlag Italia 2014

After whiplash, an abrupt increase in discharge from the neck proprioceptors, usually asymmetric, might be generated by an overexcitation of the sympathetic fibres related to the B receptors of the deep cervical erector muscles [1, 2].

Several studies have reported altered postural control in people with neck pain and disturbances in static balance have been demonstrated [3].

Non-specific neck pain or whiplash-associated disorder (WAD) exhibit greater postural instability than healthy controls, signified by greater COP excursions irrespective of the COP parameter chosen. In particular, COP excursions are particularly increased in WAD compared to healthy individuals.

Further, the decreased postural stability in people with neck pain appears to be associated with the presence of pain and correlates with the extent of proprioceptive impairment, but appears unrelated to pain duration [4–6].

Post-traumatic vertigo is not a clinical entity, but this term refers only to the common aetiology of a heterogeneous collection of vestibular disorders. Even if there are many convincing signs indicating the existence of anatomical and functional connections between the neck and the vestibular system, the assessment of vertigo after whiplash is extremely complex. No reliable clinical, electronystagmographic or posturographic test exists to confirm the linkage between the neck trauma and the vertiginous symptoms.

Keeping these observations in mind, static posturography could provide useful information about the postural conditions of patients suffering from vertigo after whiplash.

Before the introduction of computerized posturography (PG), the VSR was studied using various tests (Romberg, Fukuda, Unterberger, Babinski-Weil, Ataxia test battery, etc.) which nevertheless do not permit a quantitative and objective study of postural function. Falls and difficulties in dynamic task, such as single-leg stance with eyes closed, the step test, tandem walk on a firm and soft surface, stair walking and the timed 10 m walk with and without head movement, have also been reported [7].

Routinely, posturography (PG) recording is performed under two basic conditions:

1. Patient standing on the platform with eyes open (EO)
2. Patient standing on the platform with eyes closed (EC)

Besides these basic tests to verify the presence of a latent postural disorder, other destabilizing tests are usually employed. We use two types of examinations to verify this:

1. Patient standing on the platform with EC and with the head in extreme retroflexion (EC-HER)
2. Patient standing on the platform with EC immediately after head shaking (EC-HST)

The parameters we can achieve from the computer elaboration are shown in Table 17.1. An important difference between the PG and the older techniques for the study of posture is that the former provides us with precise objective data which can be compared throughout time for each patient and each with different pathologies of balance.

In this context, PG, performed with particular types of stimuli or provocation tests, may identify a cervical origin of the dizzy symptoms. Through tests performed with rotation ("cervical dynamic activation") [8, 9], "head turned" [10] (Fig. 17.1) and retroflexion of the head [11] (Fig. 17.2), it will be possible to obtain some information on how cervical inputs can generate instability syndromes. However, positive results obtained with the above-mentioned tests must be evaluated within the entire clinical context because they cannot be considered as pathognomonic.

Table 17.1 The main parameters and the graphic elaborations obtained by computer, the role of the proprioceptive inputs in patients suffering from postural disorders

Parameters	Graphic elaborations
X min, max, mean	Displacement of pressure centre on X axis
X min, max, mean	Displacement of pressure centre on Y axis
Velocity of the sway	Its standard deviation is an index of the "homogeneity" of the postural oscillations
Length L (mm)	Total sway path of centre of pressure
Surface S (mm^2)	Is indicative of the precision of the system
L.F.S.	Correlation function between L and S
Statokinesigram	Area covered by the sway
Stabilogram	Displacement on time of the sway for X and Y
Fast Fourier transform	
Romberg's index	Ratio between the same value with EC and EO

This allows a quantification of the importance of the pressoreceptor system for balance and provides us with useful information for the management of rehabilitation treatment

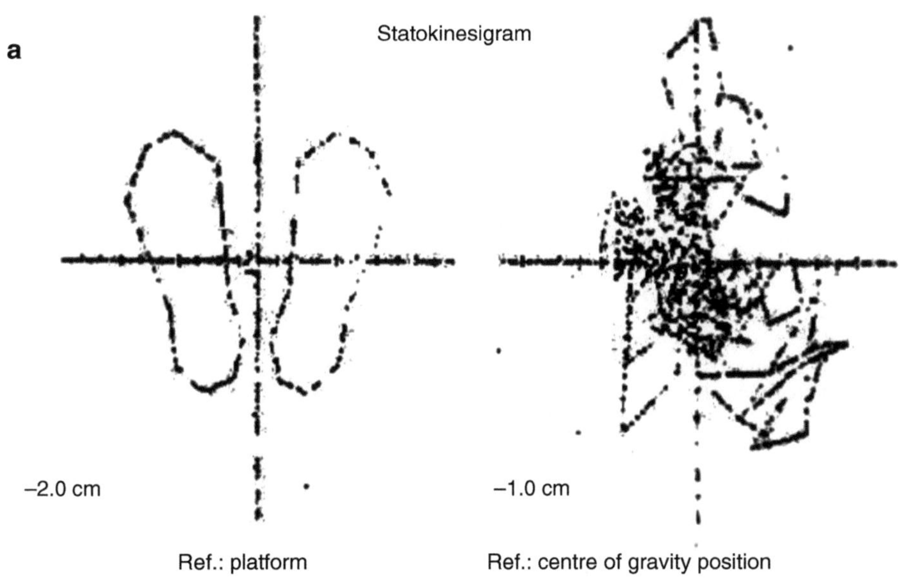

Fig. 17.1 (**a–c**) Patient suffering from vertigo from WI. (**a**) Normal result in EO. (**b**) The SKG is abnormal when the head of the patient is rotated towards the right. (**c**) A similar pattern can be observed with the head rotated to left

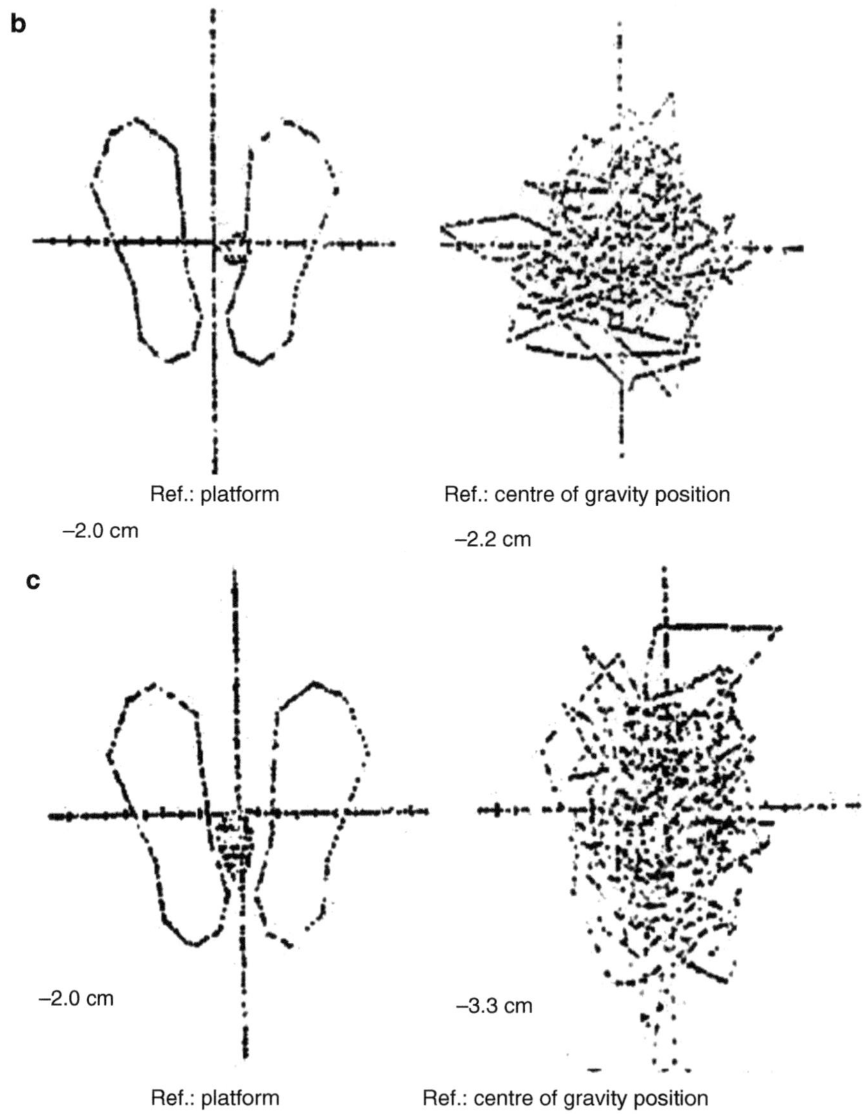

Fig. 17.1 (continued)

Armato and Ferri [12] published a study on 569 patients with whiplash, with or without associated head injuries. Of these, 21 % had either normal vestibular functioning or only static stabilometric alterations that were compatible with a modified proprioception of the cervical spine.

Cobo et al. [13] investigated 99 women. Fifty-four women had suffered whiplash within 2 weeks and 45 were included in a healthy control group. Static

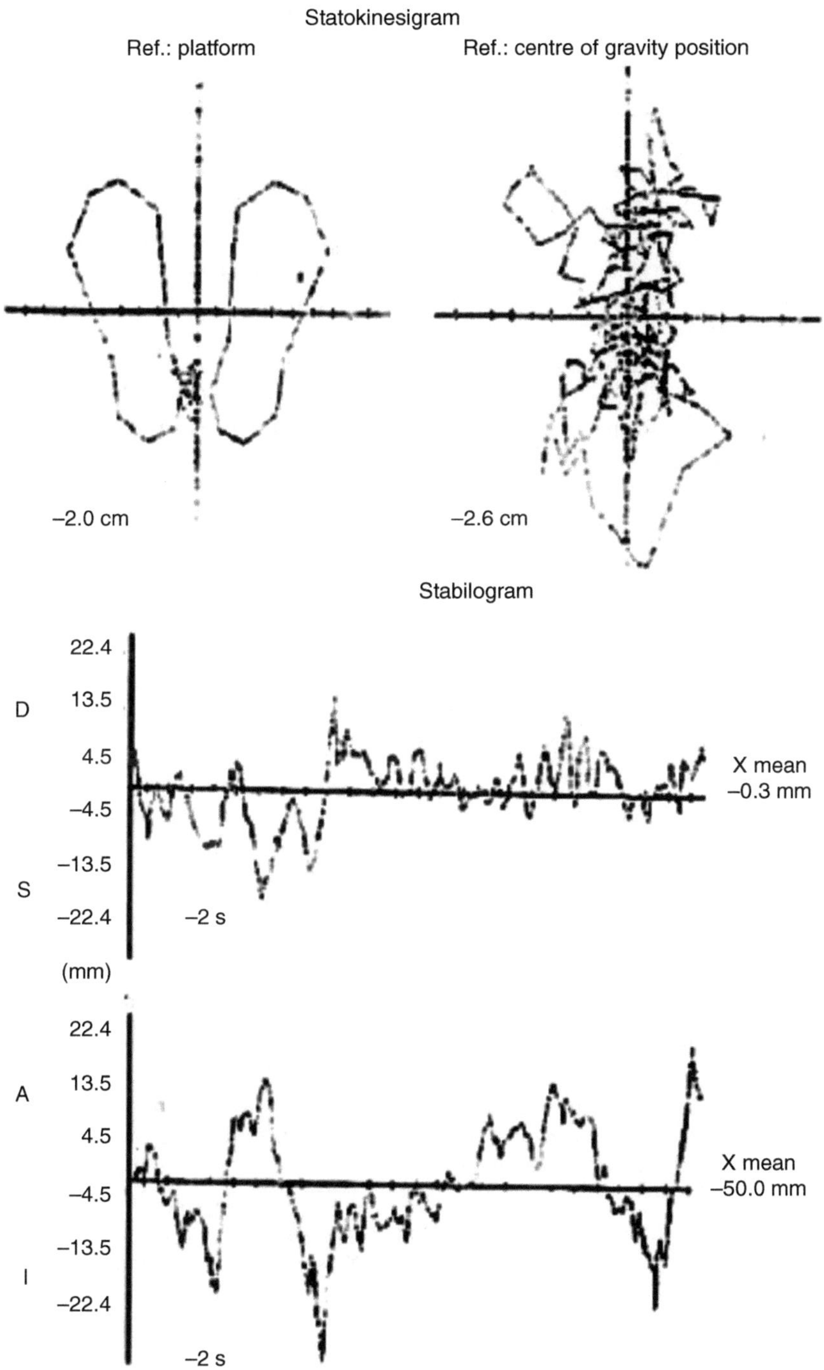

Fig. 17.2 Patient suffering from WI. *Above*, the pathological SKG in EO-HER; *below*, the SBG shows a prevalence of the oscillation on the anterior-posterior axis

posturography on a force platform was carried out in all study participants, by means of the Romberg test in four sequential phases, using the postural sway area as a dependent variable. The visual analogue scale (VAS) and Northwick Park Neck Pain Questionnaire (NPH) were used to evaluate pain and function. Postural sway area increased significantly in each of the consecutive phases in both groups. The differences of the means of the postural sway area were statistically significant in all Romberg phases ($p = .009$ to $p = .000$). No correlation was found between postural sway area and VAS or NPH scores. There was a positive correlation between the postural sway area standing on a thick foam cushion placed over the plate with closed eyes and the number of days of transitory incapacity ($r = 0.414$; $p = .009$).

Two groups of subjects have been studied by Nacci et al. [14]: Group A included 90 subjects (age range, 17–73 years; mean age, 40.8 ± 12.6; 59 females and 31 males) suffering from whiplash injury (Grades 1 and 2 of the whiplash-associated disorders classification – WAD) and Group B comprised 20 subjects (age range, 23–79 years; mean age, 42.8 ± 17.1; 10 females and 10 males) with whiplash injury (Grades 1 and 2 of the WAD) associated with minor head injury (14–15 in the Glasgow Coma Scale – GCS) [41]. All the subjects ($n = 110$) in the study complained of a balance disorder (postural instability, uncertain gait, vertigo, etc.) that had arisen after trauma. The vestibular-spinal reflex (VSR) in all patients was investigated by means of static stabilometry using the S.Ve.P. Amplifon System©. The stabilometric test (performed within 15 days of trauma, like the vestibular test) was carried out with eyes open (EO), eyes closed (EC) and closed eyes with head retroflexed (CER). To evaluate the role of cervical proprioceptive afferences, the cervical interference index corresponding to the surface (SCI) and to the length of the oscillations (LCI) was calculated from the percentage ratio between the S and L values when the eyes were closed and the head retroflexed and the same parameter when the eyes were closed but the head was erect, considering a value less than 120 as normal 43.

To eliminate any cases of simulation, stabilometry was performed twice within the same session in EO, EC and CER (retest) 25. Moreover, to exclude exaggerated or simulated postural behaviour, subjects who had intercorrelation stabilometric recordings that appeared frankly sinusoidal and/or those who had over 2,000 mm surface values in OE were excluded from the study (12 subjects) 25 44. None of the subjects in Group A ($n = 90$) or Group B ($n = 20$) showed stabilometric recordings of sinusoidal intercorrelation in all three tests (OE, CE, CER). As far as the altered posturographic recordings are concerned, while there was no specific pattern in the two groups, they were clearly pathologic, especially during CER. Both in OE and in CE, there was an increase in the surface values and in those pertaining to shifting of the gravity centre on the sagittal plane, which was even more evident during CER. As far as the indices of cervical interference are concerned in Group A, there was pathological SCI (n.v. < 120) in 59 cases (59/90; 65.6 %) and pathological LCI (n.v. < 120) in 44 (44/90; 48.8 %). In Group B, 11 cases with pathological SCI (11/20; 55 %) and 12 with pathological LCI (12/20; 60 %) were found.

Since vestibular compensation develops after whiplash, the postural performance improves progressively, even if in certain patients a persistent backward displacement of the pressure centre could be noticed [15]. Often it is only through

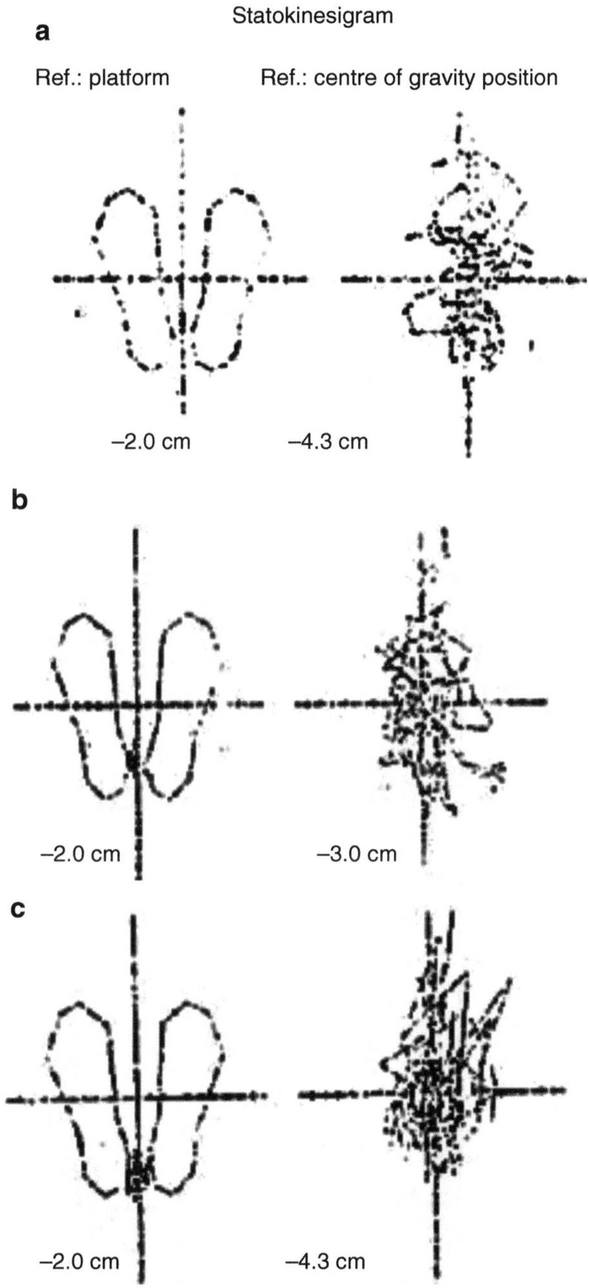

Fig. 17.3 (**a–c**) Patient suffering from UVL after a WI with EO (**a**) stabilometry is normal. Only with EO-HST (**b**) can an abnormality of SKG be detected. With EO-HER (**c**) postural stability shows a marked worsening

sensitization tests (EC–HST, EC-HER) that it is possible to detect latent static postural deficiencies not evident in basic conditions (EO and EC) (Fig. 17.3) [16]. Moreover, the PG allows assessing when some patients have reached a normal postural performance even retroflexion. Under these conditions a remarkable increase in the oscillations on the Y axis and a displacement of the pressure centre towards the critical side are detected (Fig. 17.4) [17].

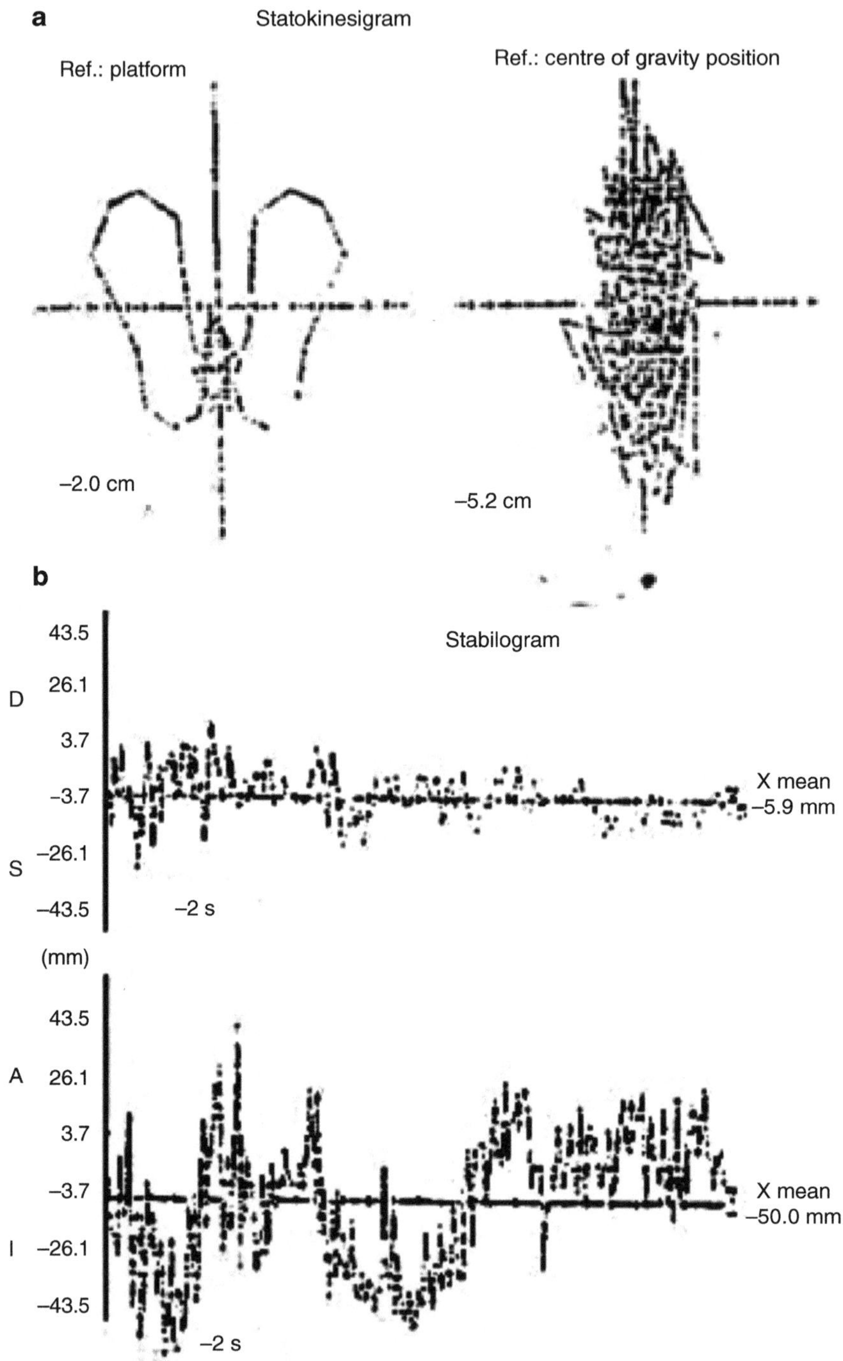

Fig. 17.4 (**a**, **b**) Patient suffering from PPV after WI. The SKG with OC-HER (**a**) is abnormal; the SBG (**b**) shows a prevalence of the oscillation on the anterior-posterior axis

Nevertheless, it must be considered that the findings may be altered or modified because of the combined actions of more than one degree of lesion.

Beside a definition of the postural damage, static PG allows visualizing and quantifying the extent of the disease and the effects of therapy on postural behaviour in patients with VSR deficiency.

This observation has to be kept in mind in the case of patients suffering from postural abnormalities following WI in whom the posturographic test performed in EC-HER plays an important role for evaluating the significance of the cervical proprioceptive input at the base of the vertiginous symptoms. In this framework, PG seems to be very useful for monitoring both postural deficiencies and the subsequent therapy.

Increased values of slow-sway component magnitude are evidenced in patients with WAD despite of neck pain as assessed by Röijezon et al. [18].

In addition to the increase of postural sway that is more evident in anteroposterior direction (Ruhe A review), a recent work has evidenced that, during balance tasks with closed eyes and one-legged stance, the relative mean activity of the anterior scalene, sternocleidomastoid, neck extensors and upper trapezius muscles, expressed as mean relative activity related to maximum voluntary electromyography (%MVE) measured by surface electromyography, was significantly increased in WADs compared with healthy controls [19].

17.2 Tetra-ataxiametric Posturography

Tetrax system (Tetrax-IBS equipment by Sunlight Medical Ltd., Tel Aviv, Israel) 25–27 (CE patent n. 93741CE02; FDA establishment registration n. 3006701790) consists of four independent mobile force plates, two for each foot. The plates are positioned in order to measure any equilibrium disturbance from the two forefeet and two heels. Each plate contains a strain-gauge force transducer, which is sensitive to vertical force. Tetrax provides independent output from the four balance plates and, by taking the average of all four measurements, provides a description of body sway in terms of displacement of the patient's centre of pressure. Subjects are requested to stand quietly on the platforms in a quiet room in four different conditions: eyes open and eyes closed on a solid surface and eyes open and eyes closed on a foam pad in order to reduce somatosensorial and visual information [20–22].

The system measures the changes and fluctuations of the vertical force exerted by the corresponding heel or forefoot during the default 30-s experimental time and emits four separate wave signals at a sampling rate of 34 Hz. On the basis of these fluctuations, the system computes a general stability score (ST), normalized for body weight according to the following equation:

$$ST = t\{\Sigma n1[(an - an-1)2 + (bn - bn-1)2 + (cn - cn-1)2 + (dn - dn-1)2]\}1/2/W.N$$

where a, b, c and d are the four pressure transducers, W is body weight, t is experimental time and n is the number of signals sampled at 34 Hz.

Tetrax provides both quantitative and qualitative sway analysis.

17.3 Quantitative Sway Analysis

General stability (ST) is, therefore, calculated as an index, which refers to a mean of oscillations, recorded by each plate: the higher the value, the lower the stability. It is the quotient of the sum of the amplitudinal changes (body sway), recorded in microvolts and divided by body weight. While it is not a direct measurement of postural stability, the fluctuations of the vertical ground reaction force normalized for body weight have been found to correlate with both the static and dynamic parts of Berg's balance test and with the anteroposterior centre of pressure (COP) velocity [28]. In fact, the ST score provides information about the adequacy of postural adjustments. A lower ST indicates smaller fluctuations and therefore better postural control, and it has also been seen to be significantly correlated to the equilibrium score of the Equitest posturography system. The weight distribution index (WDI) is calculated on the basis of the relative recorded weight at each of the four supports: the higher the WDI, the higher the abnormal distribution of the weight that had to be theoretically equally divided between the four supports.

17.4 Qualitative Sway Analysis

Fourier analysis of sway frequencies is a mathematical treatment of wave signals of body oscillations on the horizontal plane produced by the patient in order to maintain an upright position.

The Tetrax system combines the signals from the left and right leg to result in one sway frequency with a sampling rate of 34 Hz, as described by Kohen-Raz [23, 24]. The four signals recorded at the four sensors are analysed with the Fourier transformation, and then Tetrax recalculates an average of the results obtained providing a unique parameter.

Fourier analysis is then carried out to determine which signal frequencies are most common. Fourier analysis of sway frequency distribution shows that a normal postural performance is characterized by a high intensity at the low range, and this appears to indicate that posture is controlled with minimal effort, not involving any activity of the semicircular canals, which are considered to be insensitive to body displacements below 0.2 Hz.31 Fourier analysis of sway frequencies is divided into eight frequency bands (F1–F8). Posturography with an interactive balance system was recorded by means of equipment with four sensors; therefore, Fourier transformations were derived from four independent wave signals and were presented in the form of a spectrum, broken down into the following eight frequency bands: F1 0.01–0.1, F2 0.1–0.25, F3 0.25–0.35, F4 0.35–0.50, F5 0.50–0.75, F6 0.75–1.00, F7 1.00–3.00 Hz and F8 above 3.0 Hz.

Previous studies on the Fourier spectral analysis of postural sway by Tetrax (25, 26, 30–33) have shown that typical ranges of postural frequency (i.e. frequency bands) express the different levels of activity of postural subsystems, the systems that affect postural sway. Study of postural frequency can provide insights into the individual's use of these postural subsystems, which include the vestibular, somatosensory and other subsystems to maintain postural stability. Thus, spectral analysis of postural sway might be a valuable tool in clinical diagnosis. Tetrax posturography has been shown to have a high test-retest reliability.

Dehner et al. [25] investigated the balance control in patients with acute QTF grade II whiplash injuries of the cervical spine by means of Tetra-ataxiametric posturography in 40 patients with acute QTF grade II whiplash injuries and 40 healthy matched controls. The stability index ST and the Fourier analysis FA (0.10–1.00 Hz) were established for eight standing positions and sum scores were calculated. The pain index was established using a visual analogue scale ranging from 0 to 100. A follow-up examination was conducted for the patients after 2 months. The patients with acute whiplash injuries of the cervical spine achieved significantly poorer results for both ST and FA than the healthy controls. There were no differences between the eight standing positions for both ST and FA. After 2 months, 17 patients had no change in the pain development, 21 patients showed an improvement in pain intensity and two patients had deteriorated. The subgroup of patients with improvement in pain intensity showed a significant improvement in balance control concerning the FA compared to patients with unchanged pain intensity. Authors concluded that patients with acute whiplash injuries have a reduced balance control as compared to matched controls. This study gives an indication that post-traumatic neck pain is associated with impairments of postural control.

Kohen-Raz (unpublished data) coordinated a multi-country study in 90 chronic WAD patients (Israel, Germany and Czech Republic) about Tetrax and WI. The research was pointed to document backward displacement of COG following WI as previously reported. Backward displacement is characterized, in Tetrax analysis, by increasing of weight on the heels particularly evident during retroflexion of the head. Heel weight displacement is due to whiplash-induced disruption of head-to-trunk coordination that is necessary to maintain stability of ground projection of COG during head movements: in normals when the head moves backward, the trunk and the pelvis moves forward in order to counteract head displacement, while in WAD patients this kind of coordination is lost. WAD patients were compared to 90 healthy subjects from the same countries. A Student's *t*-test confirmed a significant ($p<0.05$) weight displacement on the heels in WAD patients with respect to normals in the three countries when patients retroflexed their head.

17.5 Trunk Sway Measurement

In 2003 Allum et al. [26] proposed the use of body-worn sensors measuring angular velocity (gyroscopes) or the acceleration of the trunk to effectively quantify balance during stance and gait tasks to track improvements in postural control during recovery from an acute unilateral peripheral vestibular deficit (UVL) and, successively, in order to detect potential elderly fallers [27]. Postural control was quantified using simple measurements of trunk sway: amplitudes of trunk sway angle and angular velocity, in the roll and pitch directions as well as task duration, were examined for a battery of stance and gait tasks. Sjostrom et al. [28] used the same device in WAD patients. Trunk sway occurring during clinical stance and gait tasks was compared between a group of subjects with a chronic whiplash injury, resulting from an automobile collision, and a normal collective. Twenty-five subjects with history of whiplash injury and 170 healthy age-matched control subjects participated in the study. Trunk sway angular displacements in chronic whiplash patients were assessed for a number of stance and gait tasks similar to those of the Tinetti and Clinical Test of Sensory Interaction and Balance (CTSIB) protocols. Data analysis revealed several significant differences between the two groups. A pattern could be identified, showing greater trunk sway for stance tasks and for complex gait tasks that required task-specific gaze control such as walking up and down stairs. Trunk sway was less, however, for simple gait tasks that demanded large head movements but no task-specific gaze control, such as walking while rotating the head. They concluded that subjects who have a chronic whiplash injury show a characteristic pattern of trunk sway that is different from that of other patient groups with balance disorders. Balance was most unstable during gait involving task-specific head movements which possibly enhance a pathologic vestibulo-cervical interaction.

Vonk et al. [29] used trunk sway measured during several stance and gait tasks in 18 patients suspected of malingering in order to differentiate these from 20 patients who had suffered unilateral vestibular loss 3 months earlier, 20 patients with documented whiplash injuries and 34 healthy controls. Classification results ranged from 72 to 96 % and were equally accurate for task or criteria variables based on 90 % sway values. The tasks yielding the best discrimination were standing with eyes closed on a foam and firm surface, standing with eyes open on a firm surface, standing on one leg and walking tandem steps. The criteria yielding the best discrimination were standing with eyes open on a firm surface, the difference between standing with eyes closed on foam and firm surfaces, the difference between walking tandem steps and standing on one leg with eyes open and the difference between roll and pitch velocity when walking eight tandem steps. We conclude that discriminating suspected malingering balance disorder patients is possible using variables or criteria based on objective measures of trunk sway during several stance and gait tasks.

Findling et al. [30] showed a greater trunk sway for stance tasks and complex gait tasks (e.g. walking up and down stairs) in patients with whiplash injury with and without mild traumatic brain injury while they showed equal reductions in trunk sway with respect to controls for simple gait tasks (e.g. walking while rotating the head).

References

1. Bexander CS, Hodges PW (2012) Cervico-ocular coordination during neck rotation is distorted in people with whiplash-associated disorders. Exp Brain Res 217(1):67–77
2. Hinoki M (1985) Vertigo due to whiplash injury: a neurotological approach. Acta Otolaryngol (Suppl 419):9–29
3. Silva AG, Cruz AL (2013) Standing balance in patients with whiplash-associated neck pain and idiopathic neck pain when compared with asymptomatic participants: a systematic review. Physiother Theory Pract 29(1):1–18

4. Jongkees LBW (1983) Whiplash examination. Laryngoscope 93:113–114
5. Toglia IU (1976) Acute flexion-extension injury of the neck: electronystagmographic study of 309 patients. Neurology 26:808–814
6. Ruhe A, Fejer R, Walker B (2011) Altered postural sway in patients suffering from non-specific neck pain and whiplash associated disorder – a systematic review of the literature. Chiropr Man Therap 19(1):13
7. Stokell R, Yu A, Williams K, Treleaven J (2011) Dynamic and functional balance tasks in subjects with persistent whiplash: a pilot trial. Man Ther 16(4):394–398
8. Nakagawa H, Ohashi N, Watanabe Y, Mizukoshi K (1993) The contribution of proprioception in posture control in normal subjects. Acta Otolaryngol (Suppl 504):112–116
9. Norré ME (1990) Posture in otoneurology. Acta Otorhinolaryngol Belg 44:183–363
10. Roberts TDM (1973) Reflex balance. Nature 244:158–185
11. Rubin AM, Young JH, Milne AC (1975) Vestibular-neck integration in vestibular nuclei. Brain Res 96:99–102
12. Armato E, Ferri E, García Purrinos F (2001) Results of video nystagmographic (VNG) analysis in vestibular post-traumatic pathology. Acta Otorrinolaringol Esp 52(7):567–574
13. Cobo EP, Mesquida ME, Fanegas EP, Atanasio EM, Pastor MB, Pont CP, Prieto CM, Gómez GR, Cano LG (2010) What factors have influence on persistence of neck pain after a whiplash? Spine (Phila Pa 1976) 35(9):E338–E343
14. Nacci A, Ferrazzi M, Berrettini S, Panicucci E, Matteucci J, Bruschini L, Ursino F, Fattori B (2011) Vestibular and stabilometric findings in whiplash injury and minor head trauma. Acta Otorhinolaryngol Ital 31(6):378–389
15. Casani A, Ghilardi PL, Fattori B, Vannucchi R (1991) The neuro-otological findings following mild head injury. In: Claussen CF, Kirtane MV (eds) Vertigo, nausea, tinnitus and hypoacusia due to head and neck trauma. Eisevier Science Publ, Amsterdam, pp 133–136
16. Yoneda S, Tokumasu K (1986) Frequency analysis of body sway in the upright posture. Acta Otolaryngol 102:87–92
17. Diener HC, Dichgans J, Guschlbauer B, Mau H (1984) The significance of proprioception on postural stabilization assessed by ischemia. Brain Res 296:103–109
18. Röijezon U, Björklund M, Djupsjöbacka M (2011) The slow and fast components of postural sway in chronic neck pain. Man Ther 16(3):273–278
19. Juul-Kristensen B, Clausen B, Ris I, Jensen RV, Steffensen RF, Chreiteh SS, Jørgensen MB, Søgaard K (2013) Increased neck muscle activity and impaired balance among females with whiplash-related chronic neck pain: a cross-sectional study. J Rehabil Med 45(4):376–384
20. Kohen-Raz R, Hiriartborde E (1979) Some observations on tetra-ataxiametric patterns of static balance and their relation to mental and scholastic achievements. Percept Mot Skills 48:871–890
21. Kohen-Raz R, Volkmar FR, Cohen DJ (1992) Postural control in children with autism. J Autism Dev Disord 22:419–432
22. Gstöttner M, Neher A, Scholtz A, Millonig M, Lembert Kohen-Raz R (1991) Application of tetra-ataxiametric posturography in clinical and developmental diagnosis. Percept Mot Skills 73:635–656
23. Kohen-Raz R, Himmelfarb M, Tzur S, Kohen-Raz A, Shub Y (1996) An initial evaluation of work fatigue and circadian changes as assessed by multiplate posturography. Percept Mot Skills 82:547–557
24. Morad Y, Azaria B, Avni I, Barkana Y, Zadok D, Kohen-Raz R (2007) Posturography as an indicator of fatigue due to sleep deprivation. Aviat Space Environ Med 78:859–863
25. Dehner C, Heym B, Maier D, Sander S, Arand M, Elbel M, Hartwig E, Kramer M (2008) Postural control deficit in acute QTF grade II whiplash injuries. Gait Posture 28(1): 113–119
26. Allum JH, Adkin AL (2003) Improvements in trunk sway observed for stance and gait tasks during recovery from an acute unilateral peripheral vestibular deficit. Audiol Neurootol 8(5):286–302
27. Allum JH, Carpenter MG (2005) A speedy solution for balance and gait analysis: angular velocity measured at the centre of body mass. Curr Opin Neurol 18(1):15–21

28. Sjostrom H, Allum JH, Carpenter MG, Adkin AL, Honegger F, Ettlin T (2003) Trunk sway measures of postural stability during clinical balance tests in patients with chronic whiplash injury symptoms. Spine 28(15):1725–1734
29. Vonk J, Horlings CG, Allum JH (2010) Differentiating malingering balance disorder patients from healthy controls, compensated unilateral vestibular loss, and whiplash patients using stance and gait posturography. Audiol Neurootol 15(4):261–272
30. Findling O, Schuster C, Sellner J, Ettlin T, Allum JH (2011) Trunk sway in patients with and without, mild traumatic brain injury after whiplash injury. Gait Posture 34(4):473–478

Dynamic Posturography

18

S. Barozzi, B. Monti, D.C. Alpini, and F. Di Berardino

Different stable postures are possible according to the relative position of the three principal muscle-joint systems – ankles, knees and hips – between the body's COG and the base of support (Fig. 18.1).

When external perturbations happen, the COG oscillates differently according to the postural movement strategy adopted by each individual, depending on the amplitude of the body's displacement and on individual structural patterns.

The ankle strategy is most effective for small COG movements: the body acts like a rigid mass and rotates about the ankle joints. This is possible by contracting the ankle, thigh and lower trunk muscles.

The hip strategy, in contrast, is mostly used for large COG movements: the body sways, moving the hips forward and backward with little ankle movement. This generates horizontal reaction forces against the support surface opposite to the direction of hip movement. The stepping strategy operates in order to avoid a fall when the destabilizing force shifts the COG beyond the limits of stability (Fig. 18.2) [1, 2].

S. Barozzi • F. Di Berardino
Department of Clinical Sciences and Community Health,
University of Milan, Milan, Italy

Audiology Unit, IRCCS "Ca' Granda" Ospedale Maggiore Policlinico, Milan, Italy

B. Monti
Private ENT Center "Otorinolaringoiatri Associati",
Corso Stati Uniti 39, 10129 Turin, Italy

D.C. Alpini (✉)
ENT-Otoneurology Service, IRCCS "Don Carlo Gnocchi" Foundation,
Milan, Italy
e-mail: dalpini@dongnocchi.it

D.C. Alpini et al. (eds.), *Whiplash Injuries*,
DOI 10.1007/978-88-470-5486-8_18, © Springer-Verlag Italia 2014

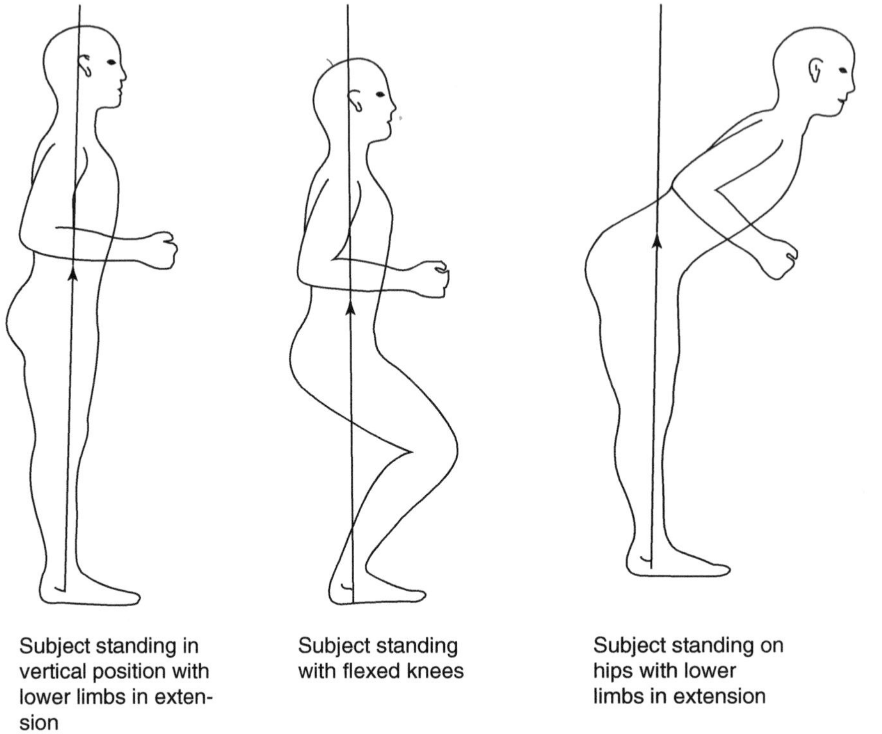

Fig. 18.1 Position of centre of gravity in different standing postures

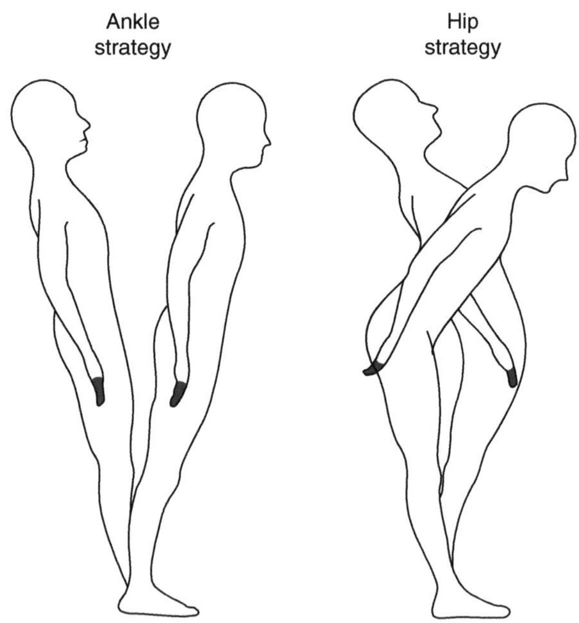

Fig. 18.2 Different strategies to counteract displacements of COG

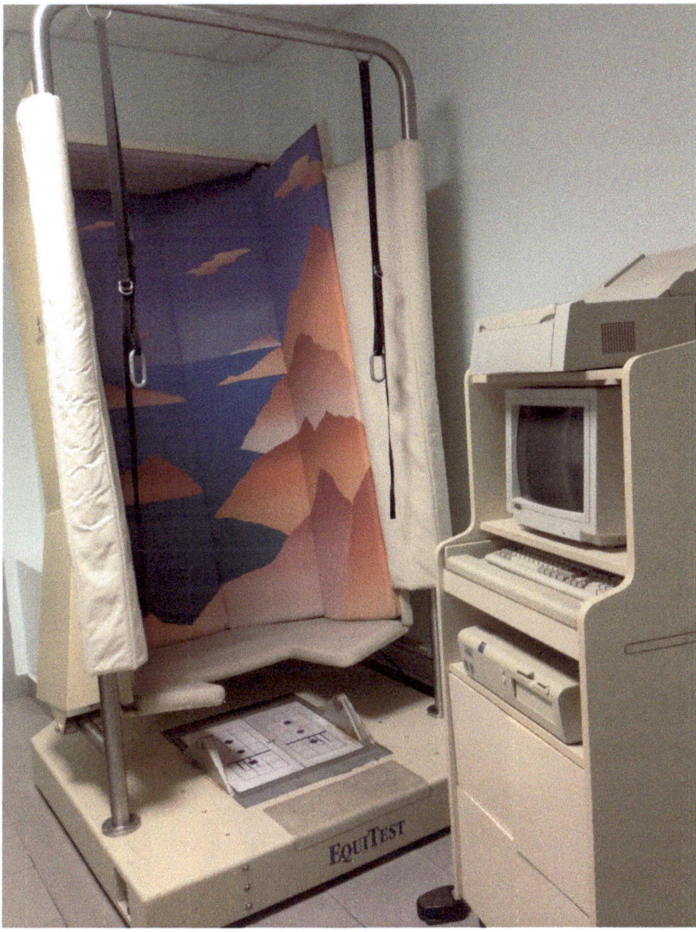

Fig. 18.3 The Equitest system

18.1 Equitest: Description of the System

The Equitest system (NeuroCom International, Inc; Clackamas, Oregon) [3, 4] is a dynamic posturography device which allows different movements of the support surface and different conditions of integration of sensory inputs (Fig. 18.3). The Equitest system consists of:

- A platform provided with pressure-sensitive strain gauges located in each quadrant. It can translate horizontally forward or backward and rotate about an axis colinear with the ankle joint.
- A movable visual surface which encloses the patient's visual surrounding and rotates about an axis colinear with the ankle joint.
- Computer, monitor and printer which analyse, visualize and print data. The Equitest standard protocol consists of two tests: (1) the sensory organization test (SOT) and (2) the motor control test (MCT).

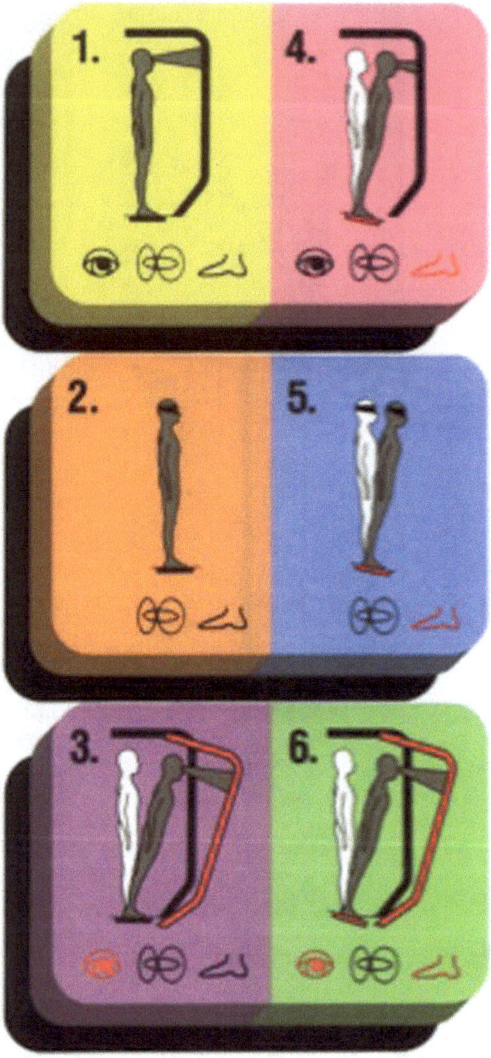

Fig. 18.4 The sensory organization test

18.1.1 Sensory Organization Test

The SOT assesses the ability of a subject to use visual, vestibular or somatosensory information to maintain upright stance under different sensory conditions [5, 6]. Tests conditions are meant to isolate the function of each equilibrium subsystem by reducing the contribution of others or by presenting conflicting sensory inputs. Thus, during the test, the platform and the visual surrounding are fixed or rotated proportionally to any forward or backward sway of the subject (sway-referenced support and sway-referenced visual surrounding) according to the following six combinations (Fig. 18.4):

1. Normal vision (fixed support)
2. Absent vision (fixed support)
3. Sway-referenced vision (fixed support)

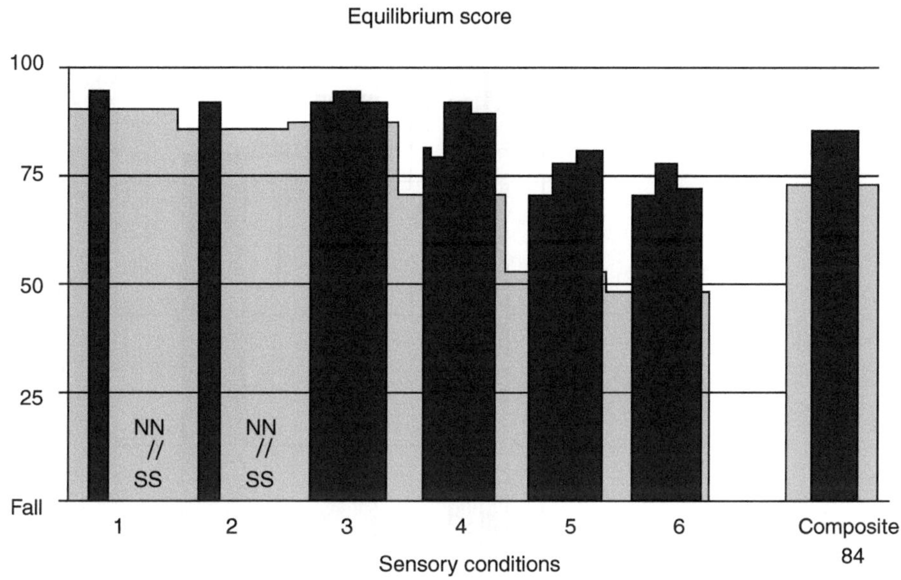

Fig. 18.5 The composite score

4. Normal vision (sway-referenced support)
5. Absent vision (sway-referenced support)
6. Sway-referenced vision (sway-referenced support)

Information from a sense subjected to sway referencing suggests that the orientation of the body's COG relative to gravity is not changing when in fact it is. Normally, individuals ignore a sway-referenced sensory input and maintain balance by using other sensory inputs.

In addition to sway referencing, eyes-closed conditions are used to further isolate the somatosensory and vestibular systems. The original test scheme does not reduce or confound the contribution of the vestibular system. Head extension may also be useful because it places the utricular otolith organs in a disadvantageous position [7, 8]. Head extension also enhances cervical proprioceptive input; therefore, it could be favourably employed in testing balance of whiplash-injured patients. To highlight the importance of dynamic posturography to detect clinical equilibrium disturbances, Fitzpatrick et al. [9] in a study on perturbed stance, showed that feedback control alone does not allow stable balancing with large disturbances. In the same way, Horak et al. [10] in 2002 observed that disturbance compensation, which is incomplete (only partial) with small disturbances, increases with increasing stimulus magnitude.

A computerized system evaluates COG sways and calculates, for each test, the equilibrium score, comparing the patient's maximum anterior to posterior COG displacement to the theoretical maximum displacement of 12.5°.

The Equitest analysis programme also calculates:

- The composite score, the average of all conditions' scores (Fig. 18.5)
- Sensory analysis, which allows identification of a sensory dysfunction and/or an abnormal sensory preference by calculating the ratios of different sensory conditions (Fig. 18.6)

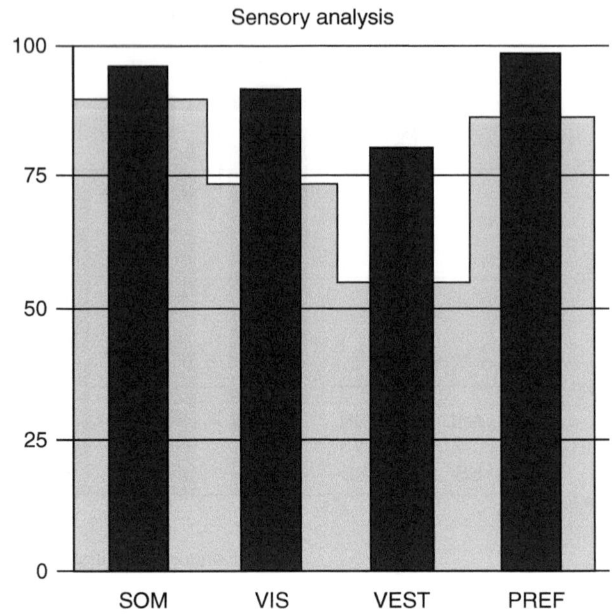

Fig. 18.6 The sensory analysis

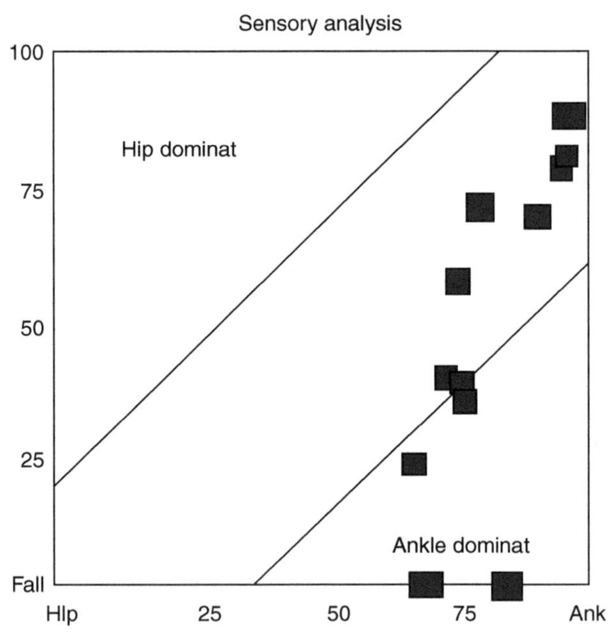

Fig. 18.7 The strategy analysis (ankle dominant)

- The strategy of movement adopted to maintain upright stance (ankle strategy, hip strategy) (Fig. 18.7)
- The COG alignment (Fig. 18.8)

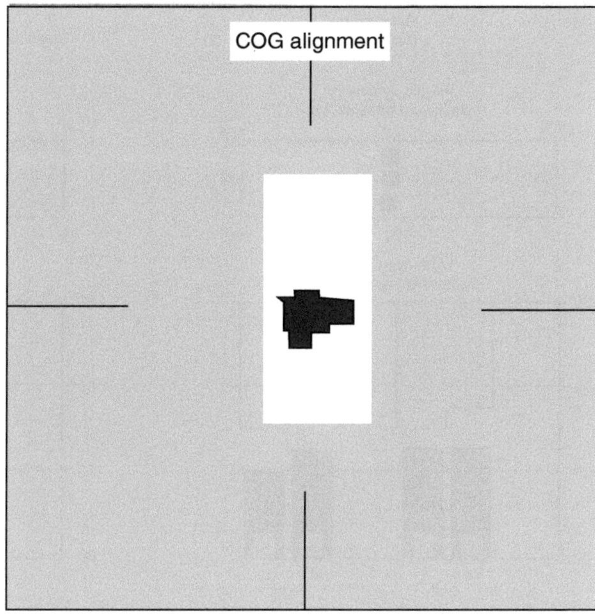

Fig. 18.8 The COG alignment

18.1.2 Motor Control Test

The MCT studies automatic postural responses to unexpected movements of the base of support: small, medium and large backward translations; small, medium and large forward translations. Each trial is analysed in terms of latency, amplitude and symmetry of response. When the support surface is unexpectedly translated forward or backward, the body initially remains stationary and becomes offset relative to the base of support. The stiffness of ankle joints initially resists to the sway but is insufficient to stabilize the COG sway.

In backward translations, when the ankle strategy is used to counteract the forward displacement, a sequential activation of distal to proximal extensor muscles is adopted (gastrocnemius, hamstrings, paraspinal muscles). These muscle activations help to stabilize knee and hip joints so that the body moves as a coordinated unit about the ankle joint [11].

When the hip strategy is used, we observe an activation of the flexor muscles of the hip joint (quadriceps and abdominals) that moves the body backward [12].

In forward translations, when the ankle strategy is used, we assist with a sequential activation of distal to proximal flexor muscles (tibialis anterior, quadriceps and abdominals).

In the hip strategy, the hip joint moves forward to activate paraspinal muscles and hamstrings. In the MCT the platform is also tilted abruptly up and down to evaluate adaptation to disruptive balance forces [13].

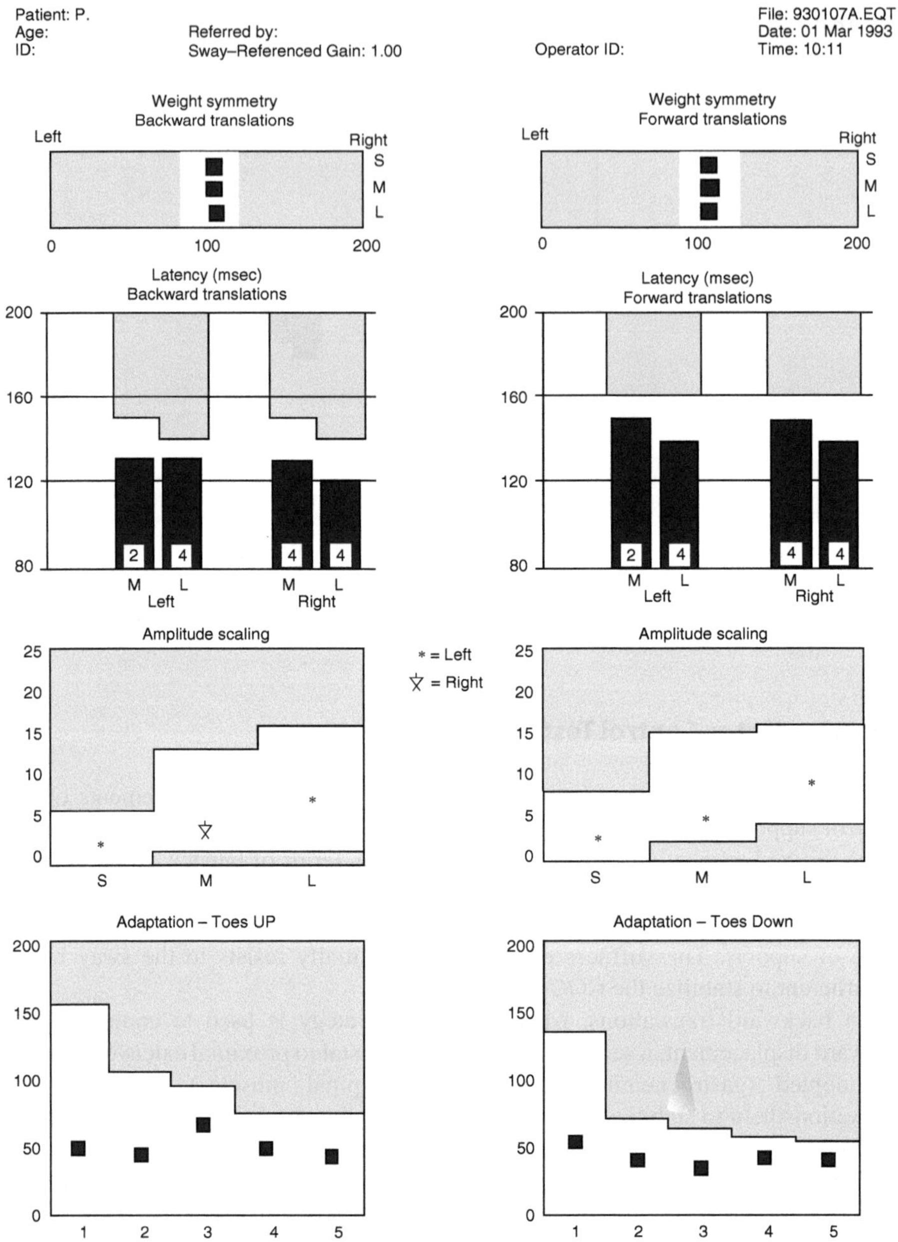

Fig. 18.9 The motor control test

Toes-up rotations of the support surface stimulate proprioceptors in the gastrocnemius muscles of both legs and elicit muscle forces which tend to destabilize posture [14, 15]. The adaptation test assesses the patient's ability to ignore these disruptive somatosensory inputs within five trials (Fig. 18.9).

18.2 Dynamic Posturography in Whiplash Injuries

The Equitest is a modern device which provides an objective assessment of balance function in its entirety. With the composite score we have an individual global equilibrium measure which can be compared to the average score of clinically normal individuals of the same age.

Several studies made in the normal population confirmed the confidence and the repeatability of computerized dynamic posturography results.

Many patients with "whiplash syndrome" experience unrelenting neck stiffness and pain. This abnormal muscular tension is postulated to be causally related to a central disorder of postural control, which has evolved secondary to injury of the inner ear labyrinthine structures.

Moving platform posturography was used by Chester [16] to demonstrate the presence or absence of a static or dynamic equilibrium disorder in 48 patients who had experienced the oscillation forces induced by a rear-end automobile collision. Other vestibular tests were used to document dysfunction of the semicircular canals and the otolith structures. A high percentage of patients were found to have faulty inner ear functioning, leading to inefficient muscular control of balance and erect posture. Active perilymph fistulas were identified at surgery in seven patients.

Kogler et al. [17] investigated a total of 32 healthy subjects (16 men, 16 women, age range 21–58 years), and ten patients age range 27–62 years (mean 44 years) with neck problems and associated balance problems since a whiplash injury were tested for postural control using the Equitest. The normal subjects were initially split into four-age groups in order to estimate the effects of age on performance. The postural stability was evaluated for dependence of support surface conditions (stable or sway-referenced), visual input (eyes open or closed) and head position (neutral, left rotated, right rotated, extended backwards or flexed forward). As expected, visual cues as well as stable support surface improve postural stability ($p<0.001$). Postural stability is statistically different in the head-extended-backward condition compared with the other four head positions ($p<0.001$ in all cases) in both patients and controls. Eliminating this test condition from the analysis, only a slight ($p<0.05$) difference between head forwards and head turned left remained. This pattern of results remained if the normal subjects were only split into two age groups instead of four. Finally, the patient group exhibited significantly lower postural performance than all the groups of normal subjects ($p<0.01$), but none of the normal groups differed significantly from each other. It is concluded that the postural control system is significantly challenged in the head-extended-backward condition in both normal subjects and patients with previous whiplash injury and persistent neck problems. The patient group differed statistically from all groups of normal subjects. This suggests that neck problems impair postural control and that the head-extended position is a more challenging task for the postural system to adapt to.

Our experience in evaluating whiplash injuries has showed that in the SOT the composite score can separate, in a confident manner, normal subjects at a conventional neurotologic evaluation from pathological ones. The only discordance was given by benign positional vertigo results which can be normal at SOT.

The opportunity to have available, objective and repeatable data is important in medical-legal cases following whiplash injuries [18].

For this purpose computerized dynamic posturography can detect patients who exaggerate symptoms of unsteadiness when test results are physiologically inconsistent. In our experience, in case of deliberate exaggeration of symptoms, we found one or more of the following inconsistent patterns:

1. Composite scores lower than 42 % in subjects who do not have ataxia and ambulate without the use of balance aids.
2. Better performances under more difficult conditions (4–5–6) then under easier ones (1–2–3).
3. Declining performances during successive trials, with a percentage of equilibrium in the first trial at least two standard deviations greater than the third.
4. Sinusoidal sway traces of COG.
5. Dispersion of the x–y plots of the initial COG alignment.
6. Sudden falls after periods of relative stability in the SOT.
7. Abnormal adaptation in toes-up and toes-down rotation. In our experience, the 70 % of patients with cervical distortional trauma and with an abnormal composite score and consistent test show vestibular dysfunction patterns on SOT sensory analysis (the sensory ratio of conditions 5/1 is abnormal).

With somatosensory and visual inputs misleading and unavailable, such as in condition 5, the upright position is allowed by otolith vestibular function which controls the extensor antigravity muscles. Therefore, vestibular inputs assessed by sensory analysis are prevalently from the otolith rather than from the canal organs. For this reason in patients with peripheral vestibular disorders, Equitest results do not always agree with caloric tests.

So, the abnormal vestibular function found in most patients with cervical trauma can be explained by a deficit in the extensor antigravity muscles [19].

The motor control strategy most commonly observed in sequences of whiplash injuries is the ankle strategy. This is evident in the strategy analysis where points fall along a nearly vertical line on the right of the plot. This finding means that patients are abnormally dependent on ankle movements even when the amplitude of sway approaches the limits of stability.

In patients who underwent whiplash injuries, trauma directed to the cervical spine usually reverberates along the whole column causing a hypofunction of the erector muscles and a prevalence of the flexors which moves forward the body's COG.

In order to resist the tendency of falling forward and to move the COG inside the base of support, some corrective postural arrangements are used: forward trunk flexion on the hip with consequent hip stiffness or flexion on the knees.

The choice of a strategy for balancing COG movements depends on personal past experiences, on the individual history of previous accidents and pre-existent muscle and joint impairments.

Therefore, although the ankle strategy is the most common pattern in cervical traumas, this does not mean that it must be found in all patients with whiplash injuries.

In interpreting Equitest results, the strategy analysis can influence the choice of rehabilitative treatment; in cases of prevailing ankle strategy, we adopt exercises aimed at potentiating the extensor muscles and only afterwards exercises with the purpose of recovering hip mobility.

In MCT the evaluation of latency offers interesting considerations: latencies within normal ranges are observed either in forward or in backward translations only in a limited number of patients with whiplash injuries. In our experience 86 % of patients have abnormal latencies either in forward (10 %) or in backward translations (12 %) or in both (64 %). Response-strength scores and weight symmetry have always been normal. In whiplash injuries abnormal latencies can be explained as disorders in the afferent somatosensory pathways.

References

1. Johansson R, Magnusson M, Àkesson M (1988) Identification of human posture dynamics. IEEE Trans Biomed Eng 35:858–869
2. Johansson R, Magnusson M (1991) Human postural dynamics. Crit Rev Biomed Eng 18: 413–437
3. Black FO, Nashner LM (1982) Workshop III – information processing in the normal and abnormal human postural control systems. Am J Otol 3(4):384–389
4. Black FO, Wall C 3rd, Nashner LM (1983) Effects of visual and support surface orientation references upon postural control in vestibular deficient subjects. Acta Otolaryngol 95(3–4):199–201
5. Nashner LM (1983) Analysis of movement control in man using the movable platform. Adv Neurol 39:607–619
6. Black FO, Nashner LM (1984) Vestibulo-spinal control differs in patients with reduced versus distorted vestibular function. Acta Otolaryngol Suppl 406:110–114
7. Nashner LM, Black FO, Wall C 3rd (1982) Adaptation to altered support and visual conditions during stance: patients with vestibular deficits. J Neurosci 2(5):536–544
8. Forssberg H, Nashner LM (1982) Ontogenetic development of postural control in man: adaptation to altered support and visual conditions during stance. J Neurosci 2(5):545–552
9. Fitzpatrick R, Burke D, Gandevia SC (1996) Loop gain of reflexes controlling human standing measured with the use of postural and vestibular disturbances. J Neurophysiol 76(6):3994–4008
10. Horak FB, Dickstein R, Peterka RJ (2002) Diabetic neuropathy and surface sway-referencing disrupt somatosensory information for postural stability in stance. Somatosens Mot Res 19(4):316–326
11. Dietz V (1992) Human neuronal control of automatic functional movements: interaction between central programs and afferent input. Physiol Rev 72(1):33–69
12. Magnusson M, Johansson K, Johansson BB (1994) Sensory stimulation promotes normalization of postural control after stroke. Stroke 25:1176–1180
13. Gabell A, Simmons MB (1982) Balance coding. Phys Ther 68:286–288
14. Brandt T (1988) Sensory function and posture. In: Posture and gait, vol 812, International congress series. Exerpta Medica, Amsterdam, pp 127–136
15. Norré ME (1990) Posture in otoneurology, vol I. Acta Otorhinolaryngol Belg 44:55–181
16. Chester JB Jr (1991) Whiplash, postural control, and the inner ear. Spine 16(7):716–720
17. Kogler A, Lindfors J, Odkvist LM, Ledin T (2000) Postural stability using different neck positions in normal subjects and patients with neck trauma. Acta Otolaryngol 120(2):151–155
18. Storaci R, Manelli A, Schiavone N, Mangia L, Prigione G, Sangiorgi S (2006) Whiplash injury and oculomotor dysfunctions: clinical-posturographic correlations. Eur Spine J 15(12):1811–1816, Epub Mar 22
19. Madeleine P, Prietzel H, Svarrer H, Arendt-Nielsen L (2004) Quantitative posturography in altered sensory conditions: a way to assess balance instability in patients with chronic whiplash injury. Arch Phys Med Rehabil 85(3):432–438

The Cervico-Cephalic Interaction 19

D.C. Alpini, V. Mattei, D. Riva, and F. Di Berardino

19.1 Introduction

While the first function of posture is an antigravity function, the second one is to provide an interface with the external world for perception and action. For this reason, body posture is built up by a set of assembled segments with own mass that are linked together by flexible joints controlled by the neuromuscular system. Posture based on the superimposed segments (the head, the trunk and legs) is under the specific automatic central and peripheral control preserving the specific orientation of each segment with respect to gravity and/or to the adjacent segment. The central organization of posture involves interactions between external forces, the mechanical properties of the body and the neuromuscular forces.

Head stabilization appears to be a necessary motor control [1] in order to provide a stable orientation platform (regarding both gravity and environment landmarks) necessary for an adequate progression of body movement. Input from different systems are essential to control posture and head stabilization and it has been postulated [2] that high motor and sensory mechanism are necessary both for simplest conditions like standing (posture control) [3] and walking (head control).

D.C. Alpini (✉) • V. Mattei
ENT-Otoneurology Service, IRCCS "Don Carlo C. Gnocchi" Foundation, Milan, Italy
e-mail: dalpini@dongnocchi.it

D. Riva
International Society of Proprioception and Posture, via Valgioie 87, 10146 Torino, Italy

F. Di Berardino
Department of Clinical Sciences and Community Health, University of Milan, Milan, Italy

Audiology Unit, IRCCS "Ca' Granda" Ospedale Maggiore Policlinico, Milan, Italy

D.C. Alpini et al. (eds.), *Whiplash Injuries*,
DOI 10.1007/978-88-470-5486-8_19, © Springer-Verlag Italia 2014

Adequate posture and head controls are specific tasks of the vestibular system [4], and they are particularly important in daily activities. Body is not a rigid block but a flexible system formed by multiple segments tied together by the muscles surrounding the joints. When a movement is performed by a standing subject, like walking, the geometry of the body is changed. Dynamic posture, in fact, can be considered as superimposed modules from feet to the head, each linked to the next by a set of muscles which have their own specific central and peripheral regulation serving to maintain the module reference position. The reference position of each the modules can be regulated independently from that of the others. Dysfunction of cervical receptors in neck disorders has been shown to lead to disturbances in postural stability, causing a disruption of the intricate coordination between eye, neck and trunk movements. These changes in cervico-cephalic coordination may underlie clinical symptoms reported by people with WAD that involve changes in function during walking [5].

The aim of the chapter is to describe specific instrumental tests able to investigate alteration of cervico-cephalic control provoked by whiplash.

19.2 CranioCorpoGraphy (CCG)

Head destabilization seems to be the specific target to investigate equilibrium disturbances in whiplash patients. Since 1968, CranioCorpoGraphy (CCG) has been used as a simple procedure to evaluate head-trunk stabilization in vestibular disorders [6]. It has proved to be one of the most efficient, quick, objective and quantitative tests for screening equilibrium function for nearly 20 years, and the West German Labour Security Surveillance Board introduced it for occupational medical ability testing in 1983. CCG records light tracings from light bulbs on the forehead, the occiput and both shoulders through a camera mounted from above (Fig. 19.1).

The recording is displayed on film (Fig. 19.1b) from an instant camera fixed above the head of the patient and directed towards a mirror on the ceiling. The results are radar-like images, and the investigator evaluates a complete movement pattern during stepping by visually inspecting the craniocorpogram. This enables the clinician to differentiate between vertigo of central and of peripheral origin [7, 8].

CranioCorpoGraphy (CCG) has been successively digitalized (dCCG) on the basis of the optoelectronic technology [9]. Digital CranioCorpoGraphy (dCCG) is a non-invasive assessment based on a 50 Hz CCD camera for acquiring the position of four markers placed on the subject who walks on the spot (Fukuda Stepping test) (Fig. 19.2).

A digital stepping analyzer (DSA.) recognizes these markers and identifies their 2D positions in the horizontal plane. These rough data are then transferred to a workstation through a universal asynchronous receiver transmitter (UART) for processing and following elaborations. The UART allows a sampling rate of 25 Hz, and so it fixes the maximum sampling rate of the whole system [9].

The output is a report that gives both analogue and quantitative information. The subject performs the test blindfolded in a semi-darkened and sound-proofed room that removes audio-visual orientation landmarks. Subjects are asked to walk on the spot at their preferred speed for at least 30 s. Claussen and Claussen [7] used a metronome in his experiments, but in our experiment the subjects walked at their preferred speed to avoid the sound of a metronome distracting them. dCCG gives qualitative information on the pattern of absolute movement and analyses the following parameters for each marker and for the coupled head and shoulder (trunk) markers:

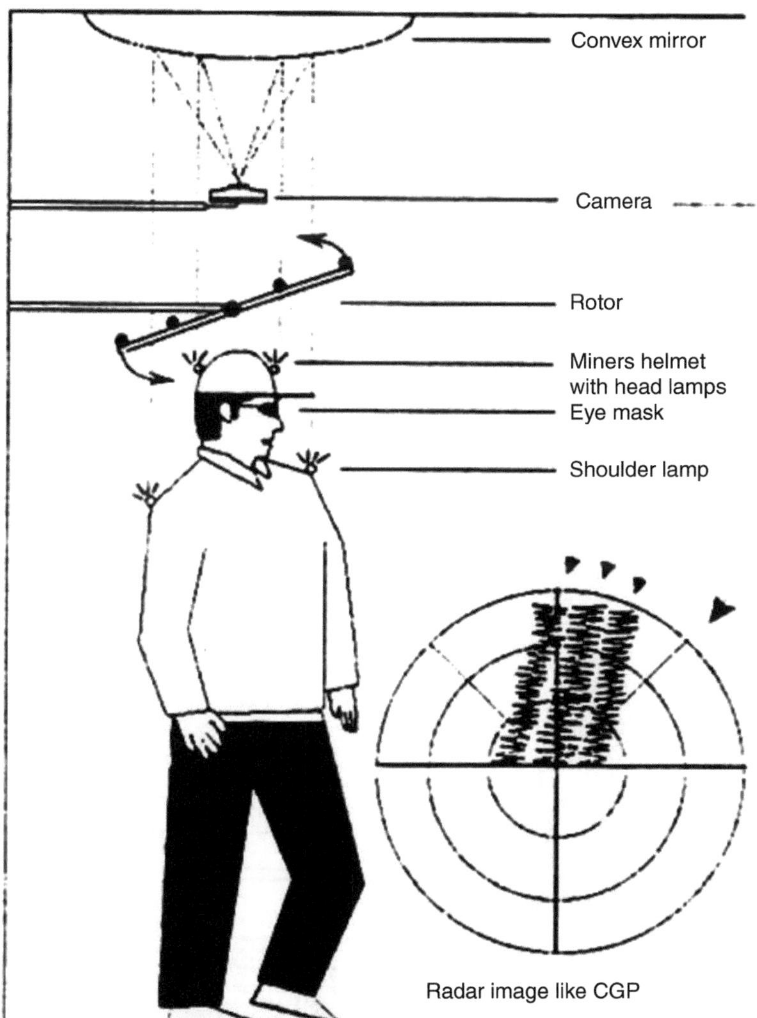

Fig. 19.1 A schematic representation of CGP (craniocorpography). Subjects walk on place in a dark room, and movements of the light bulbs placed on the head (*helmet*) and shoulder impress the film in an instant Polaroid camera in order to obtain four light traces on a *black* imagine

- Total distance: total distance (in cm) traced by the marker during body movement.
- Speed: mean marker global speed (cm/s).
- Lateral speed: mean marker lateral component speed (cm/s).
- Longitudinal speed: mean marker longitudinal component.
- Global speed (cm/s).
- Head rotation: represents the absolute difference of head rotation in the transversal plane from the beginning to the end of the test.
- Shoulder rotation: is the absolute difference of trunk rotation from the beginning to the end of the test.
- Spin body: it shows the relative position of the head with respect to the trunk during the stepping test.
- Index of coordination (%): because marker movement is composed of longitudinal (body forward projection) and lateral (body sway) components, it compares the two components to calculate lateral dispersion of body movement during forward progression.

Due to the complexity of the data analysed for each marker, a coefficient of performance (CP) was calculated to simplify the cut-off between normal and pathological tests. CP clearly identified an abnormal stepping pattern.

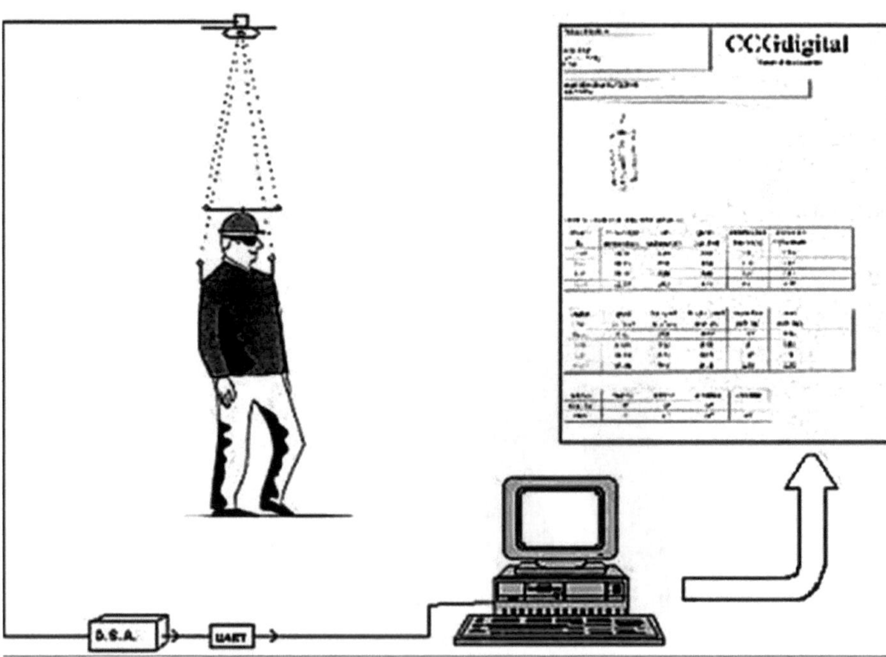

Fig. 19.2 Two passive reflective markers (*front* and *rear*) are set at the extremities of a stick attached to a worker's hardhat, while two markers (*left* and *right*) are attached on rigid shoulder supports

Fig. 19.2 (continued)

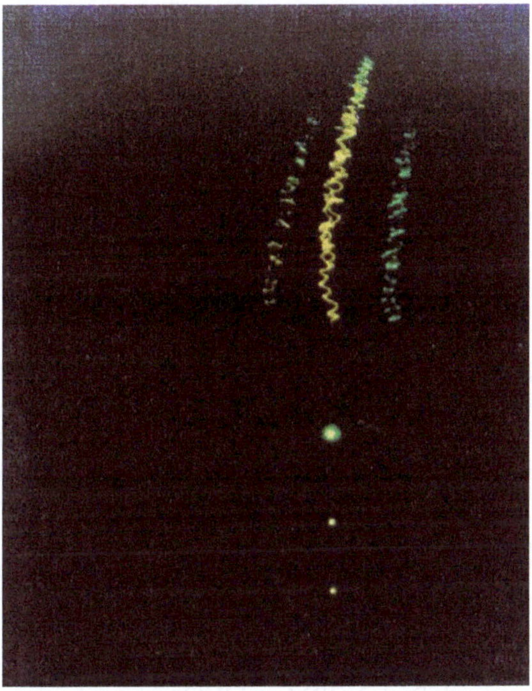

By means of dCCG, Alpini et al. [10] investigated 25 healthy subjects and 33 WAD's patients. Whiplash patients were classified as chronic (more than 6 months after injury) and recent (less than 6 months after injury). Clear differences between healthy subjects and patients were seen and three different patterns were detected:

- Pattern A: patients appeared similar to normals but quantitative analysis showed significant differences with paradoxical head over-stabilization (collar-effect).
- Pattern B: with decreased head stability.
- Pattern C: with decreased head stabilization and reduced displacements of the body.

Whiplash patients presented also different abnormal findings with respect to the different parameters considered, but all of those with pattern B or C showed abnormal CP, that to say whiplash patients presented a specific abnormality in head-to-trunk stabilization. Head destabilization following whiplash may be correlated to a central failure of head anticipatory stabilization. Anticipatory postural adjustments mean that the onset of postural change occurred before the onset of the postural disturbance due to the movement. Thus, a feedforward postural control is associated with movement control, which prevents the posture and equilibrium disturbances associated with movement performance from taking place. From these data, it seems that sensorimotor mechanisms progressively lose the ability to maintain head posture during movement with a progressive alteration of movement pattern of the whole body the longer the interval after trauma. Thus, while pain and neck stiffness are more frequent in the early period from trauma, complex disorganization of dynamic equilibrium seem to be a more significant feature later. Complete pattern disruption was evident in patients with pattern C in which head velocity was increased, rotation of the shoulder and body torsion increased and dynamic control of body centre of mass lacking, which lead to a nonprogressive or sometimes a backward stepping pattern.

Decreasing body forward progression may also be due to direct involvement of thoracic and cervical muscle proprioceptive disturbance. Only in patients with a 'normal' stepping pattern (A) did the complex evaluation of stepping performance indicate that the specific locomotor task was not disturbed. Thus, the CP is consistent with and can indicate normality of stepping control.

Different stepping patterns in different subjects after similar injuries may be explained by the intermodular model of postural control that may be controlled both in a bottom-up and in a top-down manner according to the task and the environment. In this way, whiplash could lead to significant alterations of dynamic postural control in those subjects preferentially organized with a top-down posture control.

In order to estimate the effects of cervical proprioception disturbance in WAD group, only 'chronic' patients, with a trauma which occurred more than 6 months before examination and still suffering neck pain and dizziness, were considered. All the subjects, with eyes closed, walked on place on rigid surface (RIG) and on foam (FOAM). In RIG test, head stabilization is depending on vestibular and proprioceptive cues, while in FOAM test, improved vestibular control of head stabilization is required. Both NORM and WAD adopted a personal frequency of steps; the duration of test depends on the cadence of the subject considered since almost 60 steps and 35 s were required. An optoelectronic system ELite (BTS Bioengineering S.p.a.) (sample rate 25 Hz) [11] composed of two CCD cameras mounting wide-angle objectives (C-Mount ¼″ with 2.8 mm focal length) was used. The two cameras captured the movement of six passive markers placed on the subject (three (front, rear, head) were fixed on an helmet referring to the head and three (left, right, shoulder) were attached on two rigid shoulder supports defining the trunk) (Fig. 19.3).

Cameras acquired the movement of the subject in the whole reference volume that is about 1.5 m^3 from a close range. The rough 3D data were filtered with an adaptative low-pass filter (Butterworth – maximum cut-off frequency: 5 Hz); then some parameters were computed, extrapolated from those used in the 2D analysis with some improvements and innovation. The following parameters were calculated:

- Global displacement [cm]: geometrical distance from the starting and the ending position of the rigid body.
- Speed [cm/s]: ratio between the path (sum of the geometrical distances between the positions assumed by the rigid body frame by frame) and the duration of the test.
- Rotation [degrees]: rotation angle of the rigid body in the horizontal plane, computed using ZYX Eulerian convention.
- Spin Body: sum of the of rotation angles of head and trunk in the horizontal plane.

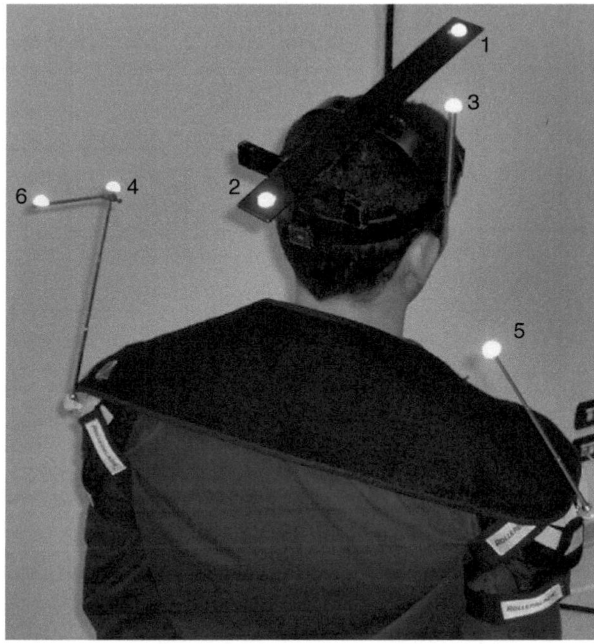

Fig. 19.3 Six markers placed on the subjects: *1* mFront, *2* mRear, *3* mHead, *4* mLeft, *5* mRight, and *6* mShoulder. *1*, *2* and *3* are fixed on a rigid helmet referring to the head, while the others are attached on two rigid shoulder supports defining the trunk

- Disharmony: it represents the capability of the subject to keep the same stepping frequency during the test. High values of this parameter indicate an incapability to keep the same pace during the test.
- Steps per minute: number of steps made in the trial normalized with the duration of the test in minutes. The number of steps was computed starting from the lateral path. In particular the change of sign of the first derivative of this variable was assumed to be a step. So the sum of all these changes normalized to the duration of the trial corresponds to the step per minute parameter.
- Index of coordination (IOC): ratio between an ideal path and the global path.
- Instability: it is the capability of the subject to maintain the same position after the double step. High values indicate the incapability to stay on the place during the test. In particular, instability is the ratio between the ideal path (previously computed) projected onto the two components lateral and longitudinal and the number of barycenters of cluster of data.
- Coefficient of performance (CP) was implemented (see Eq. 19.1). It is defined as the normalized sum of the statistically meaningful parameters (*N*).

$$\mathrm{CP} = \sum_{K=1}^{N} \frac{\mathrm{Log}\left(\dfrac{p_k}{0.05}\right)}{P_{\mathrm{TOT}}} \left(\frac{\mathrm{Parameter}_k}{\mathrm{Parameter}_{\mathrm{HEALTHY}}}\right)^{j} \tag{19.1}$$

All the parameters, with the only exception of rotations and trunk lateral displacement, show higher values in WAD than in NORM (Fig. 19.4).

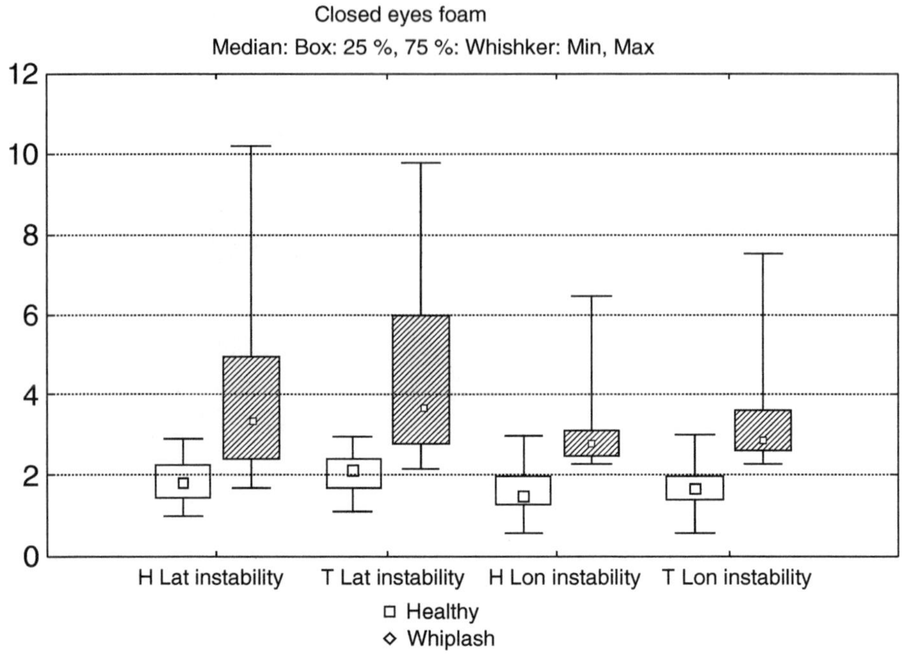

Fig. 19.4 Head and trunk lateral/longitudinal instability: comparison between healthy subjects and whiplash people. Data are expressed as median, 25th and 75th percentiles (*box*) and maximum and minimum values (*whisker*). All the differences are statistically meaningful

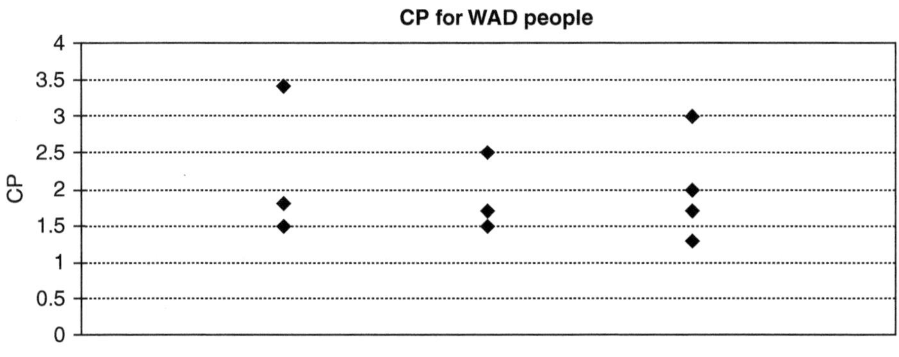

Fig. 19.5 Coefficient of performance for whiplash people: each subject presents higher value than normalcy

All the parameters that presented significant differences were used to calculate CP. Figure 19.5, shows that CP increases 57 % in WAD people with respect to NORM (the median values of the normalcy is about 1).

Stepping on a foam requires optimization of vestibular control. Generally speaking, findings show that WAD are disturbed in keeping the segment head to trunk during locomotion as a rigid body. While in healthy people sensorimotor control is as efficient despite surface conditions, in whiplash people vestibular system seems no more able to provide adequate head control if it is not sufficiently supplied by podalic cues.

The hypothesis of rigid bodies is also useful to lead the analysis on the three anatomical components of some of the described parameters since it allows to define the subject reference system. As a matter of fact, the CP is able to well characterize the two groups, with high values of CP in WAD (Fig. 19.5), making feasible a possible clinical application of this tool.

WAD present lower (not statistically significant) rotations due to their lower step frequency and to the duration of the test that is shorter than healthy people and so it is probably stopped before the beginning of rotation.

dCCG (2D and 3D) have been performed by means of prototypes. A CCG commercial equipment is CMS 70P (Zebris, Tubingen). It consists of a measuring sensor with integrated revaluation electronics and stand, a PC plug-in card. The measuring procedure is based on the exact determination of the 3D position of small ultrasound transmitters as markers, by measurement of the sound pulse time. The measuring system operates up to distance of 2 m. Markers are attached in a standard manner by means of adhesive patches to the hip, knee, ankle and ball of the foot on both sides of the body. To determine the gait phases, thin foot contact switches are stuck to the heel and the ball of the foot. The left and the right side of the body are measured in succession. After the interactive selection of the time segments to be analysed, a report is automatically prepared. Here, angles of the joints, the foot rotation and the lateral movements of the extremities are presented as time-dependent curves and as maximum values. The individual gait phases, the step length, the cadence and the average speed are evaluated. Information about instabilities is obtained from the averaged and normalized curves of all individual steps and their standard deviation.

Experiments performed with dCCG suggest that the most specific parameter able to discriminate between normal and pathological cervico-cephalic control is the ratio between head and trunk displacements. It is so possible to detect directly head and trunk sagittal (Y) and lateral (X) movements using a commercial equipment (Delos, Turin, Italy) that uses two accelerometers 2D sensitive [12], respectively, fixed to the occiput and to the sternum (Fig. 19.6).

Delos equipment records 20″ body segments movements each test. The following parameters are calculated:

- Total displacement of each segment (degrees) in X and Y plane.
- Bi-dimensional total displacements of the body segment. In this way a stabilogram-like imagine can be obtained (Fig. 19.7).
- X and Y velocities (degrees/s) for each segment.
- Head-to-trunk stability index (ratio between X or Y head and trunk displacement). A ratio <1 indicates stabilization of the head with respect of the trunk. Normal values range from 0.6 to 0.8. Values around 1 are considered border line, while ratio >1 are pathological.

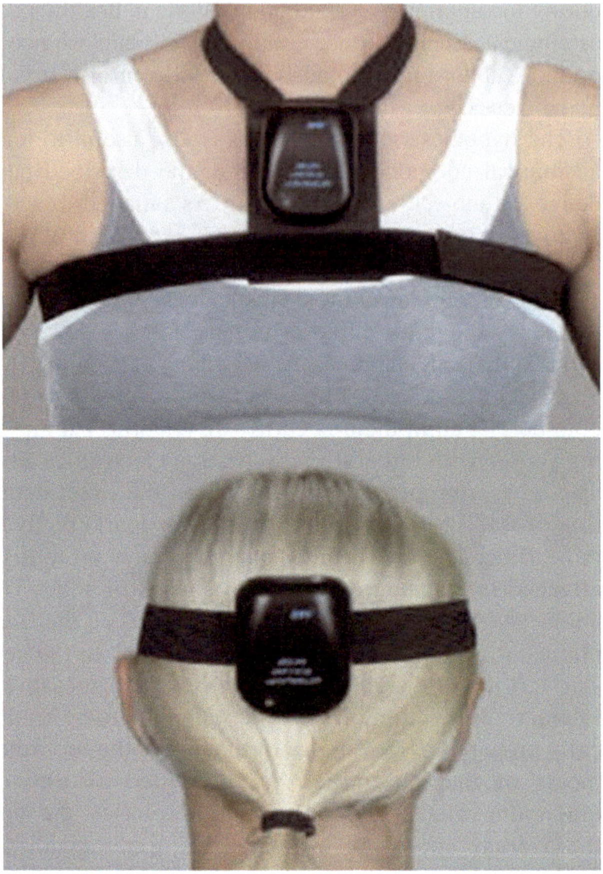

Fig. 19.6 An accelerometer is fixed on the head and the other on the trunk in order to record sagittal and lateral displacements of the two body segments

Two standard tests allow to investigate head-to-trunk stabilization:

- Head Stabilization Stance Test: evaluation of head-to-trunk stabilization during quiet steady stance (H-STAN) with eyes open and closed on firm and foam surfaces
- Stepping Test (STEP): evaluation of skill to maintain head stable with respect to the trunk during walking on place

19.2.1 H-STAN

Maintaining postural stability involves coordination of mechanical components of the limbs, the trunk and the head and sensorimotor antigravitary network, and it requires a correct perception either of the position of whole body with respect to the environment or the reciprocal position of each body segment. In quiet stance body segments are aligned along vertical axis, and they are theoretically stabilized one with respect to the other (e.g. head with respect to the trunk) during body oscillations that occur along the ankles maintaining upright position (Fig. 19.8).

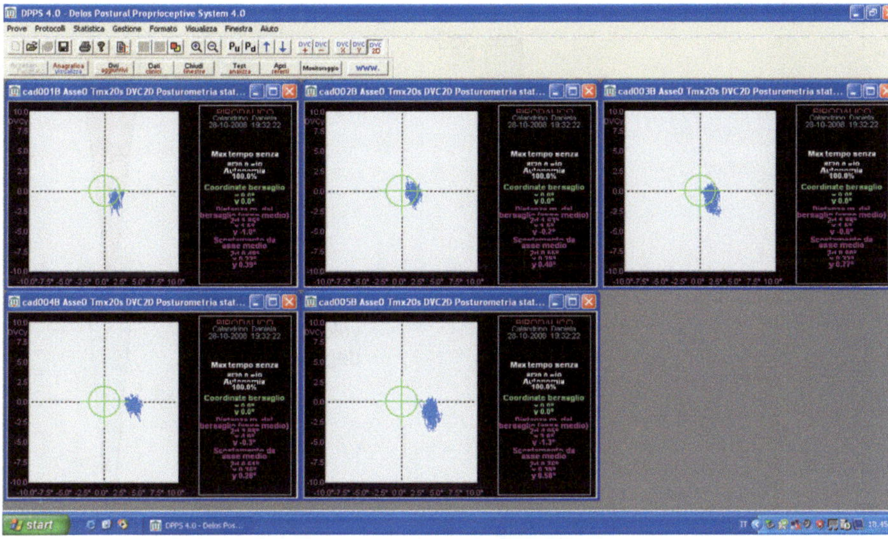

Fig. 19.7 Stabilogram-like images obtained during a standard five-conditions (eyes open and closed on firm and foam surface, head retroflexion) posturographic test by means of trunk accelerometer

In whiplash patients, this test is as frequently abnormal in eyes-closed condition on foam as the trauma is recent, that to say that cervical muscles are not able to counteract trunk sway in order to maintain body as a whole rigid inverted pendulum.

Head and trunk sway are represented as superimposed cones. In normals (left) head cone is smaller than trunk cone and head-to-trunk ratio is less than 1, while in a patient (right) the pattern is reversed.

19.2.2 STEP

Patients were requested to quietly walk on place in a quiet room in two different conditions: eyes open and eyes closed.

Different findings have been noted regarding dynamic head stabilization during walking on place. Human walking is a complex activity, and maintenance of equilibrium is a particularly challenging task for the human postural control system because our centre of mass is located a considerable distance from the supporting surface and for a major period of the walking cycle the body is supported by a single limb with the centre of gravity (CG) passing outside the base of support. During locomotion, alignment and respective balance control of each superimposed segment have to be continuatively controlled in order to provide head stabilization (Fig. 19.9).

In chronic whiplash, patient's abnormal head-to-trunk pattern in X and or Y plane can be recorded with same frequency of the experimental data obtained by dCCG.

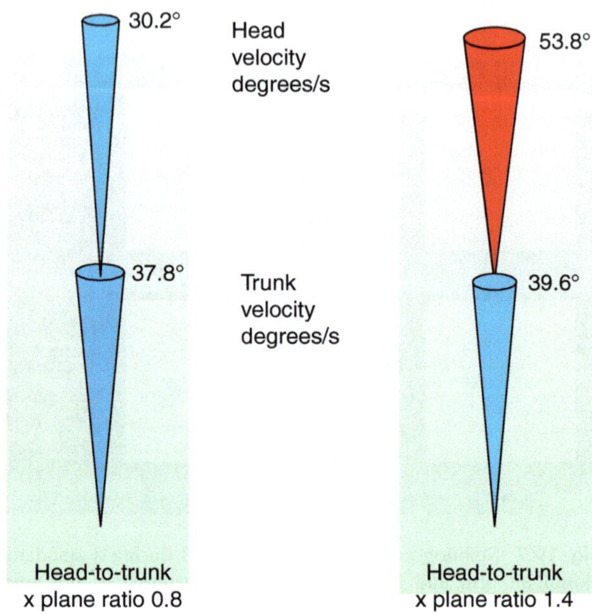

Fig. 19.8 H-STAN

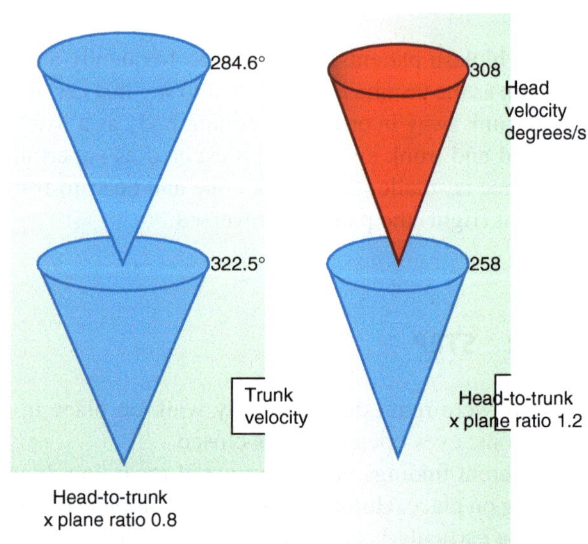

Fig. 19.9 As in Fig. 19.8 at left a normal STEP test and at right a pathological tests with increased head sway with respect to the trunk

19.3 Smooth Pursuit Neck Torsion Test (SPNT)

Whiplash produces a complex disturbance of sensorimotor control of oculomotion, balance and locomotion, involving both peripheral and central processing of eye-head-neck coordination [13].

In 1998 Tjell and Rosenhall [14] firstly described a specific oculomotor test, named *smooth pursuit neck torsion test* (SPNTT). This test was shown to possess such high sensitivity and specificity for chronic whiplash-associated disorders that it was proposed as a diagnostic test. In 2005 Treleaven et al. [15] re-proposed this oculographic test. Electrooculography (EOG) is used to measure and record eye movement while following a moving target.

The procedure we use in our laboratory is similar to those described by Tjell et al. [14] and Treleaven et al. [15]. The target consists of a light spot projected into a TV screen through a visual angle of 30°. The target is electronically controlled to provide a moving sinusoidal stimulus with a maximum velocity of 30° per second and a frequency ranging from 0.2 to 0.4 Hz. Pairs of Ag/AgCl surface electrodes are placed on the skin just lateral to the eyes bilaterally to record eye movement via changes in the corneo-retinal potential. A ground electrode is placed on the forehead. The signals are passed through a 70 Hz low-pass filter and stored on an IBM-compatible PC that continually records the change in corneo-retinal potential and eye position relative to the target during each test sequence (in our Lab EOG equipment by Toennies, Germany). The data is stored for later analysis. For each test the average velocity of the eye movements as they followed the target is calculated by subtracting the corrective movements from the total excursion of the gaze. A software program identifies and subtracts the corrective saccades (when the eyes moved more than twice as fast as the target for at least 20 ms, this was registered as a saccade). The program then formulates the corrected gain for each cycle. The signal is excluded when a blink is present, and in case of severe disturbances in the EOG signal, the entire tracking from one side of the screen to the other is excluded. Square waves and blinks (judged from recorded examples of an actual blink from each subject) are disregarded from the analysis. The mean gain (i.e. the ratio between the eye movements and of target) is the measure used to define smooth pursuit movements. Hence, the gain had the value of '1' when no corrective saccades were registered throughout the entire recording.

The smooth pursuit (SP) gain is calculated with the neck in a neutral position and also with the neck in a torsioned position. The average gain for neutral (SP neutral) and torsion to the left (SP left) and right (SP right) is calculated. The difference between the gain in neutral and the average values in torsion equalled the smooth pursuit neck torsion difference (*SPNT- diff*):

$$\text{gain}[\text{neutral}] - (\text{gain}[\text{left}] + \text{gain}[\text{right}])/2$$

The *SPNT-diff* thus equals 0 if the smooth pursuit eye movement's performance did not differ between the neutral and the rotated positions.

Tjell and Rosenhall reported that the sensitivity of the SPNTT test in the WAD group with dizziness was 90 % and the specificity was 91 %. The sensitivity in the WAD group without dizziness was 56 %. They concluded that SPNTT seemed to be useful for diagnosing cervical dizziness, at least in patients with WAD having symptoms of dizziness, because it has a high sensitivity and specificity.

Treleaven et al., on one hand confirmed the high sensitivity of the test, on the other, underlined that there was a risk of bias because eye movement analyses were performed by manual methods.

Yu et al. in 2011[16], studying the neck torsion manoeuvre used in the smooth pursuit neck torsion, have shown that there is an increased amplitude of sway when measuring in the anterior-posterior direction following neck torsion in WAD compared to healthy subjects. This cervical interference could be another bias to be taken in account in the evaluation of SPNNT.

In our experience, the use of a standardized EOG equipment with rigorous calibration procedures before each recording is enough to counteract 'technical recording bias'.

To avoid 'cervical bias' is necessary to slowly rotate the chair and to use a head rest to avoid neck fatigue and head sway.

In our laboratory, we standardized SPPNT investigating two groups of chronic WAD patients, one complaining of neck pain stiffness and one without dizziness. In both WAD groups neck torsion reduced the SP gain ($p<0.001$), and in control patients with central and peripheral or in the healthy control subjects, it did not. The sensitivity of the SPNT test in the WAD group with dizziness was 90 % and the specificity was 91 %. The sensitivity in the WAD group without dizziness was 56 %.

In our experience, SPNT test seems to be useful for diagnosing cervical dizziness, at least in patients with WAD having symptoms of dizziness. Our results in the neck torsion positions are similar to those documented by Tjell and colleagues [14] and Hildingson et al. [17] although the overall difference (SPNT) was slightly smaller on average than that of Tjell and colleagues.

Our results add support to the validity of the SPNT test to detect physiological impairments in patients following a whiplash injury. No associations were observed between smooth pursuit eye movement recordings in the neutral seated position at that time and symptoms. Furthermore, the results of the SPNT were not influenced by medication or compensation status.

High sensitivity of the test is possibly a consequence of damaged cervical proprioception, as suggested by the inventors of the test.

SPNT test suggests that the differences between the whiplash and control subjects are most likely due to disturbances to the postural control system, specifically, primary altered afferent input from the cervical spine. It could be argued that the torsion manoeuvre could stress the vertebral artery, but this is quite impossible if the movement of the neck is a pure and limited (45°) rotation without any degree of extension or flexion. Furthermore, any reduced blood flow in the vertebral artery is likely to be asymptomatic in neck torsion manoeuvres due to compensation by collateral vessels [18].

Nevertheless concomitant pathology and secondary adaptive changes in brainstem mechanisms as a result of the altered central modulation of cervical afferent input are possible, and future studies to determine the importance of these factors following a whiplash injury are necessary [19, 20].

The underlying mechanisms of the deficits measured in the SPNT test appear that both cervical proprioceptive and nocioceptive factors, as well as others, may contribute to the eye movement disturbances found in patients with persistent whiplash-associated disorders.

In conclusion, SPNTT is a simple and sensitive test even if the disturbances in patients with persistent neck pain following a whiplash injury have to be considered multifactorial and rigorous recording and torsion procedures are necessary [21].

References

1. Massion J (1992) Movement, posture and equilibrium: interaction and coordination. Prog Neurobiol 38:35–56
2. Massion J (1998) Postural control systems in developmental perspective. Neurosci Biobehav Rev 22:465–472
3. Ledebt A, Wiener-Vacher S (1996) Head coordination in the sagittal plane in toddlers during walking: preliminary results. Brain Res Bull 40(5–6):371–373
4. Allum JH, Adkin AL (2003) Improvements in trunk sway observed for stance and gait tasks during recovery from an acute unilateral peripheral vestibular deficit. Audiol Neurootol 8(5):286–302
5. Blokhorst M, Swinkels M, Lof O, Lousberg R, Zilvold G (2002) The influence of "state" related factors on focused attention following whiplash associated disorder. J Clin Exp Neuropsychol 24:471–478
6. Claussen CF (1999) Cranio-Corpo-Graphy (CCG) – 30 years of equilibriometric measurements of spatial and temporal head, neck and trunk movements. In: Claussen CF, Haid CT, Hofferberth B, Exerpta Medica, International Congress Series 1201 (eds) Equilibrium research, clinical equilibriometry and modern treatment. Elsevier Science BV, Amsterdam, Netherland pp 245–259
7. Claussen CF, Claussen E (1995) Neurootological contributions to the diagnostic follow-up after whiplash injuries. Acta Otolaryngol Suppl 520(Pt 1):53–56
8. Claussen CF, Schneider D, Helms J (1991) Cranio-corpo-graphy patterns in patients with acoustic neurinoma. Acta Otolaryngol Suppl 481:490–493
9. Ferrigno G, Pedotti A (1985) ELITE: a digital dedicated hardware system for movement analysis via real-time TV signal processing. IEEE Trans Biomed Eng 32(11):943–950
10. Ciavarro GL, Zinnato C, Alpini D, Andreoni G, Santambrogio GC (2003) Quantitative evaluation of stepping test data of patients with whiplash through digital CranioCorpoGraphy. In: Proceedings of the 25th annual international conference of the IEEE Engineering in Medicine and Biology Society (EMBS), Cancun, 17–21 September 2003, pp 1701–1704
11. Alpini D, Ciavarro GL, Zinnato C, Andreoni G, Santambrogio GC (2005) Evaluation of head-to-trunk control in whiplash patients using digital CranioCorpoGraphy during a stepping test. Gait Posture 22:308–316
12. Alpini D, Caputo D, Cesarani A, Ciavarro GL, Bariani S, Andreoni G, Santambrogio GC (2006) Dynamic head stabilization with respect to the trunk during locomotion. In: Archives of sensology and neurootology in science and practice (ASN), vol 4, pp 1–13
13. Sjostrom H, Allum JH, Carpenter MG, Adkin AL, Honegger F, Ettlin T (2003) Trunk sway measures of postural stability during clinical balance tests in patients with chronic whiplash injury symptoms. Spine 28(15):1725–1734
14. Kongsted A, Jørgensen V, Leboeuf-Yde C, Qerama E, Korsholm L (2008) Are altered smooth pursuit eye movements related to chronic pain and disability following whiplash injuries? A prospective trial with one-year follow-up. Clin Rehabil 22:469–479

15. Tjell C, Rosenhall U (1998) Smooth pursuit neck torsion test: a specific test for cervical dizziness. Am J Otol 19(1):76–81
16. Treleaven J, Gwendolen J, LowChoy N (2005) Smooth pursuit neck torsion test in whiplash-associated disorders: relationship to self-reports of neck pain and disability, dizziness and anxiety. J Rehabil Med 37:219–223
17. Yu LJ, Stokell R, Treleaven J (2011) The effect of neck torsion on postural stability in subjects with persistent whiplash. Man Ther 16(4):339–343
18. Hildingsson C, Wenngren BI, Toolanen G (1993) Eye motility dysfunction after soft-tissue injury of the cervical-spine – a controlled, prospective- study of 38 patients. Acta Orthop Scand 64:129–132
19. Baloh R, Halmagyi G (1996) Disorders of the vestibular system. Oxford University Press, New York
20. Gimse R, Tjell C, Bjorgen IA, Saunte C (1996) Disturbed eye movements after whiplash due to injuries to the posture control system. J Clin Exp Neuropsychol 18:178–186
21. Heikkila HV, Wenngren BI (1998) Cervicocephalic kinesthetic sensibility, active range of cervical motion, and oculomotor function in patients with whiplash injury. Arch Phys Med Rehabil 79:1089–1094
22. Tjell C, Tenenbaum A, Sandstrom S (2003) Smooth Pursuit Neck Torsion Test – a specific test for whiplash associated disorders? J Whiplash Relat Disord 1:9–24

Neurotology in Whiplash Injuries: Vestibulo-ocular Reflexes and Visuo-vestibular Interaction

20

L.M. Odkvist, A. Cesarani, and F. Di Berardino

20.1 Introduction

Apart from the most serious neurological disturbances, otoneurological clinical features are very important elements in cervical whiplash. Approximately 10 % of patients [1] who have suffered with whiplash injury will develop otological symptoms such as tinnitus, hearing loss, dizziness and vertigo. Some of these are purely subjective symptoms; nevertheless, for the majority there are specific tests that can be undertaken. According to Claussen and Claussen [2], about 15–20 % of subjects involved in a traffic accident develop the so-called late whiplash injury syndrome in which the individual patterns of functional lesions may be documented through appropriated neuro-otological tests.

Vertigo – which can be of different types – is one of the most common symptoms if not the most frequent one. On the other hand, whiplash-associated hearing loss is not frequent: Rowlands et al. [3] did not release any patients with otological lesion in the acute phase following their whiplash injury. This suggests that caution should be exercised when attributing these symptoms to such an injury. Before whiplash injuries are admitted as an aetiological factor in the development of such symptoms, other causes should be excluded.

L.M. Odkvist
Department of Otolaryngology, University Hospital, S-58185
Linkoping, Sweden

A. Cesarani • F. Di Berardino (✉)
Department of Clinical Sciences and Community Health,
University of Milan, Milan, Italy

Audiology Unit, IRCCS "Ca' Granda" Ospedale Maggiore Policlinico, Milan, Italy
e-mail: antonio.cesarani@unimi.it; federica.diberardino@unimi.it

D.C. Alpini et al. (eds.), *Whiplash Injuries*,
DOI 10.1007/978-88-470-5486-8_20, © Springer-Verlag Italia 2014

20.2 Peripheral Whiplash-Associated Vestibular Involvement

For balancing, motor control and keeping visual objects steady on the retina, the vestibular system and the interaction with the visual system are of paramount importance. Balance is maintained via cooperation between the vestibular afferents, proprioception, podalic pressure receptors and vision [4]. For diagnostics postural tests are important, but the easiest and most accurate way to study the vestibular system is recording of spontaneous and provoked eye movements and the interaction with the visual system. Often the cause for vertigo can be unveiled with these methods. For eye-movement recording, the most widely used methods are electronystagmography (ENG) [5] and videonystagmography (VNG) [6].

Whiplash-associated vestibular symptoms are variable in relation to either the type and intensity or the temporal course of clinical manifestations. These symptoms include positional vertigo, which can also last for 2 years [7, 8]; latent nystagmus which appeared in about 30 % of the patients either within or after a year following the trauma [9]; and spontaneous nystagmus in more than 50 % of the subjects, in most cases of positional type. In many subjects the positional nystagmus was direction-fixed, in others direction-changing, and the results of Dix-Hallpike manoeuvre suggested the possibility of otolithic damage with cupulolithiasis of the posterior semicircular canal [10]. We must also remember that latent nystagmus, pathological monolateral caloric test and anomalous rotatory test, even later than a year after the trauma, may be observed in a great number of patients.

Despite clear symptoms, it is difficult to find objective standards to produce evidence for the presence of the ailment in patients with WAD. However, Kelders et al. [11] recently found that the gain of one of the ocular stabilization reflexes, the cervico-ocular reflex (COR), was elevated in patients with whiplash injury compared with an age-matched control group.

The COR acts in conjunction with the vestibulo-ocular reflex (VOR) and the optokinetic reflex (OKR) to preserve stable vision on the retina during head motion. It is elicited by rotation of the neck, thereby stimulating proprioceptive afferents from deep neck muscles and joint capsule from C1 to C3 to the vestibular nucleus, leading to eye movements that oppose the direction of the head movement [12].

The VOR can be subdivided into rotational and translational components induced by stimulation of the semicircular canals and the otolithic organs, respectively. When the head is turned, the VOR moves the eyes in the opposite direction, responding optimally to high frequencies. The OKR is stimulated by visual motion and uses the relative velocity of the image on the peripheral retina to generate eye movements in the same direction. OKR and COR reflexes respond best at low head movement velocities. Gain values of the COR are increased over a broad range of velocities (1.2–12.8°/s) in patients with whiplash injury, though the largest difference was found at lower velocities [13].

In healthy persons, COR gain can be modified after 10 min of concurrent visual and cervical stimulation. In patients with absent vestibular function, COR gain is also increased, as it is with age (older than 60 years). Meanwhile, in elderly persons, the gains of the VOR and OKR are decreased.

20.3 Vestibulo-Oculomotor Reflex (VOR)

Examination of ocular movements in response to stimulation of the vestibular part of the inner ear is important for evaluation of the state of the vestibular system in patients. The vestibulo-ocular reflex (VOR) connects the sensory transducers, the hair cells in the semicircular canals and the otolithic organs in the vestibular part of the labyrinth with the extrinsic ocular muscles. Stimulation of the inner ears results in movements of the eyes. With VOR, during head movements the visual target is always centred on the fovea. Vestibular stimulation is achieved either by rotatory movements of the head or, in the caloric test, thermal irrigation of the ear canal. The advantage of the caloric test is that it tests each labyrinth separately. Caloric irrigation is, however, a crude and unphysiological stimulus. The rotatory test, on the other hand, uses a more physiological stimulus, however exciting both ears simultaneously.

A thermic stimulation of the labyrinth is usually achieved using water with a temperature 7° above or below body temperature. The patient lies down with the head elevated 30° from horizontal. The test is based on the fact that the calorie stimulation induces a movement of the endolymph in the semicircular canals [14]. A nystagmus is elicited and calculated concerning different qualities of the reaction. Sometimes the duration of the nystagmus response is recorded, but the most valid parameter is the speed of the slow phase of the elicited nystagmus beats. The duration of the reaction is an uncertain measurement of the calorie response and can be normal although a diminished calorie response may be present, which is unveiled only by measuring the speed of the slow phase of the nystagmus beat.

Rotatory testing has been in use since the turn of the century. The main drawback with the rotatory test is that the stimulation affects both labyrinths simultaneously. The equipment for rotatory testing is usually expensive and complicated. One advantage with the rotatory test is that the eye movement responses are not dependent on the individual anatomical variations and the recordings can be performed on subjects who do not tolerate caloric irrigation.

One additional advantage is that rotatory test provides a natural physiological acceleration stimulus. Different stimulus patterns have been used in rotatory testing – trapezoidal, triangular and damped sinusoidal. A vast amount of data has been collected from rotatory testing using broad frequency swings (0.5–5 Hz) [14].

The autorotation test, an interesting VOR test, uses the equipment for ENG, but the patient himself sinusoidally turns the head to the right and left rhythmically [15]. A calculation is made of the difference between the head movements and the eye movements. The equipment is inexpensive and easy to handle, but the drawback is that cervical influences cannot be avoided. Thus the test is not useful in cases of cervical vertigo or whiplash injuries [16–18].

The head shaking test is a simple way of testing the vestibulo-oculomotor system: The patient shakes his head with a frequency of 1–2 Hz for 10 s. Immediately after stopping the movement, eye movements are observed under Frenzel glasses or preferably recorded by ENG. A post-head shake nystagmus for several seconds indicates that there is an asymmetry in the peripheral or central part of the vestibular system [19].

The otolithic influence on VOR may be evaluated by eccentric rotatory testing that can unveil unilateral or bilateral function loss in the otolithic organs. During the rotation the subject experiences an illusion of tilt and in the darkness places a bias light bar at an angle to true horizontal and even has a tilt of the eyeballs. This type of investigation is still not fully validated [20, 21].

20.4 Vestibulo-Visual Interaction

The directioning of the eyes is a function of the cooperation of the vestibular organs, neck proprioception and vision. In cases of conflict, the visual reflexes override VOR at least in the low-frequency area. In high-frequency swings, the ocular motion is driven mainly by VOR. The cerebellar flocculus and nodulus mediate the interaction. Patients with cerebellar lesions may have a defunct visual suppression ability. Some patients with brainstem lesions may have the same functional defect. The neck proprioceptors also help maintain gaze direction during movements of the neck, body and towards visible targets. In some cases of neck lesions, a simple turning of the head to the right or left may elicit a nystagmus, which can be studied preferably with ENG. Cervical influence on the vestibulo-oculomotor system may also be unveiled if the patient is sitting in a swing chair, the head is held steady by the examiner and the eye movements are observed while the chair with the patient is turned rhythmically clockwise and counterclockwise.

20.5 Visual Suppression of VOR

The vestibulo-ocular reflex cancelling or visual suppression mechanism can be tested during the caloric response in darkness when a lamp is lit for 10 s, allowing ocular fixation. The induced eye-movement speed should decrease to 30 % of its value in darkness (Fig. 20.1). The visual suppression test becomes even more

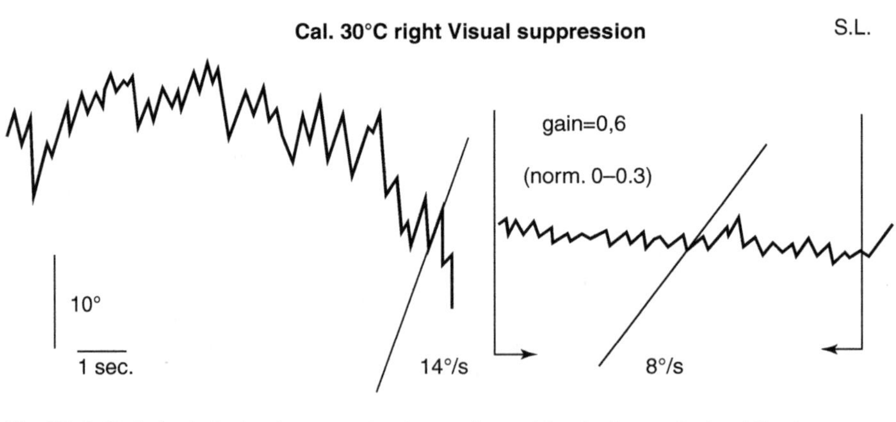

Fig. 20.1 Pathological visual suppression in a patient with a brainstem lesion. Fixation nystagmus is still present at different velocity

sensitive if it is performed in the rotatory chair with the instruction to the patient to fixate on a target by moving with the chair [22, 23] (Fig. 20.2).

20.6 COR Recordings

By passively rotating the body while fixating the subject's head (trunk-to-head rotation), isolated COR responses were recorded in the absence of visual or vestibular input. The subject's head was fixed in space by means of a custom-made bite board, and the trunk was fixed to the chair by a double-belt system at shoulder level. A cervical range-of-motion device was used to demonstrate that the head was sufficiently stabilized in space, with negligible head movement induced by chair motion.

Nacci et al. [24] evaluated subacute whiplash-associated labyrinth involvement. They submitted a group of patients within 15 days of the trauma to the following tests: liminal tone audiometry, investigation for spontaneous nystagmus (positional and positioning, with or without Frenzel glasses) and the head-shaking test (HST). In addition, all subjects underwent a vestibular bithermal caloric balance test according to Fitzgerald-Hallpike and videonystagmographic investigation. Analysis of videonystagmographic investigations showed that it is possible to find both peripheral (non-compensated/compensated labyrinth deficit and PPV) and central (vertical nystagmus) vestibulopathy. Data collected in this study confirm that PPV is possible in cervical whiplash trauma as well, even though it is more frequent in cases of minor head injury (3 % vs. 10 %).

MacNab [25] attributes tinnitus, hypoacusia and pathological nystagmus following an indirect injury in the cervical spine to a spasm in vertebral arteries. According the author, the majority of neuro-otological injuries seen after an episode of whiplash are probably attributable to ischaemic or haemorrhagic events in the labyrinth

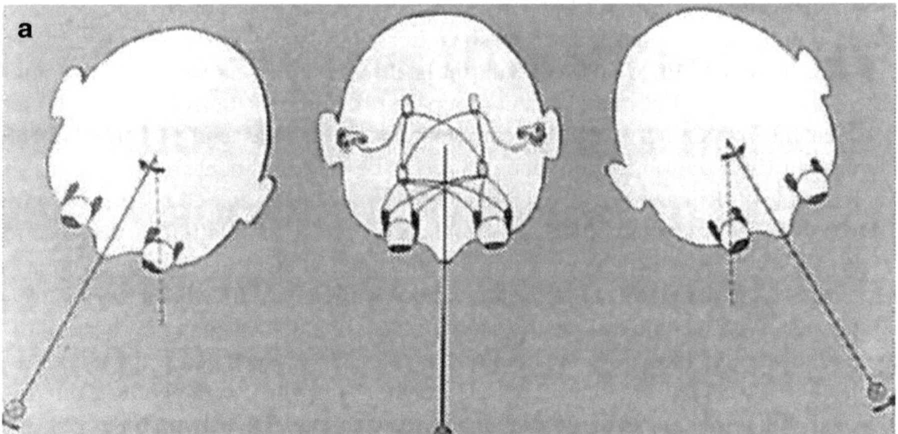

Fig. 20.2 Visual suppression test in the rotatory chair. Head movements are recorded with accelerometer on the bite-board. Eye movements are recorded with electronystagmography. The instruction is to fixate on the dot on the screen moving by the chair. Thus the target is always right in front of the eyes

Fig. 20.2 (continued)

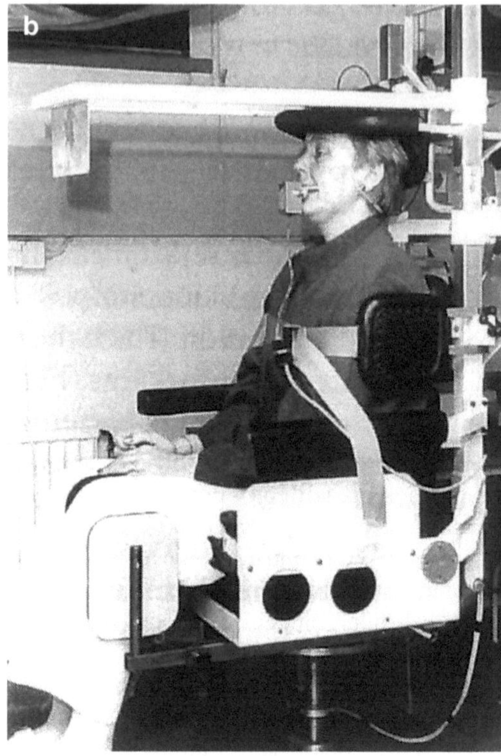

membrane (peripheral vestibulopathy, tinnitus, sensorineural hypoacusia) or to concussion and/or brainstem stretching (central vestibulopathy, tinnitus).

COR gain values in patients with WAD are significantly increased compared with those in healthy controls [26]. An age-related increase was not seen in patients, which could indicate that the whiplash injury cancels out this age-related effect [27–29]. In contrast to what was found in healthy controls, no synergy was found between COR and VOR in the patient group. Furthermore, no correlation was found between the remaining eye reflex combinations in patients and in controls. The increase in COR gain in elderly patients might be an adjustment for the decline in VOR gain [30]. Rijkaart et al. [28] showed that the COR is able to adapt after only 10 min of incongruent simultaneous visual and cervical stimulation. A decrease in VOR gain might have been responsible for an increase in COR gain in our whiplash patients, as seen in elderly subjects and in those with labyrinthine defects. However, a higher COR gain could also be the cause of a decline in VOR gain. Earlier experiments showed that the VOR gain could be adapted in 1 h by noncorresponding vestibular and visual information. Contrary to the latter theory, the COR gain was elevated with no decline in the VOR gain in WAD patients. Three hypotheses [28, 30] can provide an explanation for this lack of synergy in patients with whiplash injury:

First, it may be that decreased mobility of the neck leads to alteration in proprioception of the neck, which in turn results in an augmented gain of the COR without any problems in the VOR pathway.

Second, it may be that adaptation of the VOR requires sufficient head motion and, because of impaired neck motion, the patient has too little adaptive input for the VOR to induce a negative adaptation in VOR gain. It is known that the VOR responds best at high velocities, whereas the COR is most responsive at low frequencies. This could explain the lack of decrease in VOR gain.

Third, it may be that there is a disorganization in the process of VOR plasticity because of microtrauma in the VOR pathway, such as in the flocculonodular area of the cerebellum. The latter hypothesis will be subject to more research in the near future when we perform VOR adaptation experiments in patients with whiplash injury.

It can be speculated to what degree abnormalities in COR gain are responsible for the reported signs and symptoms. Although the correlation between them is striking, correlation does not prove causation. However, the results might explain some symptoms. Improperly tuned VOR and COR may lead to symptoms such as dizziness and to visual problems such as reading impairment. The absence of synergy between COR and VOR combined with head and neck pain may induce symptoms of fatigue.

20.7 Peripheral Whiplash-Associated Auditory Involvement

Hearing loss is frequent in general population, but it is not particularly frequent in whiplash-associated disorders. Tjell et al. [31] investigated 153 ambulatory WAD patients by means of pure-tone audiometry. Their audiograms were compared with ISO standards. Fourteen percent of patients with WAD had a hearing impairment exceeding the 90th percentile of the ISO standards. However, in most cases the hearing was not associated with whiplash injury. A subgroup (33 patients) – with normal hearing or slight hearing impairment according to the audiogram – was selected from the total group of patients with WAD. The 33 selected patients and 33 matched controls were tested with the speech-in-noise test (SRN test). However, 40 % of this subgroup of patients with WAD reported hearing problems. As many as 30 % of the patients with WAD had an abnormal SRN test result, as against 5 % of the controls. Significant relations were found between the SRN test and self-assessed hearing loss.

Thus the speech-in-noise test (SRN test) seems the most specific test to document hearing involvement in WAD.

The specific involvement of the peripheral auditory system is confirmed by Segal et al. [32] that conducted a retrospective review of clinical, pure tone and speech audiometric findings. The first evaluation was obtained within 3 months and the follow-up ones between 6 and 12 months after injury. Eighty-three patients (166 ears) reported hearing impairment after blunt neck trauma: Twenty of the 166 ears (12 %) had normal hearing and 137 ears (81.3 %) showed an acoustic trauma-like hearing impairment. Eight ears (4.8 %) had a hearing loss of at least 30 dB in the speech frequencies (500–2,000 Hz), and two ears (1.2 %) had additional impairment in the higher frequencies. Only one ear (0.8 %) had a conductive hearing loss. No speech discrimination score was poorer than 80 %. Forty-six subjects (55.4 %) reported tinnitus.

Whiplash-associated tinnitus was extensively investigated by Kreuzer et al. [33] by means of demographic data, tinnitus-related clinical data, audiological data, the Tinnitus Handicap Inventory, the Tinnitus Questionnaire, the Beck Depression Inventory, various numeric tinnitus rating scales and the World Health Organisation Quality (WHOQOL). The results indicate differences between tinnitus patients with and without trauma at tinnitus onset: Patients suffering from trauma-associated tinnitus suffer from a higher mental burden than tinnitus patients presenting with phantom perceptions based on other or unknown etiologic factors. This is especially the case for patients with whiplash and head trauma. Patients with posttraumatic noise-related tinnitus experience more frequently hyperacusis, were younger, had longer tinnitus duration and were more frequently of male gender.

On the other hand, a benign cause of otological disorder, at least as acute onset, has to be excluded as suggested by Ferrari [34] that investigated 86 whiplash patients affected with earache, fullness in the ear, diminished hearing and tinnitus. Out of 71 subjects reporting no acute onset (within 7 days of the collision that caused their whiplash), 62 had little or no cerumen occlusion, but of eight subjects reporting one or more of acute-onset earache, fullness in the ears, diminished hearing and tinnitus, seven had complete cerumen occlusion in the affected ear. This author underlines that his findings suggest high-grade cerumen occlusion frequently occurs in the ear affected by acute auditory symptoms and that a number of acute-onset auditory symptoms reported in whiplash patients may have a benign cause not whiplash associated.

References

1. Tranter RM, Graham JR (2009) A review of the otological aspects of whiplash injury. J Forensic Leg Med 16(2):53–55
2. Claussen CF, Claussen E (1995) Neurootological contributions to the diagnostic follow-up after whiplash injuries. Acta Otolaryngol Suppl 520(Pt 1):53–56
3. Rowlands RG, Campbell IK, Kenyon GS (2009) Otological and vestibular symptoms in patients with low grade (Quebec grades one and two) whiplash injury. J Laryngol Otol 123(2):182–185
4. Boyle R, Pompeiano O (1981) Convergence and interaction of neck and macular vestibular inputs on vestibulospinal neurons. J Neurophysiol 45:852–868
5. Jongkees LBW, Maas JPM, Philipszoon AJ (1962) Clinical nystagmography: a detailed study of electro-nystagmography in 341 patients with vertigo. Pract Otorhinolaryngol (Basel) 24:65–93 [PubMed]
6. van der Geest JN, Frens MA (2002) Recording eye movements with video-oculography and scleral search coils: a direct comparison of two methods. J Neurosci Methods 114:185–195
7. Pearce JMS (1989) Whiplash injury: a reappraisal. J Neurol Neurosurg Psychiatry 52: 1329–1331
8. Oosterveld WJ, Kortshot HW, Kingma GG (1991) Electronystagmographic findings following cervical whiplash injuries. Acta Otorhinolaryngol (Stockh) 11:201–205
9. Magnusson T (1994) Extracervical symptoms after whiplash trauma. Cephalalgia 14: 223–227
10. Eck JC, Hodges SD, Humphreys SC (2001) Whiplash: a review of a commonly misunderstood injury. Am J Med 110:651–656

11. Kelders WP, Kleinrensink GJ, van der Geest JN (2005) The cervico-ocular reflex is increased in whiplash injury patients. J Neurotrauma 22:133–137
12. Peterson BW, Baker JF, Goldberg J et al (1988) Dynamic and kinematic properties of the vestibulocollic and cervicocollic reflexes in the cat. In: Pompeiano O, Allum JHJ (eds) Vestibulospinal control of posture and locomotion, Progress in brain research. Elsevier, Oxford, pp 163–172
13. Montfoort I, Kelders WP, van der Geest JN, Schipper IB, Feenstra L, de Zeeuw CI, Frens MA (2006) Interaction between ocular stabilization reflexes in patients with whiplash injury. Invest Ophthalmol Vis Sci 47(7):2881–2884
14. Aschan G (1966) Clinical vestibular examinations and their results. Acta Otolaryngol (Suppl) 1224:56–67
15. Larsby B, Hydén D, Odkvist LM (1984) Gain and phase characteristics of compensatory eye movements in light and darkness. A study with a broad frequencyband rotatory test. Acta Otolaryngol 97:223–232
16. O'Leary DP, Davis LD, Kitsigianis GA (1989) Analysis of vestibulo-ocular reflex using sweep frequency active head movements. Adv Otorhinolaryngol 41:179–183
17. Schwarz DWF, Tomlinson RD (1979) Diagnostic precision in a new rotatory vestibular test. J Otolaryngol 8:554
18. Tabak S, Collewijn H, Boumans LJ, van der Steen J (1997) Gain and delay of human vestibulo-ocular reflexes to oscillation and steps of the head by a reactive torque helmet, I: normal subjects. Acta Otolaryngol 117:785–795
19. Ledin T, Deblén J, Noaksson L, Odkvist LM (1992) The head shaking test in the electronystagmography investigation. In: Claussen CF, Kirtane MV, Schneider D (eds) Conservative versus surgical treatment of sensorineural hearing loss, tinnitus, vertigo and nausea, Nachf edn. Dr Wemer Rudat, Hamburg
20. Gripmark M, Odkvist LM, Larsby B (1995) The subjective horizontal in eccentric rotation. In: Proceedings of the XXIth ordinary meeting of the Neorotologic and Equilibriometric Society, Hakone, Japan
21. Curthoys S, Halmagyi GM, Dai M (1991) The acute effects of unilateral vestibular neurectomy on sensory and motor tests of human otolithic function. Acta Otolaryngol Suppl 1481:5–10
22. Hydén D, Larsby B, Odkvist LM (1983) Visual suppression tests in diagnosis of diseases of the centrai nervous system. Adv Otorhinolaryngol 30:205–209
23. Dichgans I, von Reutem GM, Rommelt V (1978) Impaired suppression of vestibular nystagmus by fixation in cerebellar and non-cerebellar patients. Arch Psychiatr Nervenkr 226: 183–199
24. Nacci A, Ferrazzi M, Berrettini S, Panicucci E, Matteucci J, Bruschini L, Ursino F, Fattori B (2011) Vestibular and stabilometric findings in whiplash injury and minor head trauma. Acta Otorhinolaryngol Ital 31(6):378–389
25. MacNab I (2002) Acceleration injury of the cervical spine. J Bone Joint Surg 84:807–811
26. Armato E, Ferri E (2002) Analyse video-nystagmographique sur 569 cas de syndrome vertigineux post-traumatique: rèvision critique et étude du nystagmus vertical supérieur. In: Lacour M (ed) Controle postural, pathologies et traitements, innovations et rééducation. Solal Éditeur, Marseille, pp 105–118
27. Bronstein AM, Hood JD (1986) The cervico-ocular reflex in normal subjects and patients with absent vestibular function. Brain Res 373:399–408
28. Rijkaart DC, van der Geest JN, Kelders WP (2004) Short-term adaptation of the cervico-ocular reflex. Exp Brain Res 156:124–128
29. Mergner T, Schweigart G, Botti F, Lehmann A (1998) Eye movements evoked by proprioceptive stimulation along the body axis in humans. Exp Brain Res 120:450–460
30. Lovell ME, Galasko CS (2002) Whiplash disorders – a review. Injury 33:97–101
31. Tjell C, Tenenbaum A, Rosenhall U (1999) Auditory function in whiplash-associated disorders. Scand Audiol 28(4):203–209
32. Segal S, Eviatar E, Berenholz L, Vaiman M, Kessler A, Shlamkovitch N (2003) Hearing loss after direct blunt neck trauma. Otol Neurotol 24(5):734–737

33. Kreuzer PM, Landgrebe M, Schecklmann M, Staudinger S, Langguth B, TRI Database Study Group (2012) Trauma-associated tinnitus: audiological, demographic and clinical characteristics. PLoS One 7(9):e45599
34. Ferrari R (2006) Auditory symptoms in whiplash patients – could earwax occlusion be a benign cause? Aust Fam Physician 35(5):367–368

Vestibular Evoked Potentials in Relapsing Paroxysmal Positional Vertigo

21

F. Di Berardino, D.C. Alpini, L. Pugnetti, V. Mattei, and B. Franz

21.1 Introduction

Paroxysmal positioning vertigo (PPV) is a major cause of vertigo accounting for 14 % of all equilibrium disorders with an annual incidence of about 100 per 100,000 of population [1]. It starts suddenly and is usually first noticed in bed, when waking from sleep. Any turn of the head seems to bring on violent but brief bursts of dizziness. Patients often describe the occurrence of vertigo with tilting of the head, looking up or down, or rolling over in bed. It is not unusual for nausea and vomiting to accompany the vertigo. Even if a spell is brief, a feeling of queasiness may last several minutes or even hours, and those who suffer from this kind of vertigo are distressed and incapacitated for several days severely impacting on social costs due to lost working days. PPV is a common vestibular disorder leading to significant morbidity, psychosocial impact, and medical costs. PPV accounted for 8 % of individuals with moderate or severe dizziness/vertigo. Is commonly accepted that PPV is due to displacement of otoconia and/or to vestibular macula/maculae lesion.

PPV is very common after whiplash head trauma, while it is very rare in cases with a pure cervical involvement. In these cases, maybe through inner ear

F. Di Berardino (✉)
Department of Clinical Sciences and Community Health, University of Milan, Milan, Italy

Audiology Unit, IRCCS "Ca' Granda" Ospedale Maggiore Policlinico, Milan, Italy
e-mail: fdibe@fastwebnet.it

D.C. Alpini • L. Pugnetti • V. Mattei
ENT-Otoneurology Service, IRCCS "Don Carlo C. Gnocchi" Foundation, Milan, Italy
e-mail: dalpini@dongnocchi.it

B. Franz
Department of Anatomy and Cell Biology, Tinnitus Research and Balance Clinic, University of Melbourne, Wantirna, VIC, Australia

D.C. Alpini et al. (eds.), *Whiplash Injuries*,
DOI 10.1007/978-88-470-5486-8_21, © Springer-Verlag Italia 2014

concussion or vertebral artery spasm, prolonged PPV, atypical PPV, or relapsing PPV are the most observed forms [2].

Vestibular evoked myogenic potentials (VEMPs) are nowadays the specific test to investigate vestibular maculae function, that is to say the site of origin of PPV.

They have been described [3, 4] as short-latency potentials from an active electrode placed just below the inion in response to acoustic stimulation (the "inion response"), probably generated by reflex changes in the electromyogram of posterior neck muscles. Cody and Bickford [5] described the inion response [6] in subjects suffering from different cochlear and vestibular syndromes and provided further evidence to suggest that it depended on the activation of the saccular macula. Those authors concluded that VEMP recording depended on the activation of a specific reflex function called the vestibulocollic reflex (VCR), mediated by a pathway consisting of the saccular macula, its primary neurons, vestibulospinal neurons from the lateral vestibular nucleus, the medial vestibulospinal tract, and, finally, the motor neurons of the spinal cord reaching neck muscles.

Recent studies showed that rarefaction clicks are preferred for evoking the saccular response and that the sternocleidomastoid muscle (SCM) is the most advisable recording site [7–9]. Healthy subjects produce a biphasic response from the SCM characterized by a positive peak at a latency of some 13 ms (P1) from the stimulus followed by a negative wave peaking some 10 ms later (N2). Abnormal results, ranging from prolonged latencies to total absence of the response, disclose lesions anywhere in the VCR pathway.

Vestibular evoked myogenic potentials (VEMPs) are commonly used to assess the otolithic organ through a multineuron reflex test. A variant of VEMPs, the so-called periocular VEMPs, in which potentials are derived from periocular muscles, has been proposed as a specific test for utricolo-spinal reflexes [10, 11].

Franz et al. [12, 13] described a single neuron reflex test for the specific examination of the vestibular responses during sagittal and lateral tilts of the head (electrovestibulography, *EVG*). In this technique an extratympanic electrode is placed in the tympanic recess for the recording of evoked potentials. Tilting the head in roll and in pitch is employed to stimulate mainly the otolithic organ.

The aim of this chapter is to assess the vestibular function in patients affected by relapsing vertigo of peripheral origin through vestibular evoked potentials, using both techniques: VEMPs and EVG.

21.2 Materials and Methods

In this study, 52 patients were investigated (12 males, 40 females, mean age 43 ± 5.4 years). All patients presented with relapsing episodes of posterior semicircular canal-type benign paroxysmal positional vertigo.

Relapsing paroxysmal positional vertigo (RPV) was defined as three or more such episodes over a period of 12 months, with an interval symptom-free period of at least 2 months. Although dizziness could persist in these patients, complete resolution of the paroxysmal type of positional vertigo that followed a repositioning maneuver was a condition of the study. All subjects were free of diseases of the external ear canal and middle ear. In order to exclude involvements of the canals or the central vestibular pathways, they underwent to a complete neurootological battery, as well as neuroimaging (MRI). In all considered subjects these tests resulted as normal.

Out of the 52 patients suffering from RPV, 11 had no balance symptoms at the time of examination and 41 continued to suffer from dizziness, despite successful repositioning. The former were classified as asymptomatic (ASYM) and the latter as symptomatic (SYMP). The symptoms in SYMP group were described as a momentary instability, often associated with positioning or quick head movements. The provocative maneuvers [14–16] did not evoke nystagmus or vertigo in all subjects.

For VEMP examination, patients were requested to be seated on a comfortable chair keeping their head rotated to the opposite side of the stimulated ear to activate the SCM. The active surface EMG electrode was placed on the SCM of the stimulated side and referred to the ipsilateral clavicle, whereas a ground electrode was fixed on the upper sternum. The vestibulocollic reflex was evoked by rarefaction clicks (duration 100 ms, loudness 95 dB normal hearing level, rate 5 Hz) delivered by a pair of headphones in two series for a total of 200 sweeps. Contralateral NB masking 90 dB SPL was adopted. Four repetitions each side were performed. There was no adjustment to individual hearing loss. A continuous noise of 70 dB was presented to the contralateral ear. Recordings were performed using a standard clinical evoked potentials averager (Nicolet CA2000) with time bases of 50 ms. The responses to both series of sweeps were averaged twice to produce one grand average for each side and for each subject [17–19].

The parameters evaluated were:

- Presence/absence of the response
- Latency of the first positive (P1) and negative (N2) peaks
- Interpeak latencies (P1-N2)
- Amplitudes measured peak to peak (P1-N2)

Since the level of SCM contraction, which can vary remarkably between subjects, influences the amplitude of the response, we concentrated on the latencies between peaks. These latencies are more stable and better reflect the integrity of the vestibulospinal pathway. Our normal latency ranges (25 subjects, 13 females and 12 males, mean age 35.7 years) were 15.8 ± 1.5 ms for P1 and 25.4 ± 1.8 ms for N2 and interpeak latencies (P1-N2) 9.8 ± 0.8 ms (Fig. 21.1). Figure 21.1 shows a normal pattern of VEMPs in A compared to an abnormal diagram in B characterized by increased latency (P1 18.06 ms in B with respect to 15.57 in A) and decreased amplitude (4 μV in B and 32 μV in A).

EVG was performed while the patient was sitting on a chair. For recording evoked potentials, an extratympanic electrode was placed into the tympanic recess of the ipsilateral ear, being fixed with a tape on the pinna as to prevent any movement of the electrode during head tilts. The reference electrode was fixed on the mastoid plane and the ground electrode on the forehead just below the hairline. Tilting the head in roll and in pitch was employed to stimulate mainly the otolithic organ. Tilting the head was swift (below 1 Hz) although not forceful. During tilting raw data were collected and delivered to a data acquisition system with following analysis (Inner Ear Analyzer, Enttex Pty. Ltd., Port Melbourne, Australia). EVG is

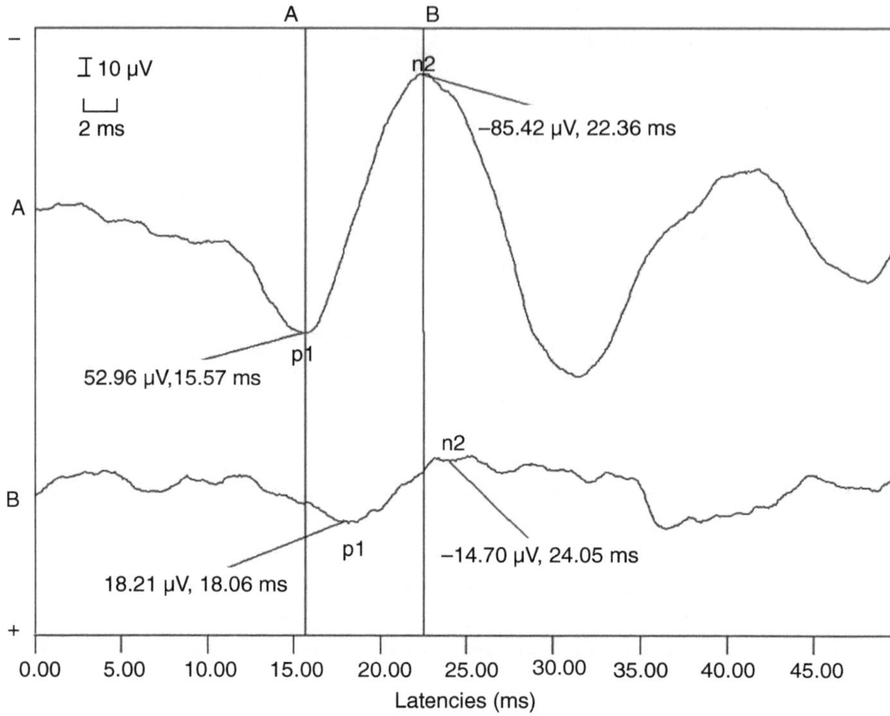

Fig. 21.1 *Left* (*A*) and *right* (*B*) VEMPs. Normal morphology and latencies in the *left* evoked VEM and reduced amplitude and increased latencies in the *righ*t evoked VEMP

based on an averaging procedure, and results are presented in boxplots, a visually suitable format for physicians that permits to easily read the results. Boxplot displays the interquartile range (seventy-fifth through twenty-fifth percentile). For a detailed explanation of the technique, see Franz et al. 2003 and Franz et al. 2006 [11, 12].

Four recordings were performed: ipsilateral tilt to the electrode ear and contralateral tilt away from the electrode ear (roll that could be mainly referred to the response of the utricle) and forward tilt and backward tilt (pitch that could be mainly referred to the response of the saccule). Each pair of tests (e.g., ipsi- and contralateral tilts and forward and backward tilt) were compared in order to calculate a coefficient, one mainly referred to sagittal responses (expressed as sacculus coefficient) and the other mainly to lateral (expressed as utricle coefficient). In normal subjects the interquartile range of ipsilateral head tilt is larger than the interquartile range of contralateral head tilt, rendering a coefficient usually below 1 (range 0.5–1.1). Similarly the interquartile range of forward head tilt is larger than the interquartile range of backward head tilt, also rendering a coefficient usually below 1 (range 0.6–1.2) as calculated in a reference group of normals (12 males and 15 females, mean age 32.5 years) (Fig. 21.2). Figure 21.2 shows a diagram of a normal EVG which shows the responses of a subject without vestibulocochlear symptoms. Each recording was preceded by a baseline assessment. This was an important measurement and allowed comparison of base level of impedance. Provided similar

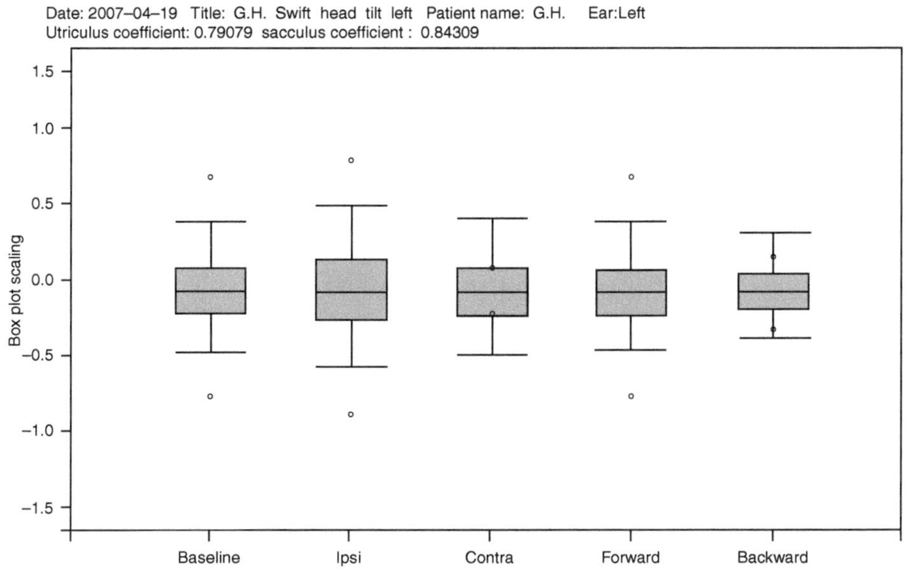

Fig. 21.2 EVG boxplots. Averaging potentials recorded in different head positions are visually compared to baseline value in order to provide an analog-scaled information regarding otolithic function

impedance in ears, very small amplitude ranges or a significant interaural difference of amplitude ranges (>30 %) is to be considered pathological.

Statistical analysis was performed with the standard student *t*-test ($p<0.05$) and the Pearson chi-square and Fisher's exact tests.

21.3 Results

VEMPs were completely normal in nine ASYM patients. Four subjects revealed an abnormal response in one ear, while only one patient revealed an abnormal response in both ears (Table 21.1).

Although the two tests did not identify individual cases as normal or pathological in the same way, the Pearson chi-square and Fisher's exact tests showed comparable results in cross correlations (Table 21.1).

The distribution of VEMPS and EVG abnormalities was comparable.

EVG was completely normal in all the ASYM patients. From the other group, eight revealed an abnormal response in both ears, whereas one revealed an abnormal response in one ear (Table 21.1).

The patients with abnormal EVG has been splitted according to the characteristic of measured abnormalities. Table 21.2 evidences that vestibular endings involvement is complex. In patients, a negative interaction between saccule and utricle thus could be supposed.

In SYMP patients, VEMPs showed a bilateral delay in nine subjects, a left-right asymmetry in 28. EVG results were more complex as pathological findings in

Table 21.1 VEMPs and EVG distribution in SYMP and ASYM patients

	SYMP	ASYMP	Number of patients
VEMPs abnormal	37	2	39
VEMPs normal	4	9	13
EVG abnormal	39	0	39
EVG normal	2	11	13

Table 21.2 EVG abnormal findings

	Number of patients
BAS (difference between baseline right and left values >30 %)	1
UTR (abnormal utricular coefficient)	11
SAC (abnormal saccular coefficient)	10
BAS+UTR (patients in which both abnormal utricular coefficient and significative baseline value difference were revealed)	4
BAS+SAC (patients in which both abnormal saccular coefficient and significative baseline value difference were revealed)	2
BAS+UTR+SAC (patients with abnormal utricular, saccular coefficients, and significative baseline value difference)	11
UTR+SAC (patients with abnormal utricular and saccular coefficients)	13

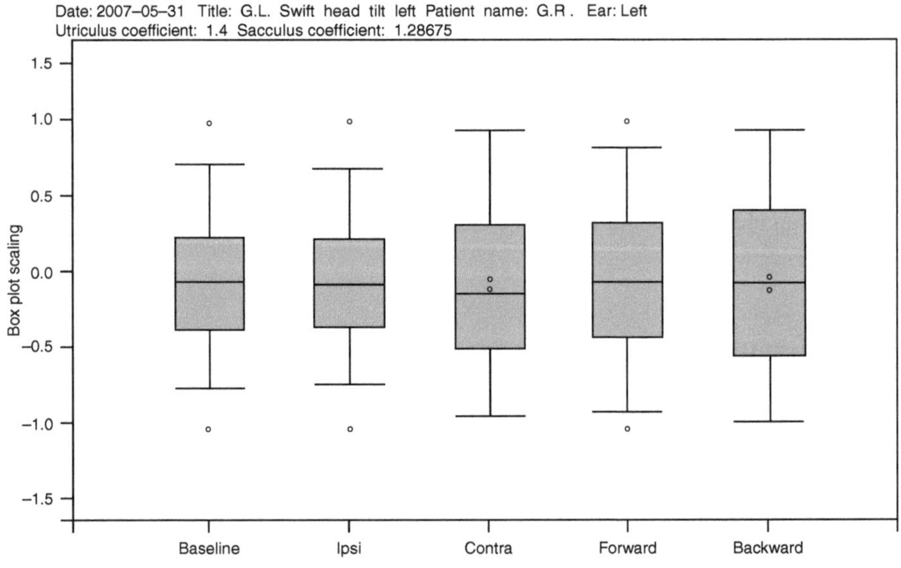

Fig. 21.3 In this case both macular coefficients are increased, specially the utricular one

SYMP patients could be subdivided into "utricular" (UTR), lateral tilt, and "saccular" (SAC), sagittal tilt, deficits (Table 21.2). In ten patients saccular responses were abnormal. UTR responses were also abnormal in 11 patients, while a combined UTR and SAC deficit was found in 13 patients (Fig. 21.3). This diagram shows an abnormal UTR and SAC responses showing that both the coefficient were increased but especially the "utricle" coefficient (1.4 compared to 1.28).

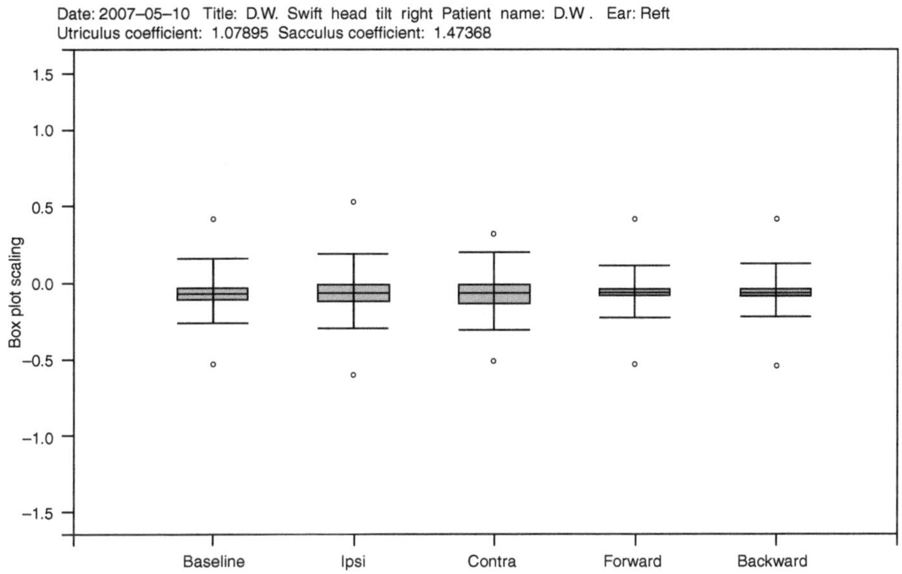

Fig. 21.4 In this case very small amplitudes of the interquartile range are detected both in the baseline assessment and in the SAC, sagittal, responses with increased coefficient (1.47). UTR, lateral, coefficient is just within normal limits (1.07)

In one female patient, a significant baseline difference was found while the UTR and SAC responses were normal. However, in two patients a significant baseline difference was found while at the same time there was a deficit in the SAC, sagittal, response, while in four patients it was the UTR, lateral, response. In 11 patients a significant baseline difference was associated with a combined UTR and SAC deficit. Figure 21.4 shows an EVG pattern characterized by very small amplitudes of the interquartile range detected both in the baseline assessment and in the SAC, sagittal, responses with increased coefficient (1.47). UTR, lateral, coefficient is just within normal limits (1.07).

21.4 Discussion

In some whiplash cases, no evidence of residual involvement of every canal can be revealed in those patients that present, during the course of their posttrauma life, relapsing episodes of benign PPV, as the subjects investigated in our study. Current neurootological tests in the diagnosis of vestibular diseases comprise electronystagmography, rotatory chair examination, caloric stimulations, and vestibular evoked myogenic potentials (VEMPs). These tests have been refined over the years, but among them VEMPs have become the most popular regarding vestibulospinal assessment. Although it is a multineuron reflex test, suggesting little specificity, there is general consensus that it gives accurate data regarding the saccule in the otolithic organ.

VEMPs when altered allow to explain residual and relapsing symptomatology with a remaining macular deficit as the most obvious cause or as an inferior vestibular nerve or vestibular nuclei involvement. In some cases, as in the patients that we were interested in, both neurootological and neuroimaging test are normal.

VEMPs may be considered a specific test of sacculo-spinal pathway even they are not able to distinguish between peripheral (saccule, inferior vestibular nerve, vestibulospinal tract) and central (vestibular nuclei) involvement [20–22].

In our patients VEMPs showed abnormalities in the largest part of SYMP patients (90.24 %).

EVG results in this study revealed the same percentage abnormalities, but it showed that about half of the SYMP patients had an abnormal UTR, lateral, response. This raises the hypothesis that abnormal responses of the utricle must be part of the overall response pattern in PPV, at least in the relapsing patients. It is known that during head tilt, both canals and maculae are stimulated, but Franz [12] assumed that responses collected through the extratympanic electrode were not contaminated by responses from the semicircular canals, as tilting the head is not performed in the optimal plane to stimulate this part of the inner ear. In addition, tilting the head is performed below a frequency of 1 Hz, which will avoid contamination by responses from the semicircular canals [23].

Anyway, a cross-coupled interaction may be not excluded due to the plasticity of the vestibular end organs, but this is out of the clinical interest regarding RPV functional assessment. In fact the main aim of vestibular investigation in this field of application is to document a disorder of the vestibular end organs as basis of the relapsing vertigo and residual unsteadiness. These data suggest that RPV could not be purely depending on sagittal tilt-sensitive receptors (mainly the saccule), and we can speculate, at least for what our experience attains, that in some patients there is also a disorder of the lateral tilt-sensitive receptors (mainly the utricle).

With the introduction of EVG, a single neuron reflex test has become available promising more information regarding vestibular end organs function.

As it is difficult for some whiplash patients to tilt the head, artifacts by muscle activity could become a problem. These are also avoided by using a very slow tilt of the head. Otherwise looking at the raw-recorded data these artifacts can be recognized. Typically muscle activity is detected by excessive voltage changes far beyond the regular appearing responses of the vestibular nerve. These excessive voltage responses can be easily removed before the analysis.

Limitation of EVG application can be a discomfort while inserting the electrode into the tympanic recess. If necessary, the discomfort can easily be overcome by placing a small cotton ball soaked with cophenylcaine into the tympanic recess for 5 min. This will give enough anesthesias to go ahead with EVG testing, and it does not interfere with the vestibular nerve response. Conductive hearing loss has no influence on EVG recording and, even if it was not our cases, EVG may be performed also with tympanic membrane perforation. Attention in the evaluation of data has to be paid if granulomatosis or cholesteatoma is present into the eardrum because impedance may be disturbed.

Conclusions

Vestibular potentials, in general, are specifically necessary to investigate residual vestibular impairment in still symptomatic patients when presenting relapsing benign PPV [24, 25]. VEMPs are well-established technique able to document vestibular involvement in the largest part of patients. EVG, an innovative examination technique, promises specific information about the status of the utricle and saccule, and possibly allowing detection of vestibular nerve degeneration. Comparison between VEMPs and EVG provides specific differential diagnosis between pure peripheral (EVG abnormal) and mixed involvement (VEMPs abnormal and normal EVG). Furthermore, the combination of both vestibular potentials may suggest useful information regarding vestibular end-organ function, at least in patients.

References

1. Caruso G, Nuti D (2005) Epidemiological data from 2270 PPV patients. Audiol Med 3(1): 7–11
2. von Brevern M, Radtke A, Lezius F, Feldmann M, Ziese T, Lempert T, Neuhauser H (2007) Epidemiology of benign paroxysmal positional vertigo: a population based study. J Neurol Neurosurg Psychiatry 78:710–715
3. Bickford RG, Jacobson JL, Cody DTR (1964) Nature of averaged evoked potentials to sound and other stimuli in man. Ann N Y Acad Sci 112:204–223
4. Cody DT, Jacobson JL, Walker JC, Bickford RG (1964) Averaged evoked myogenic and cortical potentials to sound in man. Ann Otol Rhinol Laryngol 73:763–777
5. Cody DTR, Bickford RG (1969) Averaged evoked myogenic responses in normal man. Laryngoscope 79:400–416
6. Townsend GL, Cody DTR (1971) The averaged inion response evoked by acoustic stimulation: its relation to the saccule. Ann Otol Rhinol Laryngol 80:121–131
7. Halmagyi GM, Curthoys IS, Colebatch JG, Aw ST (2005) Vestibular responses to sound. Ann N Y Acad Sci 1039:54–67
8. Welgampola MS, Colebatch JG (2005) Characteristics and clinical applications of vestibular-evoked potentials. Neurology 64:1682–1688
9. Isaradisaikul S, Strong DA, Moushey JM, Gabbare SA, Ackley SR, Jenkins HA (2008) Reliability of vestibular evoked myogenic potentials in healthy subjects. Otol Neurotol 29: 542–544
10. Wang SJ, Jaw FS, Young YH (2013) Optimizing the bandpass filter for acoustic stimuli in recording ocular vestibular-evoked myogenic potentials. Neurosci Lett 542:12–16
11. Rosengren SM, Kingma H (2013) New perspectives on vestibular evoked myogenic potentials. Curr Opin Neurol 26(1):74–80
12. Franz B (2003) Electro-otolithography: new insight into benign paroxysmal positioning vertigo. Int Tinnitus J 9:92–96
13. Franz B, Jones C, Chetcuti W (2006) Amplitude range analysis of otolithic organ responses. Int Tinnitus J 2:31–39
14. Semont A, Sterkers JM (1980) Reeducation vestibulaires. Les Cahiers D'Orl 15:305–376
15. Epley J (1996) Particle repositioning for benign paroxysmal positional vertigo. Otolaryngol Clin North Am 29(2):323–331
16. Lempert T, Wolsey C, Davies R, Gresty MA, Bronstein AM (1997) Three hundred sixty degree rotation of the posterior semicircular canal for the treatment of benign positional vertigo: a placebo-controlled trial. Neurology 49(3):729–733

17. Alpini D, Caputo D, Pugnetti L, Giuliano DA, Cesarani A (2001) Vertigo and multiple sclerosis: aspect of differential diagnosis. Neurol Sci 22(Suppl 2):S84–S87
18. Alpini D, Pugnetti L, Caputo D, Cesarani A (2004) Vestibular evoked myogenic potentials in multiple sclerosis: clinical and imaging correlations. Mult Scler 10:316–321
19. Alpini D, Pugnetti L, Caputo D, Cesarani À (2005) Vestibular evoked myogenic potentials in multiple sclerosis: a comparison between onset and definite cases. Int Tinnitus J 11:48–51
20. Colebatch JG, Halmagyi GM, Skuse NF (1994) Myogenic potentials generated by a click evoked vestibulocollic reflex. J Neurol Neurosurg Psychiatry 57:190–197
21. Wilson VJ, Schor RH (1999) The neural substrate of the vestibulocollic reflex. What needs to be learned. Exp Brain Res 129:483–493
22. Imai T, Takeda N, Ito M, Nakamae K, Sakae H, Fujioka H, Matsunaga T, Kubo T (2006) Benign paroxysmal positional vertigo due to a simultaneous involvement of both horizontal and posterior semicircular canals. Audiol Neurootol 11:198–205
23. Mackensen G (1955) Clinical use of electronystagmography, analysis of an unusual movement disorder by means of electric recording. Klin Monatsblätter Augenheilkunde Augenärzl Fortbildung 126:685–693
24. Murofushi T, Shimizu K, Takegoshi H, Cheng PW (2001) Diagnostic value of prolonged latencies in the vestibular evoked myogenic potential. Arch Otolaryngol Head Neck Surg 127: 1069–1072
25. Karino S, Ito K, Ochiai A, Murofushi T (2005) Independent effects of simultaneous inputs from the saccule and lateral semicircular canal. Evaluation using VEMPs. Clin Neurophysiol 116(7):1707–1715

Whiplash Effects on Brain: Voluntary Eye Movements

22

M. Spanio, S. Rigo, and D.C. Alpini

22.1 Introduction

Saccades and smooth pursuit eye movements play an important role in the balance system. Essentially their aim is to free foveate animals from the slavery of oculomotor reflexes, such as vestibulo-ocular reflex (VOR) and optokinetic nystagmus (OKN). These voluntary eye movements enable the gaze to be rapidly redirected (saccades) or to slowly follow (smooth pursuit movements) new targets even when the head or surroundings are moving.

Saccades usually occur during VOR and OKN in order to automatically reset slow eye drift caused by vestibular or optokinetic stimuli and bring the gaze to the incoming scene, thus they have come to be known as nystagmus quick phases. Moreover, saccades can help an oculomotor system which has been impaired by a pathology and override its resulting limitations. For instance, an abnormal smooth pursuit may present with saccades, seen on the eye record as a cogwheel shape, which enhance global oculomotor response gain [1]. Even in labyrinth defective patients, saccades represent a compensatory mechanism, taking on the role of the defective VOR [2].

The smooth pursuit system is perhaps involved in evoked nystagmus visual suppression, a function frequently investigated in clinical assessment of visual-vestibular interaction.

M. Spanio (✉)
"Salus" Private Hospital, via Bonaparte 4-6, 34123 Trieste, Italy
e-mail: cdc@salustrieste.it

S. Rigo
Otorhinolaryngology, Via del Coroneo, 32, 34133 Trieste, Italy
e-mail: rigostefano2@libero.it

D.C. Alpini
ENT-Otoneurology Service, IRCCS "Don Carlo C. Gnocchi" Foundation, Milan, Italy
e-mail: dalpini@dongnocchi.it

D.C. Alpini et al. (eds.), *Whiplash Injuries*,
DOI 10.1007/978-88-470-5486-8_22, © Springer-Verlag Italia 2014

Therefore saccadic and smooth pursuit systems assist correct behaviour of the balance system, and, when affected by neurological lesions, they might lead to balance impairment, causing blurred vision and dizziness.

Saccadic and smooth pursuit are very complex oculomotor systems whose mechanisms have not yet been completely understood. As already stated the aim of a saccade is to quickly move the gaze onto a new visual target, therefore the stimulus consists in a gap between fovea and retinal target position, whereas the aim of a smooth pursuit movement is to follow a moving object, and here the stimulus consists in a velocity retinal slip between fovea and target.

The neural pathways of the two systems are completely different, but essentially they extend from cerebral cortex to brainstem oculomotor nuclei, passing through the cerebellum.

Therefore abnormalities of saccades or smooth pursuit movements are considered a precise and sensitive marker of a central nervous system (CNS) pathology [3].

To record and analyse these ocular movements, we require special investigative techniques and a well-equipped laboratory.

In a clinical environment, visual stimulation is usually provided by a LED array, and horizontal binocular movements are collected by means of DC-EOG and Ag-AgCl electrodes. As for the saccadic test, the subject is presented with predictable or unpredictable target jumps of several amplitudes (5–40°) in both directions (rightwards and leftwards).

As for smooth pursuit the subject is studied by using continuous target movements with triangular, sinusoidal or ramp patterns. Normally stimulus peak velocities of 20–40°/s are utilized.

Eye movements in saccadic tests are usually low-pass filtered at 50 Hz and sampled at 250 Hz, whereas data from smooth pursuit tests are low-pass filtered at 10 Hz and sampled at 50 Hz. Butterworth 18 dB/oct low-pass filters and 12-bit AIO conversion are used.

The most modern eye movement recording is video-oculography (VOG). A video camera records directly the movements of the eyes and a computer analyses the data obtained in this way. According to Pietkiewicz et al. [4]., with respect to the EOG, VOG should be recommended in preference as the valuable method to assess vertigo and to discriminate between the peripheral and the central vestibular lesions but, for the purpose of WAD evaluation, informations about oculomotor system involvement are comparable.

Analysis of saccadic movements is in two steps: first, a morphological evaluation of the global eye movement response to each target jump (overshoots, postsaccadic drifts, etc.) and, second, an automatic/interactive identification of the start and end points of each saccade, followed by an automatic evaluation of the saccadic parameters (latency, amplitude, duration and peak velocity) for statistical analysis. Saccadic abnormalities are evaluated taking into account the direction and the amplitude of target displacement.

Analysis of the smooth pursuit responses is also in two steps: first, a morphological evaluation of the global eye response (both the smooth and saccadic components are investigated) and, second, evaluation of the gain and the temporal shift of the smooth component by cross-correlating the velocity of this component with that of the stimulus.

Although there is still debate as to its significance, a widespread clinical application of investigating the smooth pursuit system consists of a per-rotatory nystagmus visual suppression test. The subject is rotated in darkness and asked to fix on a dim light rotating with him. With a healthy CNS the visual system can suppress per-rotatory nystagmus down to 30 % of the initial value or even lower.

22.2 Whiplash-Associated Saccades and Pursuit Disturbances

In whiplash injuries, it has been calculated that the sudden jerk of the neck can cause an elongation of the cervical columna up to 5 cm and thus an elongation of the brainstem [5]. This event can lead to, besides a wide range of lesions in the columna, nerve roots and medulla, even lesions in the brain stem, cerebellum and oculomotor system. Several authors have investigated the saccadic and smooth pursuit systems in whiplash patients.

Oosterveld et al. [6] submitted 262 patients, chronically suffering from the after-effects of whiplash to an extensive vestibular and oculomotor examination. Some 85 % of the patients complained of light-headedness, spinning or floating sensations. Disturbances in visual pursuit movements were found in 113 patients (43 %) and in visual suppression tests in 97 patients (37 %), proving the presence of both cerebellar and brainstem pathology. However, a large number of patients (63 %) also had a spontaneous nystagmus of more than 5° *Is*, interpreted by the authors as a sign of central origin, which might interfere with smooth pursuit performance. In 41 patients oculomotor tests repeated 1 year later showed no significant improvements.

A high correlation between symptoms and oculomotor abnormalities has been found by Hildingsson et al. [7]. They examined the oculomotor function in 39 consecutive whiplash patients 6 months or more after the trauma. Twenty patients complained of chronic and disabling symptoms, such as neck ache, neck stiffness, headache, shoulder and arm pain. Two patients had vertigo or dizziness. Visual symptoms, often blurring of vision, as well as auditory symptoms were present in 15 patients. No difference in visual tracking was noted between 19 asymptomatic patients and control group subjects, whereas an oculomotor dysfunction was noted in 18 of 20 patients with persisting symptoms of a soft-tissue injury of the cervical spine. Four patients had pronounced abnormalities, and 14 had moderate oculomotor dysfunction.

In particular, smooth pursuit was abnormal with reduced velocity gain in 14 patients (in 12 asymmetrically) and with an increase in superimposed saccades in 16 patients (in 13 unilaterally). The saccades were hypometric in nine patients. Six patients had poorer accuracy and maximal velocity of the saccades, and five of these patients also showed latency prolongation. In general, patients with chronic symptoms had prolonged saccadic latency ($p < 0.001$).

Patients with more pronounced smooth pursuit abnormalities presented with saccadic dysfunction. None of the patients with saccadic dysfunction had normal pursuit. The authors suggest that the proprioceptive system in the cervicocranial area is affected in 14 patients with moderate oculomotor impairment and that in four patients with pronounced oculomotor abnormalities, the brainstem and cerebellum are affected.

Observations of Hildingsson et al. [7] demonstrate that sometimes oculomotor system disorders can occur at a later date. The authors investigated 40 consecutive whiplash patients. The most frequent acute symptoms after injury were aching and stiffness in the neck and headaches, followed by dizziness and shoulder pain. The initial oculomotor tests, performed within 3 months of the accident, were pathologic in eight patients. The follow-up test, on average 15 months after the accident, remained pathologic in the eight patients and a further five patients had changed from normal to pathologic test results. All the 13 patients with oculomotor dysfunction had disabling symptoms. In six patients smooth pursuit eye movements were abnormal with reduced velocity gain and with increased superimposed saccades.

In all 13 patients the saccades showed low peak: velocity and prolonged latencies. Three patients suffered pronounced abnormalities affecting both smooth pursuit and saccades.

Wenngren et al. [8] investigated the prevalence of brain/brainstem dysfunction after acute whiplash trauma (grades II and III according to the Quebec Task Force Classification on whiplash-associated disorders) and the possible correlation between the development of chronic symptoms and objective findings from eye motility tests. They used oculomotor tests in a sample of prospective whiplash trauma patients who were followed up for 2 years after the trauma. The initial test results did not reveal any prognostic clinical signs for the tested group as a whole, but they could discriminate some patients with clinical symptoms and signs paired with pathologic test results. Over time, some patients normalized clinically and their test results improved, while others deteriorated clinically and their test results were worse at the 2-year investigation.

Further support to the involvement of oculomotor systems in whiplash comes from the Kogler et al. study [9]. The authors investigated 25 acute whiplash patients using, among other tests, smooth pursuit tests, saccadic tests and per-rotatory nystagmus visual suppression tests. The patients were consecutive which meant that even lighter trauma could be included in the study.

They were checked after 3, 6 and 9 months. At the first consultation about half of the patients had disturbances. The results are interpreted as indicating that pathological visual suppression and especially defective smooth pursuit ability may point to a chronic lesion of the brain stem. The patients concerned also had vertigo and unsteadiness. However there was no correlation between symptoms and pathological saccade tests.

In patients referred to our hospital for whiplash symptoms, we began a study of the VOR, and of a possible cervico-ocular component, by means of active and passive head movements. Out of these patients 14 were also submitted to saccade and smooth pursuit tests. The age of the patients ranged from 51 to 24 years (mean age

Table 22.1 Whiplash patients: oculomotor results

	Saccades				Smooth pursuit (gain)		VOR/Hz (gain/phase)	
	Main sequence	Latency	Metricity	Shape	20 %	40 %	Horiz.	Vert.
1	N	Increased	N	N	0.88	0.83	0.82/–5	1.05/–3
2	N	N	N	N	0.97	0.85	0.75/3	0.95/–5
3	N	N	N	N	0.98	0.80	0.73/–9	0.98/–6
4	PV ⇑ d ⇓	N	N	N	0.90	0.75	0.96/–6	0.91/–15
5	N	N	N	N	0.89	0.82	0.75/–6	1.10/–11
6	N	N	N	Overshoots	0.97	0.87	0.75/–6	1.15/–13
7	N	N	N	N	0.90	0.82	0.80/2	1.15/–40
8	N	N	N	N	0.98	0.86	0.67/–5	0.65/–8
9	PV ⇑ d ⇓	Increased	N	N	0.99	0.68	1.07/–6	1.10/–10
10	N	N	Hypometria	N	0.94	0.62	0.93/–8	0.95/–13
11	PV ⇓	Increased	Hypometria	N	0.90	0.59	0.90/–2	0.89/–9
12	PV ⇓	N	N	N	0.78	0.65	0.65/–9	1.05/–10
13	N	N	N	N	0.85	0.78	0.69/–5	0.52/–10
14	PV ⇑ d ⇓	Increased	N	N	0.70	0.55	0.50/3	0.89/–4

PV peach velocity, *d* duration, *N* normal parameters

32.8 years); older patients were excluded in order to avoid impairment of saccadic and smooth pursuit performances due to aging or pathologies. Seven patients complained only of cervicobrachialgia or headache; seven complained also of dizziness and unsteadiness. All the patients were examined within a week of the accident. Even light trauma was included. The test results are reported in Table 22.1.

Saccade abnormalities appeared mostly in the symptomatic group, but even in some asymptomatic patients. A lower smooth pursuit gain was present only in symptomatic patients. The symptomatic group often presented a lower VOR gain. Only one asymptomatic patient presented a large phase lag of vertical VOR.

The number of patients examined is too small to draw a definite conclusion; nevertheless a relevant difference between our groups is the presence, in symptomatic patients, of an abnormality in at least one out of the three systems investigated. This might justify the balance disturbances the patients complained of. Nevertheless, the absence of a precise correlation between saccade abnormalities and symptoms, as found also by Kogler et al. [9], reduces the weight of saccade abnormalities on the balance. Even an isolated, but marked, saccade slowness cannot completely account for patients' complaints. Actually a low gain in the VOR or smooth pursuit has, on balance, greater effect than saccade slowness. A summary of the above-mentioned studies on whiplash injuries shows that saccade and smooth pursuit abnormalities are often present in symptomatic patients.

If the impairments of saccades and smooth pursuit movements are considered a marker of a CNS pathology, how can their presence be explained in subjects affected by a soft-tissue injury of the cervical spine without assuming a contemporary head injury? Patients who received head trauma must have been excluded from data analysis. Therefore oculomotor abnormalities reveal damage of the CNS probably due to pull, stretch and pressure of the medulla oblongata, brainstem and cerebellum during the sudden jerk of the head [10–12].

A different hypothesis has been proposed by Hinoki [13]. In patients with whiplash injury, there might be an overexcitation of the cervical and/or lumbar proprioceptors on the one hand and a dysfunction of the CNS, such as the hypothalamus, the brainstem and the cerebellum, on the other hand.

These two factors cause imbalance by means of a trigger-and-target relationship in which the above proprioceptors act as a trigger and the CNS acts as a target. This hypothesis of a proprioceptive trigger, according to Hildingsson et al. [7], could explain even saccade and smooth pursuit abnormalities.

Nevertheless, a further element should be taken into account with regard to this type of oculomotor test. Saccades and smooth pursuit performances depend on cognitive functions to a large extent. Radanov et al. [14] evaluated the cognitive functions in whiplash patients and found they were impaired in terms of attention and speed of information processing. [15, 16].

These observations could justify some abnormalities: for instance latency increase in the saccades and gain decrease in smooth pursuit movements.

In conclusion, the high incidence of saccades and smooth pursuit abnormalities in whiplash patients highlights the importance in investigation of whiplash injuries of oculomotor voluntary tests in order to prove the seriousness of the trauma. Nevertheless, these tests must be integrated into a larger clinical protocol aimed at the assessment of vestibular and optokinetic systems and postural control. Abnormalities in both saccadic and smooth pursuit systems may account for patients' complaints about balance only when the other tests provide normal results. The outcome of patient follow-up using these tests can be very useful both for patient control and medical legal purposes.

References

1. Dell' Aquila T, Inchingolo P, Spanio M (1989) An analysis of the smooth and the global eye response to a periodic target motion in mano In: Schmid R, Zambarbieri D (eds) Proceedings of the fifth European congress on eye movements. University of Pavia, Pavia, pp 76–78
2. Kasai T, Zee DS (1978) Eye-head coordination in labyrinthine-defective human beings. Brain Res 144:123–141
3. Leigh RJ, Zee DS (1991) The neurology of eye movements. Davis, Philadelphia
4. Pietkiewicz P, Pepaś R, Sułkowski WJ, Zielińska-Bliźniewska H, Olszewski J (2012) Electronystagmography versus videonystagmography in diagnosis of vertigo. Int J Occup Med Environ Health 25(1):59–65
5. Hildingsson C, Wenngren BI, Bring G, Toolanen G (1989) Oculomotor problems after cervical spine injury. Acta Orthop Scand 60(5):513–516
6. Oosterveld WJ, Kortschot HW, Kingma GC, de Jong AA, Saatci MR (1991) Electronystagmographic findings following cervical whiplash injuries. Acta Otolaryngol Stockh 111:201–205
7. Hildingsson C, Wenngren BI, Toolanen G (1993) Eye motility dysfunction after soft-tissue injury of the cervical spine. A controlled, prospective study of 38 patients. Acta Orthop Scand 64(2):129–132
8. Wenngren BI, Pettersson K, Lowenhielm G, Hildingsson C (2002) Eye motility and auditory brainstem response dysfunction after whiplash injury. Acta Otolaryngol 122(3):276–283

9. Kogler A, Lindfors J, Odkvist LM, Ledin T (2000) Postural stability using different neck positions in normal subjects and patients with neck trauma. Acta Otolaryngol. 120(2):151–155.
10. Sances A, Weber RC, Larson SJ, Cusick JS, Myklebust JB, Walsh PR (1981) Bioengineering analysis of head and spine injuries. CRC Crit Rev Bioeng 6:79
11. Gimse R, Tjell C, Bjørgen IA, Saunte C (1996) Disturbed eye movements after whiplash due to injuries to the posture control system. J Clin Exp Neuropsychol 18(2):178–186
12. Matsui T, Ii K, Hojo S, Sano K (2012) CervicoNeuro-muscolar syndrome: discovery of a new disease group caused by abnormalities in the cervical muscles. Neurol Med Chir 52:75–80
13. Hinoki M (1985) Vertigo due to whiplash injury: a neurotological approach. Acta Otolaryngol Stockh 419(Suppl I):9–29
14. Radanov B, Dvorak J, Valach L (1992) Cognitive deficits in patients after soft tissue injury of the cervical spine. Spine 17(2):127–131
15. Di Stefano G, Radanov BP (1995) Course of attention and memory after common whiplash: a two-years prospective study with age, education and gender pair-matched patients. Acta Neurol Scand 91(5):346–352
16. Kessels RP, Keyser A, Verhagen WI, van Luijtelaar EL (1998) The whiplash syndrome: a psychophysiological and neuropsychological study towards attention. Acta Neurol Scand 97(3):188–193

Whiplash Effects on Brain: Optokinetic Nystagmus and Visuo-Vestibular Interaction

23

A. Salami, M.C. Medicina, and M. Dellepiane

23.1 Introduction

Different papers [1–5] suggest the existence of complex peripheral and, overall, central alterations in the vestibular system as a consequence of a trauma in the cervical portion. Thus we studied optokinetic and visual vestibular system behavior in subjects who previously underwent a cervical whiplash injury. The results of our research could be both interesting from a clinical point of view and useful for medicolegal goals. Our methods could be suitable for pointing out alterations in central sites as it is known that the nystagmus resulting from the contemporary optokinetic and roto-acceleration stimulation with counterdirectional nystagmus is significantly weakened in brain stem and cerebellar lesions and more widely in the presence of lesions in the posterior cranial fossa [6–9]. The visuo-vestibular interaction has not yet been adopted in the study of cervical whiplash injury.

23.2 Methods

The investigation was carried out on 32 subjects of age between 21 and 48 (18 men and 14 women) who had undergone a cervical trauma for a traffic accident with whiplash injury (Table 23.1). Thirteen subjects were examined within the third month following the accident (1st group), six subjects between the third and the sixth month (2nd group), and 13 subjects later than 6 months up to 24 months (3rd group). It is important to note that we observed a spontaneous horizontal nystagmus in three subjects (one for each group) with an incidence of 9.3 % out of the total.

The recording of ocular movements was done by the usual method using an eight-channel Tonnies electronystagmograph. The subjects were sitting with their heads still, on a Tonnies rotatory chair Pro model, which was placed in the middle

A. Salami (✉) • M.C. Medicina • M. Dellepiane
Otorhinolaryngology, "San Martino" Hospital, Largo Rosanna Benzi 10, 16132 Genoa, Italy
e-mail: http://www.otorinoangelosalami.com/contatti

D.C. Alpini et al. (eds.), *Whiplash Injuries*,
DOI 10.1007/978-88-470-5486-8_23, © Springer-Verlag Italia 2014

Table 23.1 Complaints after cervical whiplash injuries in 32 patients

	Number	%
Headache	21	65.6
Subjective vertigo	13	40.6
Objective vertigo	4	12.5
Floating sensation	15	46.8
Tinnitus	14	43.7
Tinnitus and hearing impairment	5	15.6
Neck pain	13	40.6

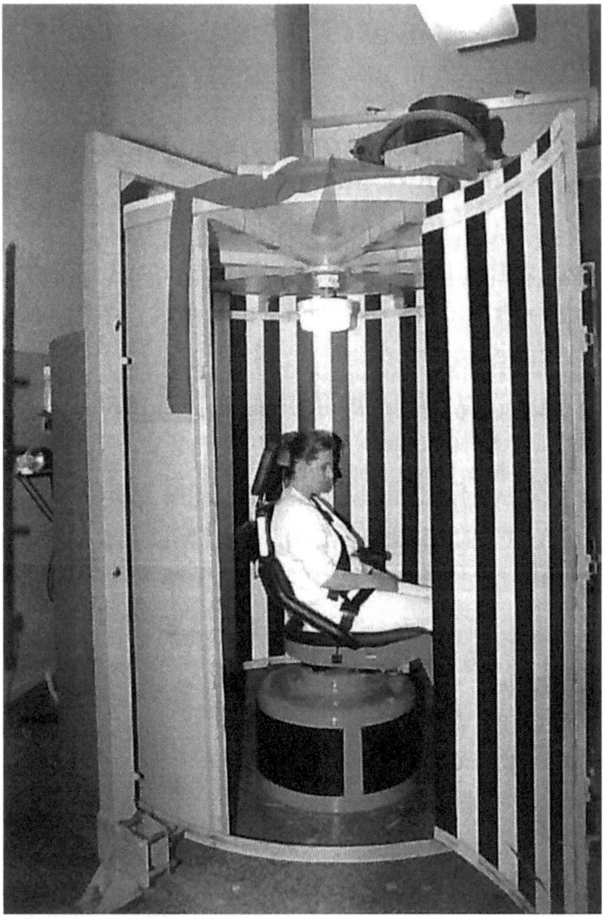

Fig. 23.1 Rotatory cylindrical chamber. The Tonnies rotatory chair system Pro in the middle

of a rotatory cylindrical chamber with a diameter of 2 and 1.9 m high. Its white internal area was covered with 32 black vertical contrasts (Fig. 23.1), each one 9.32 cm wide and with an angle of 5.61°.

The rotatory cylinder was lighted from above by a 100 W lamp and was driven by a direct current engine able to reach the desired turning speed (clockwise and counterclockwise of up to 2,000/s maximum speed, with preset acceleration ranging from 1° to 20°/s2).

Each patient was exposed to:

1. Postrotatory vestibular stimulation (VOR, vestibular ocular reflex): with stop test, eyes open in the dark at an angular velocity of 900/s which was subliminally reached clockwise and counterclockwise.
2. Optokinetic stimulation (OKN, optokinetic nystagmus) "stare type" with a cylinder rotation velocity of 300/s for 60 s with clockwise and counterclockwise rotation.

   The length of 60 s was chosen because we thought that VOR could sometimes prevail over OKN. In this respect, our previous research on visuo-vestibular interaction [10] had shown that in cases of lack of VOR substitution by OKN, sometimes it took more than 20 s for the appearance of OKN.
3. Contemporary postrotatory vestibular and optokinetic stimulation (VVOR, visuo-vestibular ocular reflex) at the postrotatory stop: the light was turned on and we effected optokinetic stimulation with a cylinder (and optical contrasts) rotation capable of inducing an OKN which was beating on the opposite side of the postrotatory vestibular nystagmus.

We took into account the fundamental parameter nystagmus "gain" as the ratio between the angular velocity of nystagmus slow phase and the stimulation velocity. VOR mean gain was calculated on the first three beats; OKN mean gain was calculated on the beats in the first 20 s; VVOR mean gain was calculated:

1. On the first three beats during the first 20 s of optokinetic stimulation, when the resulting nystagmus was beating in the OKN direction.
2. Only on the first three beats, when the resulting nystagmus was beating in the VOR direction.

The results were compared with the ones we obtained in a group of seven normal subjects, ages 28–36, and statistically evaluated (mean difference) by *t*-test.

23.3 Results

The results (Tables 23.2 and 23.3 and Figs. 23.2, 23.3, 23.4, and 23.5) can be summed up as follows:

- VOR: none of the normal or pathological subjects showed any significant differences between the sides ($p > 0.05$). In pathological subjects mean gain decreased

Table 23.2 Mean with standard deviation of the mean gain

	VOR	OKN	VVOR OKN DIR[a]		VVOR VOR DIR[b]
	(3 beats)	(20 s)	(3 beats)	(20 s)	(3 beats)
Normal subjects	0.47±0.08	0.46±0.07	0.25±0.09	0.32±0.02	(–)
1st group (0–3 month)	0.34±0.11	0.64±0.18	0.15±0.05	0.25±0.08	0.12±0.08
2nd group (3–6 month)	0.45±0.12	0.73±0.09	0.22±0.14	0.29±0.19	0.18±0.13
3rd group (over 6 month)	0.38±0.11	0.71±0.11	0.28±0.11	0.3±0.10	0.18±0.14

[a]OKN DIR, nystagmus beating in the OKN direction
[b]VOR DIR, nystagmus beating in the VOR direction

Table 23.3 Significance test (*t*-test) between normal subjects and whiplash patients

	VOR	ON	VVOR OKN	Direction
	(3 beats)	(20 s)	(3 beats)	(20 s)
Normal vs. 1st group	$p<0.05$	$p<0.05$	$p<0.01$	$p>0.05$
Normal vs. 2nd group	$p>0.05$	$p<0.01$	$p>0.05$	$p>0.05$
Normal vs. 3rd group	$p>0.05$	$p<0.01$	$p>0.05$	$p>0.05$

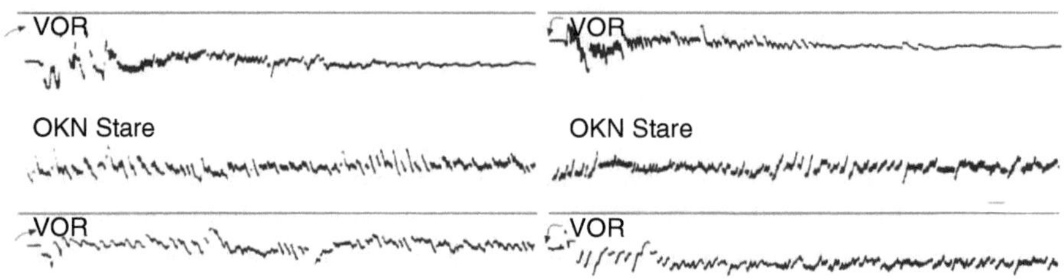

Fig. 23.2 Normal subject. From *top* to *bottom*: the postrotatory nystagmus (VOR) in the dark at the constant angular velocity of 90°/s with clockwise and counterclockwise chair rotation; optokinetic nystagmus "stare type" (*OKN*) with the cylinder rotatory constant velocity of 30°/s for 60 s; and visuo-vestibular ocular reflex (*VVOR*) with a cylinder rotation which caused an OKN beating on the opposite side of the postrotatory vestibular nystagmus. VVOR with counterdirectional VOR and OKN always evokes a nystagmus beating in the OKN direction

in all three groups compared with normal ones (Table 23.2), but it was statistically significant ($p<0.05$) only in the subjects of the first group (Table 23.3), that is, in those subjects who underwent the trauma more recently.

- OKN: none of the normal or pathological subjects showed any significant differences between the sides ($p>0.05$). In pathological subjects mean gain increased—with respect to normal ones—in all three groups (Table 23.2), with a significant increase ($p<0.05$) in the first group and highly significant increase ($p<0.01$) in the second and third groups (Table 23.3).
- VVOR: in normal subjects VVOR always beats OKN direction, with a mean gain on the first three beats slightly inferior to the one calculated during the first 20 s (Table 23.2).

In 16 cases the pathological subjects' VVOR beats in the same direction of normal subjects (six in the first, four in the second, six in the third group), with a mean gain on the first three beats which only in the first group showed a statistically significant variation (decrease) ($p<0.01$) compared with normal subjects (Table 23.3). In the three groups of pathological subjects, the mean gain, during the first 20 s, showed a decrease compared to normal, but it was not statistically significant (Table 23.3).

In the remaining 16 cases (seven in the first, two in the second, seven in the third group), VVOR beats in the same direction as VOR for a variable length of 3–15 s (Figs. 23.3 and 23.4) with a mean gain on the first three beats always highly inferior to VOR ones; VVOR beating in the VOR direction was followed by a variable

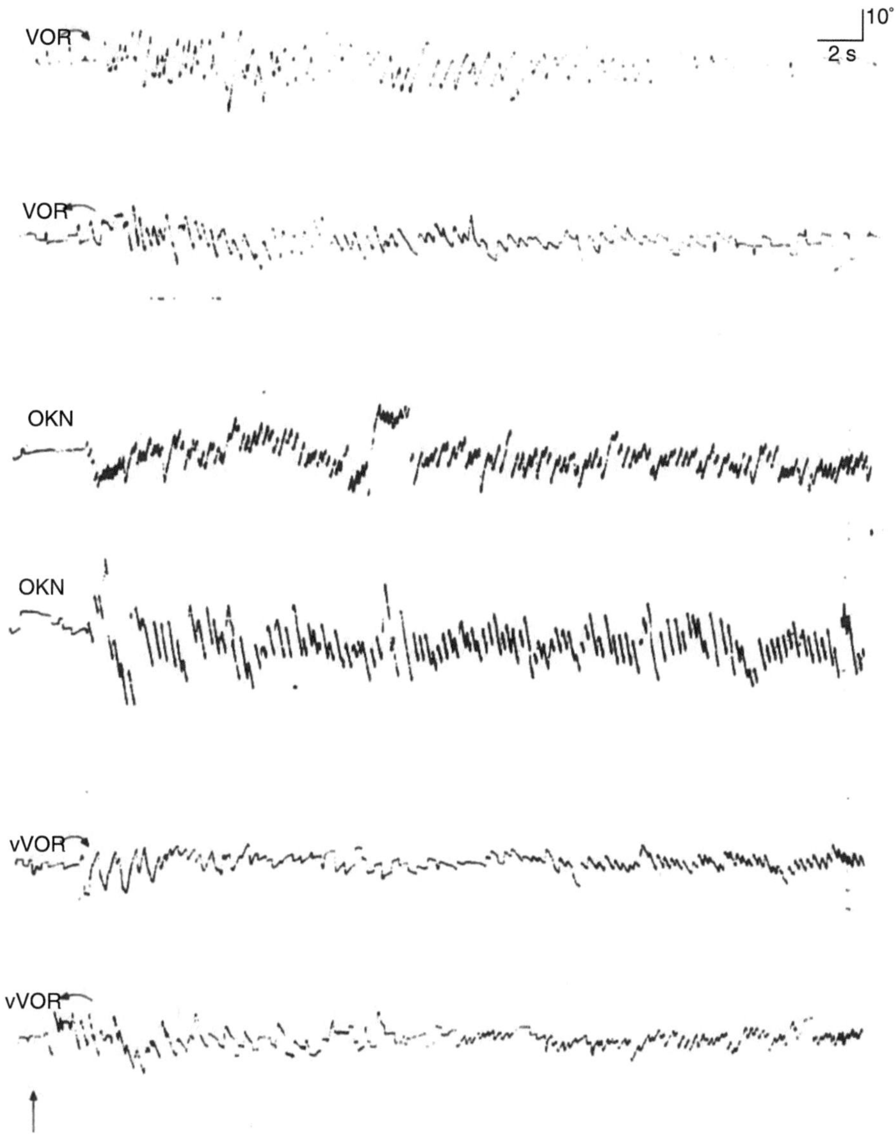

Fig. 23.3 Patient of the first group. From top to bottom: postrotatory nystagmus (VOR) and optokinetic nystagmus "stare type" (OKN and visuo-vestibular ocular reflex). Note increase of OKN; VVOR is characterized by a nystagmus beating in the VOR direction for about 10 s. After a varying period of ocular immobility, a nystagmus beating in the OKN direction appeared. The vertical arrows point out the chair stop. For further information, see Fig. 23.2

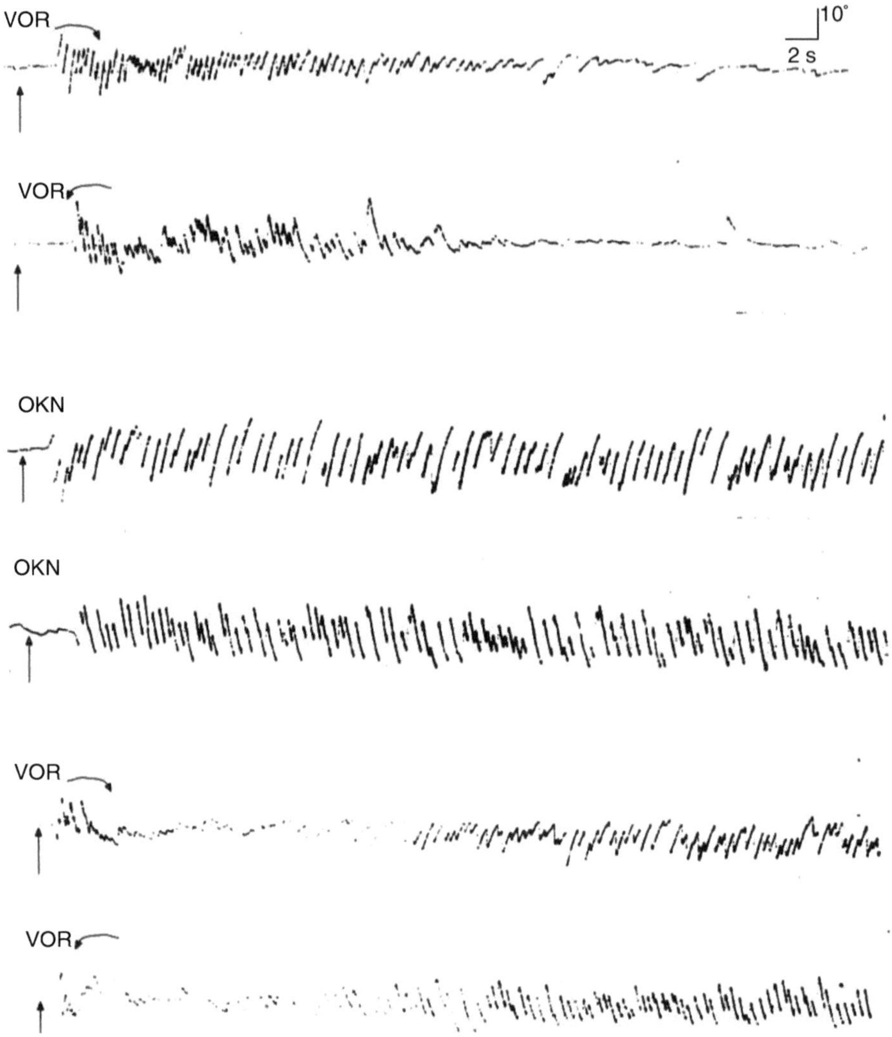

Fig. 23.4 Patient of the second group

period (a few seconds) of ocular immobility and then by a nystagmus beating in the OKN direction (Fig. 23.5).

23.4 Discussion

The results of our research pointed to a statistically significant decrease of VOR and VVOR mean gains (beating in the OKN direction calculated on the first three beats) compared with normal subjects in the patients of the first group and a significant

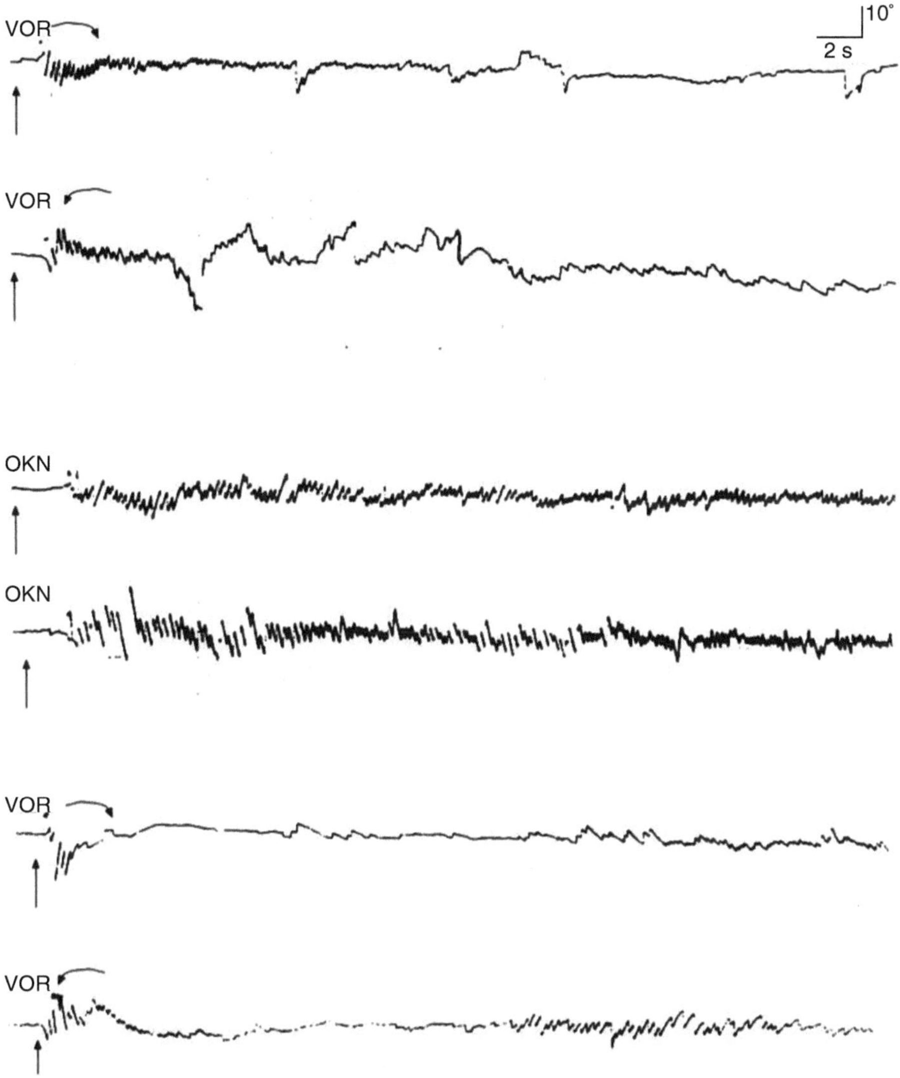

Fig. 23.5 Patients of the third group

increase of OKN mean gain in the patients of all the three groups. Furthermore, at VVOR, immediately after the stop, we observed a nystagmus beating in the VOR direction which lasted from 3 to 15 s in 16 patients out of 32 (seven in the first, two in the second, seven in the third group).

In 1968 and in 1970, Miura et al. [11, 12] observed that cervical trauma of a certain extent (about 7 G) which was experimentally induced in rabbits determined either microcirculatory alterations of brain stem and the superior portion of the spine or circulatory disturbances of the peripheral labyrinth. By analogy we can assume that the significant decrease of VOR mean gain that we observed in patients with cervical whiplash injury belonging to the first group could be due to labyrinthic alterations subsequent to circulatory labyrinthic alterations.

The possibility of damage, also minor, to peripheral vestibular structures as a direct consequence of cervical whiplash injury is also suggested by Chester [13] and by Brandt [1], as well as on the basis of the experimental data of Schuknecht and colleagues [14], who found a degeneration of Corti's organ and secondary of the pertaining acoustic fibers; these data could be taken into account in trying to explain, partially at least, the vestibular and audiological complaints (particularly hearing loss and tinnitus) referred to by some of our patients (Table 23.1).

As to the significant increase of OKN mean gain that we observed in all three groups, our results agree with those obtained by other authors [15]. Therefore, taking into account the importance either of vestibular nuclei in the production of OKN [45, 35] or of the pathway (even if it is not completely known) which is crossed by optokinetic impulses at the subcortical site (tectum region and pontinus tegmen) [16, 17] and if we also consider that the cerebellar nodulus and flocculus receive visual and proprioceptive vestibular inputs [18–20], we may conclude that OKN increase in cervical whiplash injury is determined by (a) pathological reactivity of vestibular nuclei caused by cervical proprioceptors "overexcitation" [21]. The connections of cervical proprioceptors with brainstem and particularly with vestibular nuclei and reticular structure are already known [22], and (b) an altered microcirculation of brain stem [23] and/or by a neurological-vascular friction which may cause functional disorders of CNS and in particular of brain stem structures in cervical whiplash injury [24].

As to VVOR, it is known that the optokinetic-vestibular interaction with counterdirectional VOR and OKN evokes, in normal subjects, a nystagmus which is always beating in the OKN direction, with a mean gain decrease in relation to OKN.

Our present results confirm these data as a further demonstration that a peripheral labyrinthic excitation, evoked by any technique and even if it is intense, induces, in normal subjects, a nystagmus which is always overcome by a contrasting OKN.

Nevertheless in six cases out of 13 patients belonging to the first group, VVOR appeared with a nystagmus beating in the OKN direction, but with a mean gain—on the first three beats—which was significantly decreased compared with normal subjects. Finally in 16 out of 32 cases of the three groups (seven in the first, two in the second, and seven in the third group), VVOR was characterized by a nystagmus beating in the VOR direction.

Numerous studies of animal anatomy and physiology showed the importance of the cerebellar flocculus in the working out of visual vestibular interaction [25] and its influence on central velocity storage mechanism [26–28]. Therefore this structure is likely to be involved as a consequence of cervical whiplash injury, and an alteration may occur in the transmission of inputs coming from the caudal portion of inferior olive nucleus. We may also face an alteration of the flocculus control function on vestibular inputs, as Miles and Fuller [29] have already showed.

From a clinical point of view, these data confirm the importance of ENG examination in cervical whiplash injury. The alterations of OKN (statistically significant increase of mean gain in all three groups of patients) and of VVOR (nystagmus beating VOR direction) show—without reference to its pathogenetical origin—the presence of lesions, especially of central type and more specifically regarding brain stem and cerebellum. It is evident that these results are interesting from a medicolegal point of view. Therefore we can repeat Oosterveld and colleagues' words: "In cases where legal medicine is involved, the outcome of an extensive nystagmographic examination can be of utmost importance both for the doctor and for the patients."

References

1. Brandt T (1984) Clinical evidence for cervical vertigo? In: Vertigo: its multisensory syndromes. Springer, London, p 281
2. Compere WE (1966) Electronystagmographic findings in patients with "whiplash injuries". Laryngoscope 78:1226
3. Gay JR, Abbott K (1953) Common whiplash injuries of the neck. JAMA I52:1698
4. Hildingsson C, Wenngren B, Bring G, Toolenen G (1989) Oculomotor problems after cervical spine injury. Acta Orthop Scand 60:513
5. Hildingsson C, Wenngren B, Toolanen G (1993) Eye motility dysfunction after soft-tissue injury of the cervical spine. Acta Orthop Scand 64:129
6. Hinoki M (1972) Vertigo due to whiplash injury from the standpoint of neurootology. In: Itemi K (ed) Whiplash injury. Kanehara, Shuppan, Tokyo, p 100
7. Hinoki M (1985) Vertigo due to whiplash injury: a neurotological approach. Acta Otolaryngol Stockh 419(Suppl I):9
8. Hinoki M, Hine S, Tada Y (1971) Neurotological studies on vertigo due to whiplash injury. Equilib Res 28(Suppl 1):5
9. Kano MS, Kano M, Maekawa K (1990) Receptive field organisation of climbing fiber afferents responding to optokinetic stimulation in the cerebellar nodulus and flocculus of the pigmented rabbit. Exp Brain Res 82:499
10. Salami A, Medicina MC, Dellepiane M, Mora R, Guglielmetti G (1996) Optokinetic nystagmus and visual-vestibular interaction in subjects with "whiplash injuries". Acta Otorhinolaryngol Ital 16(2):91–98
11. Miura Y (1968) Functional disorders of the blood vessels in the brain and spinal cord due to experimental whiplash injury. 27th annual meeting of the Japan Neurosurgical Society. Cited by Hinoki M (1985) Vertigo due whiplash injury: a neurotological approach. Acta Otolaringol Stockh 419(Suppl 1):9
12. Miura Y, Tanaka M (1970) Disturbance of the venous system in the head and neck regions in rabbit with whiplash injury. Brain Nerve Inj 2:217
13. Chester JB (1991) Whiplash, postural control, and the inner ear. Spine 7:716
14. Schuknecht HF, Neff WD, Perlman HB (1951) Experimental study of auditory damage following blows to the head. Ann Otol 60:273
15. Oosterveld WJ, Kortschot HW, Kingma GG, De Jong HAA, Saatci MR (1991) Electronystagmographic findings following cervical whiplash injuries. Acta Otolaryngol Stockh 111:201
16. Henn V, Young L, Finley C (1974) Vestibular nucleus units in alert monkey are also influenced by moving visual fields. Brain Res 71:144
17. Bon L, Corazza R, Iinchingolo P (1982) Oculomotor velocity efferent copy in the nucleus of the optic tract in the cat pretectum. Annual general meeting of the European Brain and Behaviour Society, Parma
18. Simpsom J, Alley K (1974) Visual climbing fiber input to rabbit vestibulo-cerebellum: a source of direction-specific information. Brain Res 82:302

19. Precht W, Strata P (1980) On the pathway mediating optokinetic responses in vestibular nuclear neurons. Neuroscience 5:777
20. Carleton SC, Carpenter MB (1984) Distribution of primary vestibular fibers in the brainstem and cerebellum of the monkey. Brain Res 294:281
21. Ikeda K, Kobayashi T (1967) Mechanisms and origin of so-called whiplash injury. Clin Surg 22:1655
22. le Boy R, Pompeiano O (1981) Convergence and interaction of neck and macular vestibular inputs on vestibulospinal neurons. J Neurophysiol 45:852
23. Mc Nab I (1982) Acceleration extension injuries of the cervical spine, vol II. The Spine/WB Saunders, Philadelphia, p 515
24. Ommaya AK, Fass F, Yarnell P (1968) Whiplash injury and brain damage: an experimental study. JAMA 204:285
25. Baloh RW, Jenkins HA, Honrubia V, Yee RD, Law GY (1979) Visual-vestibular interaction and patients with cerebellar atrophy. Neurology 29:116
26. Nagao S (1983) Effects of vestibulocerebellar lesions upon dynamic characteristics and adaptation of vestibulo-ocular and optokinetic responses in pigmented rabbits. Exp Brain Res 53:498
27. Waespe W, Cohen B, Raphan T (1984) Dynamic modification of the vestibuloocular reflex by the nodulus and uvula. Science 228:199
28. Hasegawa T, Kato I, Harada K, Ikarashi T, Yoshida M, Koike Y (1994) The effect of uvulonodular lesions on horizontal optokinetic nystagmus and optokinetic after nystagmus in cats. Acta Otolaryngol Suppl 511:126
29. Miles FA, Fuller JH (1974) Visual tracking and the primate flocculus. Science 189:1000

Abducting Interocular Ophthalmoplegia After Whiplash Injuries

24

D.C. Alpini, A. Cesarani, and E. Merlo

24.1 Introduction

Internuclear ophthalmoplegia (INO) is a well recognisable disorder of horizontal eye movements, and it is a common finding in neurological disorders [1]. INO is due to a functional impairment of the medial longitudinal fascicle (MLF) ipsilateral to the medial rectus paresis. Generally INO is characterised by the impairment of adduction of the eye on the side of the impaired MLF and abduction overshoot. The electro-oculographic saccadic and gaze nystagmus patterns are typical.

In whiplash injuries, ocular motor disturbances are frequent also in those patients in whom a head trauma did not occur [2–4]. In rare cases [5] eye movement disorders are characterised by ocular conjugate movement impairment sometimes as typical INO, sometimes as isolated abducens palsy.

With a certain frequency, we observed "atypical" abducting ophthalmoplegia pattern, characterised by bilateral impairment of the velocity of the abducting eye [6–8].

This finding was described by Lutz [9], who proposed the existence of an abduction paresis of prenuclear origin (posterior internuclear ophthalmoplegia, pINO).

D.C. Alpini (✉)
ENT-Otoneurology Service, IRCCS "Don Carlo C. Gnocchi" Foundation, Milan, Italy
e-mail: dalpini@dongnocchi.it

A. Cesarani
Department of Clinical Sciences and Community Health, University of Milan, Milan, Italy

Audiology Unit, IRCCS "Ca' Granda" Ospedale Maggiore Policlinico, Milan, Italy
e-mail: antonio.cesarani@unimi.it

E. Merlo
ENT Department, Azienda Ospedaliera Ospedale di Circolo di Busto Arsizio, Saronno e Tradate, Milan, Italy

Department of Otolaryngology, Tradate Hospital, Piazza 24 Maggio, 1, 21049 Tradate Varese, Italy

D.C. Alpini et al. (eds.), *Whiplash Injuries*,
DOI 10.1007/978-88-470-5486-8_24, © Springer-Verlag Italia 2014

As his basic neuroanatomical assumptions were erroneous, the existence of this kind of INO remained controversial, and papers in the literature are quite rare.

Abduction INO differs from abducens nerve palsy in several aspects, such as absence of strabismus and diplopia in the primary position and adduction nystagmus of the contralateral eye [10–14].

The aim of this chapter is to report the frequency of abducting INO that occurred in a group of patients after whiplash injuries without head trauma and to discuss possible etiopathogenic mechanisms.

24.2 Material and Methods

Twenty-three consecutive subjects were investigated: 16 women and seven men with mean ages of, respectively, 31.35 and 34.7 years (from 16 to 70 years).

Eye movements were recorded in DC by a computerised Nicolet Biomedical Nystar electro-oculograph, using monocular electrodes. Eye movements were elicited by means of a semicircular LED bar, and the following tests were performed:

- Horizontal and vertical random saccades from 6° to 32°
- Sinusoidal 0.2 and 0.4 Hz horizontal smooth pursuit and 0.2 vertical smooth pursuit
- 400/s bidirectional horizontal OKN and 200/s vertical OKN

The following parameters were calculated:

- Saccades: delay, accuracy, number, performance index, and mean velocity at each amplitude
- Smooth pursuit: gain, DC offset, total harmonic distortion, and maximum velocity
- OKN: number of beats, frequency, maximum velocity, and gain
- Sinusoidal provoked nystagmus (0.5 Hz at 11.5 and 5.75°/s2) in the dark (VOR) and in the light (VVOR): nystagmus frequency and mean slow phase velocity (SPV) and VVOR gain (VVOR-SPVNOR-SPV)

24.3 Results

The presence of bilateral abducting eye slowing was evaluated comparing accuracy, performance index and saccadic eye velocity with the normal values previously calculated in a group of 25 normal adults. No patients showed slowing of the adducting eye or another pattern like typical INO.

Horizontal saccades revealed slowing of the abducting eye in eight patients (ABD) (34.7 %): two men and six women with mean ages of 35.87 years (from 16 to 58 years).

The mean age of the group of patients without abducting slowing was 33.67 years (from 19 to 70 years).

In Table 24.1 the distribution of altered neurological tests is shown. The percentages of altered tests regarding patients with abducting eye slowing are referred to alterations of parameters other than eye velocities, such as latency, accuracy, offset, and directional preponderance.

Table 24.1 Percentages of pathological tests in patients with (ABD) and without (no-ABD) abducting interocular ophthalmoplegia

	ABD (%)	No-ABD (%)
Horizontal saccades	62.5	20
Vertical saccades	25	26.6
Horizontal smooth pursuit	37.5	40
Vertical smooth pursuit	25	33.3
Horizontal OKN	25	20
Vertical OKN	0	6.6
VOR	37.5	40
VVOR gain	25	66.6

Horizontal saccades are altered in 62.5 % of ABD patients versus 20 % of the other group. All the other ocular motor tests are altered in the same manner in the two groups of patients (with exception of VVOR).

24.4 Discussion

Internuclear ophthalmoplegia can be attributed to a lesion of the MLF between the levels of the third and sixth nucleus [15]. It has been assumed that the lesion affects axons arising from cells in the paramedian pontine reticular formation (PPRF), but this is not an accepted explanation for every case. In fact the impairment of movement is variable, the most severe lesions causing complete loss of adduction beyond the midline during contralateral gaze; in some cases the impairment also affects the convergence mechanism, while in others convergence is normal.

Cogan [14] divided INO into anterior and posterior types according to whether the convergence was normal or not, while Lutz [9] divided INO into anterior and posterior according to whether the medial or the lateral rectus muscle was paralysed. If convergence is still possible, it seems to be difficult to distinguish monolateral INO of abduction from abducens paralysis, while bilateral abducting INO may refer only to a lesion of the internuclear fibres.

There has been little agreement on the location of the responsible lesion and the pathophysiological explanation of abducting INO. Some authors [16], rejecting the existence of a prenuclear abduction paresis, attributed such cases to the pontine involving the abducens nerve along its infranuclear intrapontine course. Others [17] postulated decreased excitation of the lateral rectus motor neurons due to a lesion of prenuclear structures, that is, aberrant "pyramidal tract" fibres to the abducens nucleus or the connection between the PPRF and the ipsilateral abducens nucleus. An impaired inhibition of the antagonistic medial rectus muscle was discussed by Collard et al. [18] suggesting an MLF lesion contralateral to the paretic eye.

Thomke et al. [13] demonstrated that the lesion is ipsilateral to the abduction paresis at the upper pons or midbrain level. They also showed the existence of a fasciculus near the MLF specific for inhibition of medial rectus. They stated that ABD ophthalmoplegia is due to impaired inhibition of medial rectus tonic resting activity following interruption of this para-MLF fasciculus.

In our opinion, despite the controversy about the physiopathology of abducting ophthalmoplegia, the term of "abducting interocular ophthalmoplegia" is preferable rather than the classical "internuclear". In our experience this pattern is not rare, and

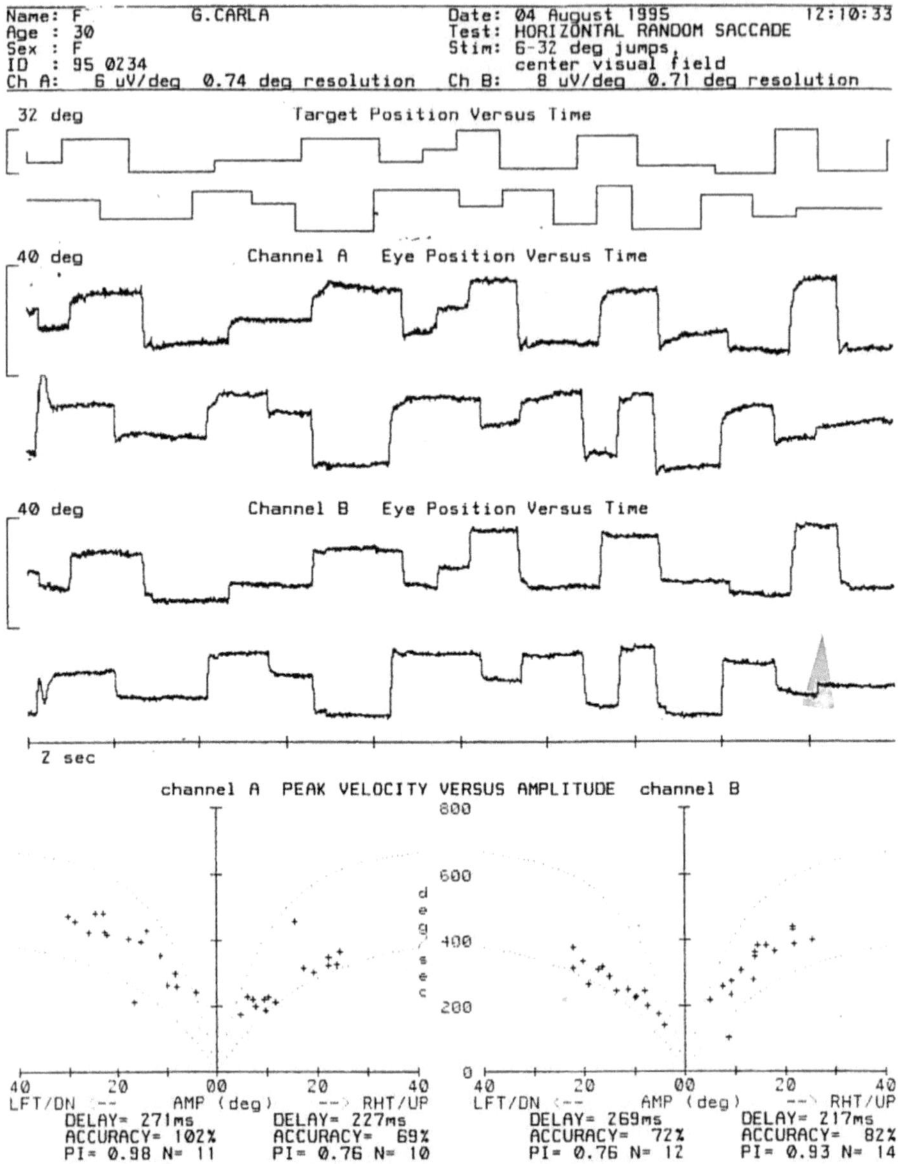

Fig. 24.1 A case of abducting interocular ophthalmoplegia following whiplash

if monocular ENG recording is routinely performed, it describes a third of the patients suffering vertigo and/or dizziness after whiplash injuries, even without minor or major head trauma.

In Fig. 24.1 a case of abducting interocular ophthalmoplegia following whiplash is showed. The involved parameters are peak velocities/movement amplitude ratio (the butterfly diagram) and the percentages of accuracy, comparing abducting and adducting movements.

The PI (performance index) refers to patient peak velocities compared to normal values previously stored in the programme.

It is interesting to reveal that neuro-otological differences in the two groups of patients concern, in an opposite way, horizontal saccades and VVOR. In fact in the ABD group, horizontal latencies or adducting accuracies (parameters different from those correlated to abducting eye slowing) were altered in 62.5 % versus 20 % of the other subjects, while VVOR was normal in 75 % and altered in 66.6 % of no-ABD patients.

In no case was adducting slowing recorded, and we know only one paper in the literature describing INO after whiplash without head trauma [6].

If we hypothesise a brainstem lesion with para-MLF involvement due to neck hyperextension, there will be no need to exclude the possibility of the neurologically most frequently occurring adducting ophthalmoplegia. Our cases are not misdiagnosed bilateral abducens palsy as described either on the basis of the clinical considerations reported in the introduction or on the basis of ophthalmological examination excluding abducens palsy.

In our opinion abducting interocular ophthalmoplegia has to be considered a disorder of ocular coordination correlated to head-eye, according to Treleaven et al. and Montfoort et al. [19, 20], and/or head-neck coordination disorders, according to Kongsted at al. and Treleaven et. al. [21, 22], caused by whiplash. It must not necessarily be correlated to a brainstem lesion.

References

1. Bronstein AM, Rudge P, Gresty MA, Boulay G, Morris J (1990) Abnormalities of horizontal gaze. Clinical, oculographic and magnetic resonance imaging findings. II. Gaze palsy and internuclear ophthalmoplegia. J Neurol Neurosurg Psychiatry 53:200–207
2. Baker RS, Epstein ADD (1991) Ocular motor abnormalities from head trauma. Surv Ophthalmol 35:245–267
3. Wenngren BI, Pettersson K, Lowenhielm G, Hildingsson C (2002) Eye motility and auditory brainstem response dysfunction after whiplash injury. Acta Otolaryngol 122(3):276–283
4. Hildingsson C, Wenngren BI, Bring G, Toolen G (1989) Oculomotor problems after cervical spine injury. Acta Orthop Scand 60:513–516
5. Shifrin LZ (1991) Bilateral abducens nerve palsy after cervical spine extension injury. A case report. Spine 16:374–375
6. Jammes JL (1989) Bilateral internuclear ophthalmoplegia due to acute cervical hyperextension without head trauma. J Clin Neuroophthalmol 9:112–115
7. Lee J, Flynn JT (1985) Bilateral superior oblique palsies. Br J Ophthalmol 69:508–513
8. Hopf HC, Thomke F, Gutman L (1991) Midbrain vs. pontine medial longitudinal fasciculus lesions: the utilization of masseter and blink reflexes. Muscle Nerve 14:326–330
9. Lutz A (1923) Ueber die Bahnen der Blickwendung und deren Dissocierung. In: Sanders EACM (ed) Syndromes of the medial longitudinal fasciculus. Klin Monatsbl Augenh 70: 213–235
10. Sanders EACM, De Keizer RJW, Zee DS (1987) Eye movement disorders. MartinusNijhoff/ Dr W Junk, Dordrecht
11. Kommerell G (1975) Internuclear ophthalmoplegia of abduction. Arch Opthalmol 93: 971–980
12. Larmande AM (1969) La paralysie supranucleaire du VI (dite ophtalmoplegie intemucleaireposterieure). Arch d'Ophtalmol 29:521–530

13. Thornke F, Hopf HC, Kramer G (1992) Internuclear ophthalmoplegia of abduction: clinical and electrophysiological data on the existence of an abduction paresis. J Neurol Neurosurg Psychiatry 55(2):105–111
14. Cogan DG, Kubik CS, Smith WL (1950) Unilateral internuclear ophthalmoplegia; report of eight clinical cases with one postmortem study. Arch Ophtalmol 44:783
15. De Keizer RJW, Zee DS (1987) Eye movement disorders. In: Eye Movement Disorders (Monographs in Ophthalmology) Sanders EACM, De Keizer RJW, Zee DS (eds) Martinus Nijhoff/Dr W Junk, Dordrecht, p 186
16. Bakheit AM, Behan PO, Melville ID (1991) Bilateral internuclear- ophthalmoplegia as a false localizing sign. J R Soc Med 84:627–630
17. Sanders EACM (1987) Syndromes of the medial longitudinal fasciculus. In: Sanders EACM, De Keizer RJW, Zee DS (eds) Eye movement disorders. MartinusNijhoff/Dr W Junk, Dordrecht, p 183
18. Collard M, Eber AM, Streicher D, Rohmer F (1979) L'ophtalmoplegieintemucleaireposterieure-existe-t-elle? A propos de onze observations avec oculographie. Rev Neurol 135: 293–312
19. Treleaven J, Jull G, Grip H (2011) Head eye co-ordination and gaze stability in subjects with persistent whiplash associated disorders. Man Ther 16(3):252–257
20. Montfoort I, Van Der Geest JN, Slijper HP, De Zeeuw CI, Frens MA (2008) Adaptation of the cervico- and vestibulo-ocular reflex in whiplash injury patients. J Neurotrauma 25(6): 687–693
21. Kongsted A, Jørgensen LV, Leboeuf-Yde C, Qerama E, Korsholm L, Bendix T (2008) Are altered smooth pursuit eye movements related to chronic pain and disability following whiplash injuries? A prospective trial with one-year follow-up. Clin Rehabil 22(5):469–479
22. Treleaven J, Jull G, LowChoy N (2006) The relationship of cervical joint position error to balance and eye movement disturbances in persistent whiplash. Man Ther 11(2):99–106

Part IV

Treatment

25 Pharmacological Treatment of Whiplash-Associated Disorders (WAD)

E.A. Pallestrini, E. Castello, G. Garaventa, F. Ioppolo, and F. Di Berardino

25.1 Introduction

The term 'whiplash' has been used to describe a mechanism of injury and the various clinical manifestations as a consequence of the injury. Moreover, signs and symptoms have been designated the 'whiplash syndrome'. In 1995, the Quebec Task Force (QTF) on Whiplash-Associated Disorders (WAD) adopted the following definition of whiplash: 'whiplash is an acceleration-deceleration mechanism of energy transfer to the neck. It may result from rear-end or side-impact motor vehicle collisions, but can also occur during diving or other mishaps. The impact may result in bony or soft-tissue injuries (whiplash-injury), which in turn may lead to a variety of clinical manifestations called Whiplash Associated Disorders' [1].

Whiplash patients can be classified according to severity of signs and symptoms. The QTF-WAD classification system consists of five levels: WAD 0 indicates no complaints or physical signs; WAD I indicates neck complaints but no physical signs; WAD II indicates neck complaints and musculoskeletal signs (such as a decreased range of motion or muscle tenderness); WAD III and IV indicate neck complaints and neurological signs (WAD III) or fracture/dislocation (WAD IV), respectively. The most common presenting symptoms following an acute motor

E.A. Pallestrini • E. Castello • G. Garaventa
I Division of Otolaryngology, Head and Neck Surgery,
"San Martino" Hospital, Genoa, Italy

F. Ioppolo (✉)
Department of Physical Medicine and Rehabilitation,
"Sapienza" University, Piazzale Aldo Moro 5,
00185 Rome, Italy
e-mail: francescoioppolo@yahoo.it

F. Di Berardino
Department of Clinical Sciences and Community Health, University of Milan,
Milan, Italy

Audiology Unit, IRCCS "Ca' Granda" Ospedale Maggiore Policlinico, Milan, Italy

D.C. Alpini et al. (eds.), *Whiplash Injuries*,
DOI 10.1007/978-88-470-5486-8_25, © Springer-Verlag Italia 2014

vehicle collision were neck pain (88–100 %) and headache (54–66 %). Other symptoms were neck stiffness, shoulder pain, arm pain/numbness, paraesthesia, weakness, dysphagia, visual and auditory symptoms and dizziness. In most cases, WAD resolves quickly; 47 % of injured people return to normal activities within 4 weeks, and only 2 % continue to be absent from pre-accident activities 1 year after injury.

Pharmacological treatment of acute WAD regards especially vertigo, dizziness, neck pain, headache, nausea and unsteadiness. Vertigo, nausea and cervical pain are very frequent in the acute and subacute [2] WADs; unsteadiness and diffuse (not only cervical) spine pain are very usual in the chronic WADs [3, 4].

25.2 Whiplash-Associated Headache and Neck Pain

The main goal of treatment must be to kill the pain in order to avoid processes of spinal and central sensitisations that may lead to chronic pain [5].

Paracetamol at the dosage of 1 g three times a day for 7/10 days is the first drug of choice for pain relief. Paracetamol has to be preferred over other nonsteroidal anti-inflammatory (NSAI) drugs, even if it has to be administered at high dosages. *Paracetamol* and, in general, NSAI have to be combined with *muscle relaxant substances.* They can be divided into: (1) drugs active on CNS (mephenesin, carisoprodol), (2) drugs with spinal actions (baclofen), (3) drugs active on the muscular system (dantrolene) and (4) drugs active on the different systems (thiocolchicoside). *f3-blockers* also reduce muscular hypertonicity of cervical spine, and they can be employed as well as proper muscle relaxant drugs. *Paracetamol* could be combined with myorelaxants such as *tizanidine,* a centrally acting $\alpha 2$ adrenergic agonist, used 2–4 mg twice a day for 7/10 days. If dizziness or true vertigo is present, this drug in not indicated due to its central effects on brainstem and thus on vestibular nuclei. In these cases, it is better to combine paracetamol with low doses of benzodiazepines (BDZ) like *diazepam* 5 mg at night time.

In presence of nausea, it is possible to use *metoclopramide* 10 mg twice a day for 7/10 days. In these cases, *L-sulpiride* at low dosage (12.5 mg twice or three times a day) also allows a good control of nausea and dizziness; it also has a mild myorelaxant action.

WAD is considered chronic if pre-accident activity levels are not gained within 6 months. Ongoing cervical pain and reduced range of motion (ROM) associated with chronic WAD constitute both a prognostic and a therapeutic dilemma. The location and severity of tissue injury and the prognosis of chronic neck pain may depend on predisposing neck pathology. In addition to peripheral input, long-standing neck pain (like other chronic pain conditions) may be associated with a central component that can modify the pain threshold. Considerable research has been dedicated to determine the direct and indirect roles of the zygapophyseal joints in the generation of pain and dysfunction in whiplash injury [6].

Blocking the sensory nerves that innervate these joints reduced symptoms in 50 % of the subjects with chronic whiplash pain. However, this finding suggests that no responders might have been suffering from a pathology related not to the joints but to soft tissue. Almost nine of ten whiplash sufferers had some degree of muscle spasm [7].

In particular, these patients had decreased ability to relax the trapezius muscles. Such a finding raises the question of whether cervical muscular dysfunction causes ongoing excess loading of the zygapophyseal joints, yielding the clinical picture of chronic whiplash, or whether muscle dysfunction is an attempt by the body to splint a subtly injured cervical spine.

Several theories about musculoskeletal pain syndromes such as WAD suggest that pain and muscle activity interact and may contribute to the chronicity of symptoms. Studies using electromyography (EMG) have demonstrated abnormal muscle activation patterns of the upper trapezius muscles in the chronic stage of WAD (grade II) [8].

Concerning chronic treatment of whiplash-associated (WA) pain, the most commonly prescribed pharmacological agents are the same: oral muscle relaxants and nonsteroidal anti-inflammatory drugs. Also in these cases, *paracetamol* has to be preferred. However, the effectiveness of these drugs in chronic patients is limited by their systemic therapeutic effect and unfavourable side effects. Physical interventions such as mobilisation, manipulation and exercises have proved beneficial for pain and dysfunction at least in the major part of the patients. Anyway, in chronic WA pain, the only treatment that has clearly shown benefit is radiofrequency neurotomy [9].

The potential benefits of relaxing selected neck muscles [10] with *botulinum toxin type-A (BTX-A)* for the treatment of muscle pain in WA chronic head and/or neck pain have been investigated by Freund et al. [11, 12].

BTX-A (*Bot*ox®) is a neurotoxin and is effective for treating a variety of disorders of involuntary muscle contraction, including spasticity, cervical dystonia, blepharospasm and hemifacial spasm. It inhibits neuromuscular signalling by blocking the release of acetylcholine at the neuromuscular junction. The biological effects of the toxin are transient with normal neuronal signalling returning within approximately 3–6 months postinjections. The injection technique used for the neck is based on experience with cervical dystonia. The sites chosen are chiefly in the large superficial muscles, specifically, the splenius capitis, rectus capitis, semispinalis capitis and trapezius. These muscles can easily be palpated in most individuals and can be injected without sophisticated techniques. Most patients exhibit tender areas in the larger muscles, often in conjunction with tight bands or knots. The neurotoxin effects are thought to act only upon motor nerve endings, while sensory nerve fibres are spared from such effects. Thus, analgesic effects are likely to occur, not as a result of blocking afferent sensory fibres at the site of injection but rather from secondary effects that may be attributed to muscle paralysis, improved blood flow and release of fibres under compression by abnormally contracting muscles. The primary action may affect alpha and gamma motoneuron function in the muscle spindles resulting in lower muscle tone. BTX-A treatment is potentially a painful procedure [13]. It is contraindicated in the presence of infection at the injection site(s) and in individuals with known hypersensitivity to any ingredient in the formulation. Individuals with peripheral motor neuropathic diseases or neuromuscular functional disorders should receive BTX-A treatment with caution. BTX-A should also be used with caution in patients receiving aminoglycosides or other agents interfering with neuromuscular transmission.

BTX-A injections are not a curative treatment. BTX-A provides a temporary paralytic effect and requires repeated injections to continue the beneficial effects. The duration of effect is longer with the initial injection and progressively gets shorter with repeated injections for most dystonic disorders. It is not known at this time whether BTX-A can be readministered indefinitely or if the effectiveness will wear off over time.

25.3 Whiplash-Associated Equilibrium Disturbances (WAED)

Whiplash injury is a very common cause of vertigo and dizziness. The physiopathological mechanisms of this kind of injury can be explained from the effect of forces applied to the head and the neck during the collision. In the first phase, the force applied to the rear end of the car during the collision results in a forward acceleration of the body while the head is pushed backwards from inertial forces causing a cervical hyperextension. In the second phase, which always occurs because of the effect of inertial forces, the head is pushed forward with subsequent hyperflexion of the neck. The whole duration of these phases is about 20 ms. This is the reason for the lack of activation of neck neuromuscular protective reflexes, whose latency is about 50 ms. During neck hyperextension the elongation of cervical rachidian tissues may even reach 5 cm [14].

The vestibular system is frequently involved in whiplash injuries; lesions may involve labyrinth and central vestibular organs and pathways.

Three lesion levels of the vestibular system can be distinguished: (1) labyrinth and organ damage, (2) central vestibular and oculomotor system damage (3) and both involvement of the peripheral and central vestibular systems. Table 25.1 reports the classification of post-traumatic vertigo (from [12], modified).

The prerequisites for successful pharmacological treatment of WAEDs are the ‘4 Ds’: correct diagnosis, correct drug, appropriate dosage and sufficient duration. First, a correct *diagnosis*, on the basis of the patient history, clinical examination and laboratory investigations; second, the correct *drug*—only a few have been

Table 25.1 Causes of post-traumatic vertigo

Damage site	Lesions	Physiopathology
Labyrinth	Labyrinthine lesions, temporal bone fractures, concussive trauma, haemorrhagia	Otolith displacement
	Maculae—semicircular canals Perilymphatic fistula	Round—oval window rupture
Vestibular nerve	Axonotmesis neurotmesis	Concussion—haemorrhage
Brainstem cerebellum	Concussion haemorrhage ischemia	Neurotransmitter release
Cervical rachis	Whiplash syndrome	Vascular—proprioceptive

proven in controlled trials to be effective in a sufficiently *large sample* of patients, but experience can suggest appropriate drug choice for every *specific patient*; third, an appropriate *dosage*—often the initial dose is too low or too high so that the treatment is either ineffective or not well tolerated; and fourth, a sufficient *duration*—often drugs are either given for too long, such as antivertiginous agents (e.g. dimenhydrinate), which delay central compensation and may cause drug dependence, or not long enough.

In the child, pharmacological treatment of vestibular post-traumatic disorders is essentially symptomatic for the early and efficient development of compensatory mechanisms. The main aspects of treatment are related essentially to the dosages and the frequency and duration of drug administration for each case. The choice of substance is based on the clinical experience of the physician and on knowledge of the pharmacological characteristics of the different categories of drugs [15].

In the elderly, pharmacological treatment of post-traumatic vertigo shows particular aspects linked to the aging processes. Several factors such as relative enhancement of fat tissue, the reduction of body mass, decreased hepatic and kidney functions and the diminution of serum albumin influence drug pharmacokinetic properties (absorbency, tissue distribution, metabolism, sensibility and clearance).

We can distinguish therapies for vertigo spells, chronic unsteadiness or relapsing vertigo.

25.4 Vertigo

Vestibular sedative drugs should be employed immediately after head-neck trauma and continued for a few days.

In benign positional vertigo (BPV) drug treatment should principally support rehabilitative training because neck pain and muscular stiffness and spasm make difficult vestibular physical treatment in the early stage of the disease

Symptomatic therapy involves vestibular suppressor and antiemetic drugs. Among the vestibular suppressor drugs, antihistamines, phenothiazines and benzodiazepines are the most widely used.

Antihistaminic drugs (dimenhydrinate, flunarizine, cinnarizine, hydroxyzine, betahistine, astemizole) act on the synapses between the first and the second neurons, on the reticular formation, on the vestibular dopaminergic pathways and on H1 receptors. The pharmacological effect is vestibule suppressive with inhibition of positional nystagmus.

Betahistine interferes with the diamine oxidase prolonging histamine action; it has a moderate agonist activity on H1 receptors and a strong activity as an H3 antagonist. Betahistine inhibits neurons of the lateral vestibular nuclei [16] and increases the basilar and cochlear flow in animal models. Betahistine has vasodilatative effects on stria vascularis, on spiral ligament and on vertebrobasilar circulation [17]. Betahistine improves microcirculatory flow of the inner ear and central vestibular system, and this can explain the positive effects in the treatment of paroxysmal peripheral vertigo, modulating effect on cerebral and labyrinthine circulation.

Astemizole has a strong inhibitory action on vertigo and nystagmus, and it is interesting from a clinical point of view because it crosses the blood-cerebrospinal-encephalic barrier only in a minimal concentration; for this reason this drug has very low sedative effects, and therefore its main action is on the peripheral vestibular system [18].

Phenothiazines (promethazine, thiethylperazine, prochlorperazine) are very effective in decreasing acute vertiginous symptoms and vegetative side effects. Pharmacological effects on the vestibular system are the inhibition of peripheral cholinergic inputs, inhibition of H1 receptors in vestibular nuclei and an effect on the bulbar chemoreceptor trigger zone. *Phenothiazines* have important side effects on the extra pyramidal system, on pressure control mechanisms and on prolactin secretion. For these reasons phenothiazines should be administrated carefully especially in the elderly.

Scopolamine shows strong anticholinergic activity on brainstem, reticular formation and vestibular nuclei. This drug cannot be used in patients suffering from glaucoma, prostatic hypertrophy and heart diseases [19–21].

Benzodiazepines (diazepam, lorazepam, clonazepam, etc.) enhance GABAergic inhibitory properties of vestibulocerebellum on vestibular nuclei and activate the internuclear inhibitory pathways. They are also active on glycinergic pathways, on substantia nigra, on the limbic system and on cholinergic activatory reticular formation. The final effect is the inhibition of the vestibulo-oculomotor reflex and nystagmus. Benzodiazepines have inhibitory effects on breathing and blood circulation and for these reasons should be carefully administered in elderly patients.

Propranolol has been successfully employed in the treatment of whiplash injury-related vertigo. This drug reduces hypertonicity of spinal muscles lowering the discharge frequency of neuromuscular

fusicellular endings, with a subsequent diminution of cervical pain [22].

25.5 Chronic Unsteadiness and Relapsing Vertigo

Damage to the vestibular apparatus due to whiplash injuries produces acute symptoms, which gradually improve as central compensation occurs. The aim of the pharmacological strategy in peripheral vestibular lesions is to improve CNS restorage mechanisms; for this reason vestibulo-suppressive drugs, even if effective in reducing vertigo and imbalance, worsen the CNS compensation and should be administered only in the first stage of the disease. On the other hand with the employment of CNS excitatory drugs or drugs with decompensating effects during rehabilitative training, compensation processes will be stimulated with acceleration of healing.

Among drugs which enhance compensation processes, the *amphetamines, ginkgo biloba* and *calcium antagonists* are the most used [23–25]. Amphetamines theoretically could be employed in the treatment of peripheral vestibular lesions based on their positive effects on compensation processes. Their use is limited because of significant side effects. *Pemoline* and *fipexide* belong to this category of

Table 25.2 Neuroactive drugs not specifically acting on vestibular neurotransmitters

Metabolic enhancers	Citicoline, deanol, piracetam, oxiracetam, ginkgo biloba, protirelin, L-acetylcarnitine
Neurotrophics	Gangliosides
Excitants	Amphetamines, fipexide, pemoline
Antidepressants	Tricycles IMAO, sulpiride
Anticonvulsants	Carbamazepine
Myorelaxants β-blockers	Baclofen

Table 25.3 Neuroactive drugs specifically acting on vestibular neurotransmitters

Antihistamines	Flunarizine, cinnarizine, hydroxyzine, astemizole, betahistine, diphenhydramine, dimenhydrinate
Phenothiazines	Promethazine, thiethylperazine, prochlorperazine
Benzodiazepines	
Scopolamine	

drugs and are particularly interesting for their limited side effects; *pemoline* affects dopamine turnover and has few peripheral effects; *fipexide* affects the reticular formation and shows dopamine-like effects. *Ginkgo biloba* enhances postural and locomotor balance and oculomotor function recovery in experimental unilateral vestibular lesions.

Cinnarizine and *flunarizine* [26] selectively block calcium entry into peripheral vestibular system cells (especially cristae cells); both these drugs show antihistaminic and anticholinergic activities. In the peripheral vestibular system, calcium antagonists modulate neurotransmitter release. Flunarizine interferes in ACh release and enhances compensation processes. In elderly patients, these drugs should be administered carefully for its Parkinson's-like effects after prolonged treatment [27].

In the elderly where CNS reorganisation after vestibular damage is less effective, drugs with positive effects on compensation, as well as haemorrheologic and neuroactive drugs, should be used. Drugs which increase CNS neurotransmitter storage will be also useful in these patients [28]. In particular, neuroactive drugs are employed for their actions on CNS neurotransmitters, while vasoactive substances improving blood macro- and microcirculation enhance CNS metabolism. Neuroactive substances can be classified as drugs not specifically acting on vestibular neurotransmitters and drugs specifically acting on vestibular neurotransmitters (Tables 25.2 and 25.3).

Among the neuroactive drugs which are not specifically active on vestibular neurotransmitters, *citicoline* has dopaminergic and serotonergic activities and reduces platelet aggregability. *Deanol* and *oxiracetam* have cholinergic action; *piracetam,* a GABA derivative, has strong dopaminergic and mild GABAergic activities and improves cerebral ATP synthesis; this drug accelerates compensation phenomena and is well indicated in vertigo due to a brainstem disinhibition [29] and in post-traumatic vestibular lesions. *Protirelin* is a TRH derivative; this drug's main effect is on the cholinergic neurotransmitter system and it shows secondary effects on the dopaminergic, noradrenergic and serotonergic systems.

Among alpha-blockers, *dihydroergotoxine,* an alkaloid derivative, has vascular and metabolic activities enhancing alpha-adrenoceptor blocking activity. Dihydroergotoxine also has a dopaminergic activity and inhibits the specific cerebral phosphodiesterase response in c-AMP metabolism. Their use is however limited to selected cases. *Nicergoline* is an ergot derivative with actions on dopamine turnover, on cerebral blood flow and on cerebral glucose consumption; this drug enhances neurotransmitter storage, and for this reason its employment seems to be interesting in post-traumatic vertigo of central origin especially in the elderly.

Drugs active on the microcirculatory system have been found to have multiple actions on the neurotransmitter system, on cerebral flow and on cerebral metabolism with limited side effects. Among these substances *buflomedil* [30] has alpha-blocking, antiaggregant and haemorrheologic properties and a calcium antagonist effect. This drug acts to diminish cerebral oxygen consumption. *Pentoxifylline* has different pharmacological properties; the main one is the improvement of erythrocyte deformability (through an ATP improvement) and the diminution of blood viscosity (through a diminution of fibrinogen). This drug reduces platelet aggregation by acting on membrane phosphodiesterases, reducing thromboxane synthesis and improving at the same time the synthesis of prostacyclin. Pentoxifylline reduces platelet adhesiveness to the vessel wall and results in delaying the thrombogenic action. Among calcium antagonists, *nimodipine* improves dopa's inhibiting action.

In chronic WAD, paying attention to the patient's age and the metabolism [31], cinnarizine and flunarizine may be used, at the lowest dosage possible and for the shortest possible period. *Cinnarizine* has vasodilatatory, antihistamine and anticholinergic effects inhibiting central vestibular system activities. The main CNS action of *flunarizine*, difluorinated derivative of cinnarizine, is blocking Ca^{2+}'s entry into cells during hypoxia.

Sometimes post-whiplash headache, generally a tension-type headache, in pre-whiplash migrainous patients may evolve into the vestibular migraine. Characteristic features include recurrent attacks of various combinations of vertigo, ataxia of stance and gait, photophobia and phonophobia and other brainstem symptoms, accompanied or followed by head pressure, pain, nausea or vomiting [31]. Tricyclic antidepressants in combination with diet gave a good response. Generally, only drugs that are effective for treating migraine with and without aura can currently be recommended. For the therapy of acute attacks, aspirin and an antiemetic could be offered, whereas metoprolol (100 mg/day), topiramate (50–100 mg/day) or valproic acid (300–900 mg/day) could be offered for prophylaxis.

Very rarely, and only after a major and complex whiplash such as rear and consequently front collision, atlantooccipital strain may lead to a central vestibular lesion inducing downbeat nystagmus (DBN, a form of acquired nystagmus that is characterised by slow upward drifts with downward quick phases). Patients frequently report blurred vision or oscillopsia, which increases on lateral gaze, as well as associated unsteadiness of gait and postural imbalance. As a pathophysiological mechanism, a tone imbalance of the central vestibular pathways subserving vertical eye movements, including the otolithic pathways, such that DBN is often gravity dependent, has been proposed for DBN. *Baclofen* and *clonazepam* dosage of 0.5 mg tid or 1 mg bid, both GABA agonists, improve DBN [32].

Pharmacological therapy can be employed during rehabilitative treatment. The aim of drug treatment is to reduce hypertonic contracture of muscles of the neck to facilitate physiotherapeutic treatment and to improve the efficacy of such therapy. In these cases, *muscle relaxant substances* may be employed. Also drugs acting on central plasticity mechanisms may be useful (e.g. *piracetam*). Amantadine results to be particularly useful in WA chronic unsteadiness especially when it is due to a labyrinthine damage. Amantadine [33–35] on one hand reduces vestibular organ damage through an anti-glutamate action on NMDA labyrinth receptors and on the other hand through dopaminergic mechanism improves compensation.

In labyrinthine post-traumatic lesions (direct or indirect through labyrinth concussion or vertebral artery spasm), the preferred drugs are those with positive effects on vestibular compensation. Vestibular suppressive drugs would be helpful initially to improve vertigo and neurovegetative phenomena but should be avoided for long treatments.

In post-traumatic vertigo of central origin (generally caused by vertebrobasilar acute insufficiency), drugs which are active on neurotransmitter systems may be employed together with vasoactive substances improving CNS circulation and metabolism. In the brainstem involvement, drugs which are active on the cholinergic, histaminergic and adrenergic neurotransmitter systems (scopolamine, cinnarizine) are effective in reducing symptoms but can interfere with the processes of compensation. In cases exhibiting lack of cerebellovestibular control, drugs with GABAergic actions such as benzodiazepines may be employed successfully [30, 31].

References

1. Spitzer W, Skovron M, Salmi L, Cassidy J, Duranceau J, Suissa S, Zeiss E (1995) Scientific monograph of Quebec task force on whiplash associated disorders: redefining "whiplash" and its management. Spine 20:1–73
2. Sterling M (2004) A proposed new classification system for whiplash associated disorders-implications for assessment and management. Man Ther 9(2):60–70. Review
3. Treleaven J, Jull G, Sterling M (2003) Dizziness and unsteadiness following whiplash injury: characteristic features and relationship with cervical joint position error. J Rehabil Med 35:36–43
4. Ferrari R, Russell AS (1999) Development of persistent neurologic symptoms in patients with simple neck sprain. Arthritis Care Res 12:70–76
5. Curatolo M, Petersen Felix S, Arendt Nielsen L, Giani C, Zbinden AM, Radanov BP (2001) Central hypersensitivity in chronic pain after whiplash injury. Clin J Pain 17:306–315
6. Lord SM, Barnsley L, Wallis BJ, Bogduk N (1996) Chronic cervical zygapophyseal joint pain after whiplash: a placebo-controlled prevalence study. Spine 21:1737–1745
7. Wiley AM, Lloyd J, Evans JG (1986) Musculoskeletal sequelae of whiplash injuries. Adv Q 7:65–73
8. Nederhand MJ, Hermens HJ, Ijzerman MJ, Turk DC, Zilvold G (2000) Cervical muscle dysfunction in the chronic whiplash associated disorder grade II (WAD-II). Spine 25:1938–1943
9. McDonald GJ, Lord SM, Bogduk N (1999) Long-term follow-up of patients treated with cervical radiofrequency neurotomy for chronic neck pain. Neurosurgery 45:61–68
10. Fischer AA (1988) Documentation of myofascial trigger points. Arch Phys Med Rehabil 69:286–291

11. Freund B, Schwartz M (2000) Treatment of whiplash associated neck pain with botulinum toxin A: a pilot study. J Rheumatol 27:481–484
12. Freund B, Schwartz M (2002) Use of botulinum toxin in chronic whiplash associated disorder. Clin J Pain 18:S163–S168
13. Juan FJ (2004) Use of botulinum toxin-A for musculoskeletal pain in patients with whiplash associated disorders BMC. Musculoskelet Disord 5:5
14. Brandt T (1991) Vertigo: its multisensory syndromes. Springer, Berlin
15. Pallestrini BA, Garaventa G, Castello E (1994) Equilibrium disorders. In: Cesarani A, Alpini D (eds) Equilibrium disorders. Springer, Milano, p 183
16. Tomita M, Gotoh F, Sato TI (1978) Comparative responses of the carotid and vertebral arterial system of rhesus monkeys to betahistine. Stroke 9:382–387
17. Uemoto H, Sasa M, Takaori S, Ito J, Matsvoka I (1982) Inhibitory effect of betahistine on polysynaptic neurons in the lateral vestibular nucleus. Arch Otolaryngol 236:229–236
18. Fischer A (1991) Histamine in the treatment of vertigo. Acta Otolaryngol Stockh 479(Suppl):24–28
19. Childs A (1986) Scopolamine effects in vestibular defensiveness. Arch Phys Med Rehabil 67:554–555, 160
20. Pyykko I, Padoan S, Schalen L, Lyttkens L, Magnusson M, Henriksson NG (1985) The effects of TIS-scopolamine, dimenhydrinate, lidocaine and tocainide on motion sickness, vertigo and nystagmus. Aviat Space Environ Med 56:777
21. Shojaku H, Watanabe Y, Ito M, Mizukoshi K, Yajima K, Sekiguchi C (1993) Effect of transdermally administered scopolamine on the vestibular system in humans. Acta Otolaryngol Stockh 504:41–45
22. Rubin W (1973) Whiplash with vestibular involvement. Arch Otolaryngol 97:85–87
23. Claussen CF, Schneider D, Patil NP (1989) The treatment of minocycline induced brainstem vertigo by the combined administration of Piracetam and Ergotoxin. Acta Otolaryngol Stockh 468(Suppl):171–1741
24. Ganança MM, Caovilla HH, Ganança FF, Serafini F (1995) Dietary management for tinnitus control in patients with hyperinsulinemia-a retrospective study. Int Tinnitus J 1(1):41–45. PubMed PMID: 10753319
25. Pfaltz CR, Aoyagi M (1988) Calcium-b1ockers in the treatment of vestibular disorders. Acta Otolaryngol 460(Suppl):135–142
26. Boniver R (1979) Vertigo particularly of vascular origin, treated with flunarizine. Acta Otorhinolaryngol Belg 33:270–281
27. Wouters DV, Amery MD, Towse G (1983) Flunarizine in the treatment of vertigo. J Laryngol Otol 97:697–704
28. Zee DS (1985) Perspective on pharmacotherapy of vertigo. Arch Otolaryngol Stockh 11:609–612
29. Igarashi M, Oosterveld WJ, Thomsen J, Watanabe I, Rubin W (1983) Medical treatment of vertigo. How valutate its effect? Adv Otorhinolaryngol 30:345–349
30. Clissold SP, Lynch S, Sorkin EM (1987) Buflomedil. A review of its pharmacodynamic and pharmacokinetic properties, and therapeutic efficacy in peripheral and cerebral vascular diseases. Drugs 33(5):430–460. Review. PubMed PMID: 3297620
31. Strupp M, Thurtell MJ, Shaikh AG, Brandt T, Zee DS, Leigh RJ (2011) Pharmacotherapy of vestibular and ocular motor disorders, including nystagmus. J Neurol 258:1207–1222
32. Hegemann SCA, Palla A (2010) New methods for diagnosis and treatment of vestibular diseases. Med Rep 2:60
33. Ossola B, Schendzielorz N, Chen SH, Bird GS, Tuominen RK, Männistö PT, Hong JS (2011) Amantadine protects dopamine neurons by a dual action: reducing activation of microglia and inducing expression of GNDF in astroglia. Neuropharmacology 61(4):574–582. Epub 2011 May 11
34. Leonov H, Astrahan P, Krugliak M, Arkin IT (2011) How do aminoadamantanes block the influenza M2 channel, and how does resistance develop? J Am Chem Soc 133(25):9903–9911
35. Thömke MMW (2007) Frequently occurring forms of dizziness and their treatment. MMW Fortschr Med 149(Suppl 2):70, 72–75

Physiotherapy of Neck, Back and Pelvis 26

I. Odkvist, L.M. Odkvist, S. Negrini, and C. Mariconda

26.1 Introduction

Recent studies highlight the fact that where there is pain in a WAD patient, there is a rapid alteration of neck muscle functioning. It has been seen that within 24 h of the trauma, there is an alteration in muscle control: on the contrary, there is no proof of an automatic recovery if the pain diminishes and so special training is necessary [1, 2].

Physical exercise plays a major role in rehabilitating the patient, integrating him back to a normal life. It is possible to identify some goals to be obtained in WAD rehab:

1. Activation of the deep neck muscles (exercises with a low load)
2. Re-education of deep neck muscle resistance
3. Realignment of the activation patterns of both the deep and the superficial neck muscles
4. Posture realignment, also during functional tasks
5. Readjustment of force and resistance to functional necessities (exercises with a high load)

The basic principles of physical exercises are the segmentation, simplification and an increasing and continuous feedback. This treatment is executed with the patient in various positions, from the supine up to the orthostatic, so as to pass from a low workload to a more elevated one.

I. Odkvist • L.M. Odkvist
Physiotherapy, Risbrinksgatan 6a, Linkoping, Sweden

Department of Otolaryngology, University Hospital, Linkoping, Sweden

S. Negrini (✉)
Department of Clinical and Experimental Sciences, University of Brescia, Brescia, Italy
e-mail: stefano.negrini@med.unibs.it

C. Mariconda
Department of Physical Medicine and Rehabilitation, Gradenigo Hospital, Torino, Italy
e-mail: carlo.mariconda@gradenigo.it

D.C. Alpini et al. (eds.), *Whiplash Injuries*,
DOI 10.1007/978-88-470-5486-8_26, © Springer-Verlag Italia 2014

The motor control of the scapular girdle must not be overlooked seeing that a variation of load distribution on the spine will negatively increase the compressive load on the cervix vertebrae.

Scientific evidence [3] has been collected for a multimodal programme which foresees:

- Explanations and reassurance for the patient
- Encouragement in activities and movement
- Pain relief
- Therapeutic exercises
- Ergonomic strategies

26.2 Orthopaedic Collar

Keeping in mind the numerous clinical variables and subjective ones of WAD, more recent new studies highlight the importance and long-term efficacy of a swift mobilisation and treatment of the symptoms of distortion trauma. The mobilisation is carried out in terms of treatment and pain prevention of the disability and consequent recuperation of good specific muscle control.

In some cases we have noticed that immobilisation, where not clinically adequate, even if followed by rehabilitation treatment has led to a longer recovery time and longer absences from work. This also evidently means an increase in health and social welfare costs.

26.2.1 Physiotherapy

Decontraction is usually the very first step. It can be achieved by relaxing the patient, letting him feel confident with the therapist. This is easier, for example, in a good environment, as happens in water, but for everybody it is suggested to work gradually, with the head well fixed at the beginning resting on the table and then in the therapist's hands with a very good manual grasp. Many exercise techniques able to reduce pain do exist and can be used in conjunction with decontracting and strengthening manoeuvres when one begins to remove the collar. We can mention, for example, the McKenzie method [4], the Mézières, Souchard or Bienfait approaches, the Sohier or Maitland technique, and so on. Obviously, The Method does not exist, but only many useful techniques that must fit the pathology of a single patient and the knowledge and ability of the physiotherapist. Physiotherapy is not only muscular (and psychological) relaxation: it is also a first step in returning a part of the body to its normal daily life activities. This means that exteroception and proprioception play a role other than the simple goal of decontraction.

The evidence suggests that physical exercises [5, 6] may be beneficial in the short and long term. According to our experience, regaining enough strength to permit not only movement but usually also the ability to sustain the head is perhaps the most important goal when rehabilitation begins. In fact, the collar reduces muscular usage, provoking deactivation that combines with injury and pain to reduce strength and trophism of muscular tissue. The early stage of rehabilitation constitutes also a very important step in regaining proprioceptive input from the muscular and articular tissues.

There are some techniques that are fundamental and cannot be ignored during early stage of treatment: isometric strengthening and rhythmic stabilisation. The first one constitutes a type of contraction more than a real technique and must be done at the beginning in a neutral position along the classical axes of movement and then at different degrees of movement as well as the intermediate plane. This is very important because the muscular tonic fibres are prevalent in the neck musculature due to its physiological role and because the first step is to permit the head to be stable over its "slender column".

The second technique involves movements effectuated by the patient with the opposition of the therapist, provoking isometric and eccentric contractions along different axes of movement. This technique greatly increases both the strength and also the proprioceptive input. Having gained strength it is then necessary to gain mobility too. As we saw, it is possible to recover both together, but it is also wise to include in a good programme exercises along all the axes of movement, not ignoring the protraction-retraction movement. These exercises at the beginning will be passive and conducted by the therapist while respecting the pain. As both the patient and the therapist will become more confident, pain will be explored more, particularly using active (assisted or not) contraction to avoid overstretching. Active exercises are very useful at this stage, and also auto-mobilisation can be applied. The literature suggests that these techniques can be used as an adjunct to strategies that promote activation and that they can be beneficial particularly in the short term.

There are techniques developed to "normalise" the joint positions. These can be more or less gentle, depending on the method. They are an important way to regain good joint positioning, normalising in this way the afferents, reducing muscular hypercontraction and avoiding pain. Studies about these techniques have not been published. As has been sufficiently stressed above, proprioception plays a fundamental role in all the rehabilitation programmes, permitting good range of movements once it is possible. We do not think that neurology is the key to open the door of orthopaedic rehabilitation, as others involved in rehabilitation have proposed, but we are conscious of the importance of not neglecting this fundamental element.

The literature does not address postural control improvement as a single therapeutic element; rather, many researchers have proposed it as a part of a multimodal treatment plan.

It is not possible to only propose a cervical intervention, because the neck has a function: let the eyes look forward. This function must be accomplished independently by the various elements, and this means based on the posture of the rest of the body. This posture must be compensated by the neck. This is why it is of enormous importance to intervene and modify the posture of the body if we want to prevent other stresses on the neck. When rehabilitating a neck it is not possible to neglect the other parts of the spine. The vertebral column in fact has been defined as one articulated long bone, and an injury in one part always reflects on the other (apart from a lesion developed during the injury itself). This is why it is very important to consider the thoracic and lumbar regions too.

Active participation of the patient is a cornerstone of effective physical treatment. Therapists used to think that a patient must rely on them and that without their help the patient will not be able to work properly. Perhaps this is true, but what is much more important is what the patient loses by not working on his own. Working at home is fundamental, and particularly isometric exercises and the ones necessary to regain mobility can be done and controlled without many problems.

26.2.2 High-Frequency Proprioceptive Reprogramming

High-frequency proprioceptive reprogramming (HFPR) [7] permits intervention at an archeo-proprioceptive level, which means all the impulses sent from the peripheral structures which reach the subcortical processing structures (spinal cord, encephalic trunk and cerebellum). This instrument activates a series of stimulations which are much more complex than those perceived during a simple exercise on a self-stabilising board. The HFPR (Delos®) signifies a self-stabilising board having one or two degrees of leeway and being connected to a PC allowing monitor visualisation of the exercises with visual feedback (Fig. 26.1).

The patient has to govern a series of high-frequency proprioceptive stimulations in diverse situations of unbalance which force him to activate his archeo-proprioception to the most with particular attention to the spinal proprioceptive reflexes. These reflexes are the base of a correct functional stability of the joints. Postural command also receives benefit from proprioceptive training seeing that its quality (above all in dynamic situations) is based on the synergic action of archeo-proprioception, sight and the vestibular system. It is absolutely fundamental to create situations of disequilibrium in a monopodalic position on a self-balancing board having visual feedback to obtain an exact assessment of disequilibrium control.

26.3 Neuromuscular Taping

Neuromuscular taping (NMT) [8] is a rehabilitation system using elastic self-adhesive tape applied to the skin. It functions locally and at a certain distance through reflexes as it stimulates both the deep and superficial skin receptors through body movement by sending exteroceptive and proprioceptive stimuli to the central nervous system which generates a muscular reflex reaction.

The tape is made of water-resistant cotton which is elastic lengthwise and provides 40 % extra elasticity to the skin.

The two principal application techniques of the NMT are decompressive and compressive mode.

In both cases the effect is aimed at the vascular, lymphatic, skin, muscular and nervous structures and is used for the subsequent rehabilitative goals:

- Pain reduction
- Implementation of local vascularisation through reabsorption of oedemas and haematomas

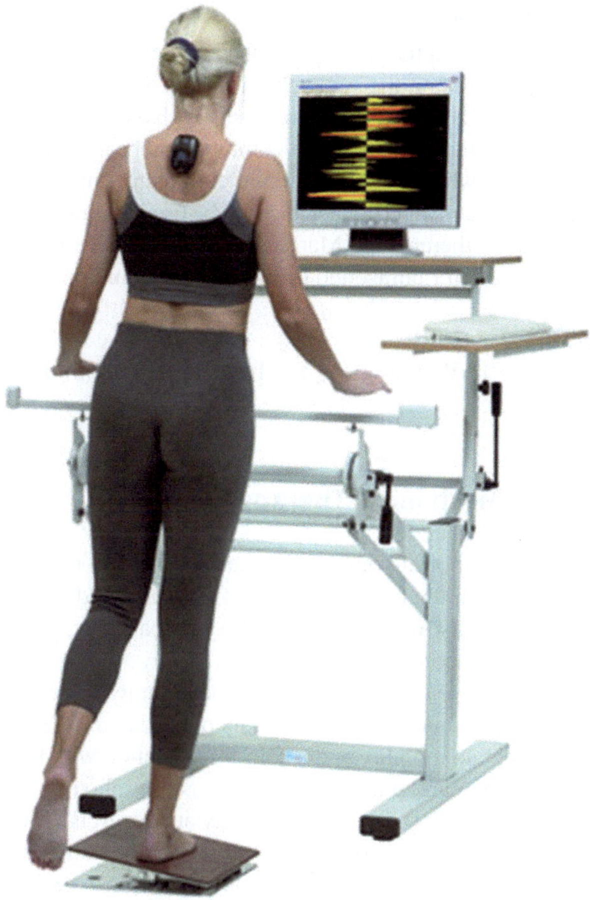

Fig. 26.1 Delos® equipment. Subject stands on the board with one or 2 ft and tries to maintain equilibrium. Body and board sway are contemporary recorded and presented as visual feedback in order to improve visual control of dynamic posture stabilisation

- Normalisation of muscular tone
- Joint realignment
- Postural improvement

Even if there is no scientific evidence of the above article, neuromodulative activity of pain impulses from the posterior horns of the spinal cord can be hypothesised. Neuromuscular taping is therefore a valid and efficient rehabilitative instrument to be integrated into WAD diagnoses, both in acute, post-acute and chronic phases.

26.3.1 Physical Therapy

The main goal of physical therapy is to promote soft tissue healing and to diminish inflammation. Few studies in literature investigated the effect of physical therapies in treating patients with whiplash-associated disorders (WAD), and their efficacy has not been demonstrated in this group of patients [9].

26.3.1.1 Heat

Many times heat has to be proscribed in the cervical region, and this is particularly true in whiplash injury: the sympathetic plexus is placed around the vertebral artery and can be influenced by this type of treatment with dangerous effect, particularly when a lesion is suspected here. Vertigo can commonly appear using heat in the cervical region, and that is why, when vertigo is a major complaint, it is better not to try this type of therapy. Infrared is very superficial and could be used, with some cautions, associated with massage. Radar therapy and Marconi rays are forbidden because of the heat that develops, as is the case for ultrasound therapy, which could micromassage the soft tissues.

26.3.1.2 Cold

This type of therapy does not have a great significance and is not usually used in such cases.

26.3.2 Mechanical Therapy

The most important danger in treating whiplash is excessive mobilisation of a structure not completely repaired. This is what could happen with all manual therapies, and this is why it is necessary to be very cautious, particularly if the healing process could not be completed.

Manipulation is a common treatment but its value has not been established till now. According to our experience it is inappropriate in whiplash patients, because it is possible to obtain mobility and a pain-free situation with less risks using simple exercises.

Massage can be applied, but it must be relaxing to reduce muscular contraction particularly just before and after physical exercise therapy.

Traction. There is only one study [9] addressing the problem of traction of pathological necks, but it did not focus on whiplash and its results were not definitive. The most important danger with this treatment is the damage to soft tissues, with overstretching of ligaments, capsule of zygo-apophyseal joints and (less important) muscles. This is always present to a lesser or greater degree, and this is why traction, according to our thought, must not be applied.

26.3.3 Electrotherapy

This type of therapy is not so useful. Transcutaneous electrical nerve stimulation (TENS) can reduce pain; iontophoresis can have an anti-inflammatory effect, but their importance is not very great in whiplash injured patients.

26.3.4 Laser Therapy

It can be useful if trigger points can be detected. Particularly useful, in our experience, are the He-Ne and the As-Ga lasers.

26.3.5 Magnetotherapy

There are results in the literature [9] about the association between the use of a collar and continued magnetotherapy with benefits in the short term. In our experience, it is possible to prescribe a 20-min application for at least 20 times: usually it is necessary to use 60 G with a frequency of five times a week.

There are only two controlled trials that examined the efficacy of *pulsed electromagnetic treatment (PEMT)* in the treatment of patients with acute WAD. The study of Foley-Nolan et al. [10] compared PEMF treatment versus sham PEMF treatment. The authors found that PEMF treatment significantly reduced pain after 4 weeks compared with sham treatment, but not after 3 months. Similarly, Thuile and Walzl [11] showed a significant reduction in pain and improvement in cervical ROM in patients treated with PEMT compared with those who received medication alone. Although there is some evidence that PEMT decreases pain intensity and increases cervical ROM over the short term, the evidence is insufficient to support the use of this treatment with confidence.

Heat, ice, massage, transcutaneous electrical nerve stimulation (TENS), pulsed electromagnetic treatment (PEMT), electrical stimulation, ultrasound, laser and shortwave diathermy may be prescribed for the treatment of Grades II and III WAD as optional adjuncts to manual and physical therapies and exercise.

26.3.6 Acupuncture

While this technique is not recommended for Quebec Grade I WAD, it can be employed in Grades II and III WAD as an optional adjunct for symptoms lasting more than 3 weeks.

See also chapters 36 and 37

Regarding laser acupuncture one controlled trial investigated the efficacy of laser acupuncture combined with cervical collar use versus treatment with collar and placebo laser [12], but this technique does not appear to be any more effective than the placebo in treating acute WAD.

26.4 CARET Therapy

The acronym CARET indicates capacitive and resistive energy transfer. This innovative rehabilitation instrument utilises the transmission of long waves within biological tissues consequently stimulating energy production in the tissues and activating repair and anti-inflammatory processes at a cellular level. The physiological effects confirming the energy transfer are:

- Reduction of the viscosity of connective tissue with a consequent increase in extensibility
- Vasodilatation with local increase in blood flow and a consequent removal of algogenic substances

- Drainage and resorption of oedemas and haematomas, resorption of excess synovial fluid
- Reduction of muscular spasms owing to reduced activity of secondary efferents
- Repair of fibril muscle damage
- Reintegration of membrane potential in nerve fibres

In processing the WAD results, we find indication both for pain control and reparative scopes, therefore permitting a better clinical response and a reduction in recovery time.

26.4.1 Treatment Planning

A collision victim becomes hypervigilant for any symptoms that before the collision might have been disregarded but because of amplification became far more intrusive. The symptom pool may increase even though the acute injury is resolving. These initially minor symptoms may be due to occupation, sports or hobbies, symptoms from medication use and importantly attributable to maladaptive postures and changes in physical fitness that arise as patients withdraw from normal activities. These various benign, physical sources do not usually cause severe or significant pain but this is where psychological factors begin to become important.

In the *acute stage* painkillers and anti-inflammatory drugs like nonsteroidal anti-inflammatory drug (NSAID) for the first 2 weeks may be given, and this can be combined with paracetamol. The physiotherapist, in the first 24 h, can use cold packs to prevent pain, unnecessary tissue swelling and oedema. A soft, supporting cervical collar should be used the first few days after injury. The collar offers support for the neck and head in a pain-free position with the neck in a favourable position. After a few days the collar should be taken off a number of times each day. During these hours the neck is trained with gradually increasing active exercises. It is important to know that the recovery is not delayed by not using the collar. Short periods of collar use are suggested by some authors [13]. The patient should avoid excessive use of the collar, which could cause bad posture and delay mobilisation. The collar may also be suitable for nocturnal use. The patient should avoid sleeping on the stomach as this causes an extreme extension and sometimes rotation of the cervical spine.

For sleeping a suitable pillow is advisable, offering support to the head with the head in a median position and the cervical muscles relaxed.

In the acute phase acupuncture has its role for pain relief starting carefully as soon as possible after the accident and increasing in intensity and number of needles as days go by. Massage may be tried.

In the *subacute phase*, after approximately 2 weeks, more active physiotherapy can be given. The physiotherapist performs a new examination concerning the range of movement and the muscular status. Mobilisation is instructed and performed with care, first free active movements and later turning, leaning and flexion movements against the resistance of the hand of the therapist. Biofeedback training is helpful. This induces muscle strengthening enabling the patient to cease using the collar.

Now is also the time for treatment of other parts of the body. Thus the physician and the physiotherapist have to examine the range of movement in the cervical, thoracic and even the lumbar parts of the spine, as thoracic and lumbar disturbances are common in traffic accidents together with neck lesions.

Hypermobility and hypomobility are looked for. Asymmetries are noted. Hypermobility is usually most common in the lumbar back, caused by traffic trauma. Muscular stabilisation training is instructed and is usually the only treatment necessary.

Hypomobility is most common in the thoracic spine. The treatment is vertebral joint mobilisation.

In this stage it is of uttermost importance to induce leg muscle strength training, as for balance, walking and returning to a normal life the use of the legs for appropriate stance and body support is mandatory. For the patients self-confidence, one basic thing is the possibility to move around freely and be able with muscle power to counteract imbalances and not have to stop walking or training due to lack of leg muscle ability.

The sacroiliac joints are very important to examine after traffic accidents. The symptoms may be obscure and delayed in appearance. Sometimes symptoms and signs appear years after the trauma. The patient is examined standing up. Differences in height between the right and left iliac crests are looked for. The *Vorlauf* phenomenon, when one spina iliaca posterior is immobile when the patient bends forward, indicates immobility in one sacroiliac joint. The patient is treated according to the findings, with mobilisation of the immobile joint. This is performed with the patient in a lateral or prone position, the sacrum fixed and the iliac bone mobilised by the physiotherapist. Massage may help some patients considerably but in others increase the pain.

In the *subchronic* and *chronic stage*, more stabilisation training is performed, including neck movements with muscle strengthening. The training is performed, supervised and instructed by the physiotherapist and also with a written home training programme. Video instructions are advisable. Both for neck training and general robustness of the whole body, training in water is of benefit.

Most whiplash patients have balance problems caused by a brainstem disturbance or being of neck origin – cervical vertigo [14, 15]. Neck treatment may help, but often true balance training is needed: walking, turning, head and eye movements and standing on one leg, on a hubcap or on foam rubber [16, 17]. The automated training in the computerised force plate, the Balance Master, is of great help. The trauma may have caused benign positional paroxysmal vertigo, which craves a specific treatment [18].

The patient may be very tired and also have mental problems, with fatigue and depressive tendencies. Hence the psychological approach has to be considered by all members of the treating team, especially the physiotherapist who has a lot of contact with the patient, repeatedly and often in long sessions. The goal is to help the patient return to a normal family life and also to work.

26.4.2 Follow-Up

For the subsequent weeks, months and even years, it is of importance to have a well programmed follow-up of the whiplash patient. This should preferably be performed by the initial treatment team, who knows the patient and has participated in the assessment. The follow-up takes into consideration all angles of the problems, the neck, back, pelvis and balance, as well as the psychological and practical problems. The treatment results are recorded by case history according to a questionnaire and clinical investigation including balance testing. Stabilometry or, even better, dynamic posturography is performed for an objective assessment of the deficit and improvement in balancing ability.

26.5 Education or Advice

Numerous studies include education [19] or advice as components of the intervention using educational videos and pamphlets. Ferrari et al. [4] found no beneficial effect of a one-page pamphlet of evidence-based whiplash prevention information on patient perceived recovery at 2 weeks or 3 months. Pamphlets emphasising the good prognosis of whiplash were distributed to all participants in the Kongsted et al. [20] trial, which found no clinically meaningful differences between rigid collar, usual care with an emphasis on fear reduction and resuming normal activities, and active mobilisation at 1 year.

By contrast, educational videos were shown to have beneficial effects on improvement in pain among acute whiplash patients. They received by mail the 20-min video that provided reassurance, home exercises and advice on early return to normal activities or watched from their bedside a 12-min psycho-educational video emphasising behavioural and home exercise interventions and breathing relaxation for muscle tension. In subjects there was relief from pain at 1, 3 and 6 months after injury, and they also used much less medication and had lower rates of health-care utilisation [21].

Conclusions

Patients that normally receive conservative interventions are those with Grades 1 and 2 WAD. Conservative treatment includes local heat and ice treatment, neck collar immobilisation, ultrasound, traction, massage, (active) mobilisation, exercises, pulsed electromagnetic therapy and multimodal rehabilitation.

Active interventions that stimulate the patient to return to daily activities as soon as possible are preferable to rest and wearing of a collar.

Physical therapy specifically aimed at the musculature (e.g. transcutaneous electrical nerve stimulation, ultrasound, heat, ice and acupuncture) improves prognosis in acute WAD.

In chronic WAD, the only treatment that has clearly shown benefit is radiofrequency neurotomy [2].

References

1. Mealy K, Brennan H, Fenelon GCC (1986) Early mobilisation of acute whiplash injuries. Br Med J 292:656–657
2. McDonald GJ, Lord SM, Bogduk N (1999) Long-term follow-up of patients treated with cervical radiofrequency neurotomy for chronic neck pain. Neurosurgery 45(1):61–67
3. McKinney LA, Doman JO, Ryan M (1989) The role of physiotherapy in the management of acute neck sprains following road-traffic accidents. Arch Emerg Med 6:27–33
4. Ferrari R (2002) Prevention of chronic pain after whiplash. Emerg Med J 19(6):526–530
5. Magee D, Oborn-Barrett E, Turner S, Fenning N (2000) A systematic overview of the effectiveness of physical therapy intervention on soft tissue neck injury following trauma. Physiother Can 52:111–130
6. Scholten-Peeters GG, Verhagen AP, Bekkering GE, van der Windt DA, Barnsley L, Oostendorp RA, Hendriks EJ (2003) Prognostic factors of whiplash-associated disorders: a systematic review of prospective cohort studies. Pain 104(1–2):303–322
7. Riva D, Trevisson P (2004) L'augmentation de la force exprimible pour l'optimisation de la performance sportive, vol 445. KS – Kinésithérapie Scientifique, Paris, pp 27–32
8. Mostafavifar M, Wertz J, Borchers J (2012) A systematic review of the effectiveness of kinesio taping for musculoskeletal injury. Phys Sports Med 40(4):33–40. doi:10.3810/psm.2012.11.1986
9. Verhagen AP, Peeters GG, de Bie RA, Oostendorp RA (2001) Conservative treatment for whiplash. Cochrane Database Syst Rev 4:CD003338
10. Foley-Nolan D, Moore K, Codd M, Barry C, O'Connor P, Coughlan RJ (1992) Low energy high frequency pulsed electromagnetic therapy for acute whiplash injuries. A double blind randomized controlled study. Scand J Rehabil Med 24:51–58
11. Thuile CH, Walzl M (2002) Evaluation of electromagnetic fields in the treatment of pain in patients with lumbar radiculopathy of the whiplash syndrome. Neuro Rehabil 17:63–67
12. Aigner N, Fialka C, Radda C, Vecsei V (2006) Adjuvant laser acupuncture in the treatment of whiplash injuries: a prospective randomized placebo-controlled trial. Wien Klin Wochenschr 118:95–99
13. Scholten-Peeters G, Bekkering G, Verhagen A, van der Windt D, Lanser K, Hendriks E, Oostendorp R (2002) Clinical practice guideline for the physiotherapy of patients with whiplash associated disorders. Spine 27:412–422
14. Àlund M, Ledin T, Odkvist LM, Larsson SE, Moller C (1993) Dynamic posturography among patients with common neck disorders. A study of 15 cases with suspected cervical vertigo. J Vestib Res 3:383–389
15. Alund M, Ledin T, Moller C, Odkvist LM, Larsson SE (1991) Dynamic posturography in cervical vertigo. Acta Otolaryngol Stockh 481(Suppl):601–602
16. Norré M, Beckers A (1988) Vestibular habituation training. Arch Otolaryngol Head Neck Surg 114:883–886
17. Odkvist I, Odkvist LM (1988) Physiotherapy in vertigo. Acta Otolaryngol Stockh 455(Suppl):74–76
18. Epley J (1992) The canalith reposition procedure: for treatment of benign paroxysmal vertigo. Otolaryngol Head Neck Surg 107:399–404
19. Brison RJ, Hartling L, Dostaler S, Leger A, Rowe BH, Stiell I, Pickett W (2005) A randomized controlled trial of an educational intervention to prevent the chronic pain of whiplash associated disorders following rear-end motor vehicle collisions. Spine 30:1799–1807
20. Kongsted A, Qerama E, Kasch H, Bach FW, Korsholm L, Jensen TS, Bendix T (2008) Education of patients after whiplash injury: is oral advice any better than a pamphlet? Spine 33(22):E843–E848
21. Oliveira A, Gevirtz R, Hubbard D (2006) A psycho-educational video used in the emergency department provides effective treatment for whiplash injuries. Spine 31:1652–1657

Manual Medicine in Whiplash-Associated Disorders (WAD)

27

G. Brugnoni, C. Correggia, and C. Mariconda

27.1 Introduction

Manual Medicine (MM) is a medical discipline devoted to diagnosis and conservative therapy of some algetic pathologies of the muscular-skeletal apparatus and in particular the rachis: such consequences are benign but extremely widespread.

In the beginning MM availed itself of numerous techniques from American osteopathy, an alternative medicine [1], which had the undeniable merit of drawing attention to the micro-mechanical problems of the rachis which had been unrecognized by traditional medicine, even if these had been considered as the cause or possible co-cause of all diseases. Osteopathy was, and still is, based on obsolete scientific conceptions and is lacking in simple and clear diagnosis repeatable by all operators seeing as it is based on deep palpation of fine intervertebral movements.

Benign vertebral pain reported in the majority of cases is more often linked to a dysfunction of neuro-motorial control of the rachis [2] and not always owing to a lesion.

A step forward was made by R. Maigne [3], through the conception of new simple and repeatable semeiotics [4, 5] based on pain-provoking manoeuvres with the aim of identifying pain in one or more mobile vertebral segments. In the absence of organic lesions, Maigne defined this situation as "painful minor intervertebral dysfunction" (PMID), an excellent definition for the majority of vertebral dysfunctional pathologies.

G. Brugnoni
Italian Academy of Manual Medicine,
Italian Institute for Auxology, Milan, Italy
e-mail: guido.brugnoni@libero.it

C. Correggia • C. Mariconda (✉)
Department of Physical Medicine and Rehabilitation, Gradenigo Hospital, Turin, Italy
e-mail: carlo.mariconda@gradenigo.it

D.C. Alpini et al. (eds.), *Whiplash Injuries*,
DOI 10.1007/978-88-470-5486-8_27, © Springer-Verlag Italia 2014

Research began by the Audiology Clinic of the University of Milan at the end of the 1990s to use the diagnosis and manipulative techniques of MM for Ménière's disease [6] and then in other vertiginous pathologies, above all those of vertebral origin.

The dysfunction of neuro-motorial control and consequent alterations of the neuromuscular patterns of the rachis, in problems of equilibrium, can cause a dysfunction to the vestibule-vertebral unit (see Chap. 7), that is, the anatomic-physiologic structure which controls the connections between the proprioceptive trigeminal and cervical-dorsal information and the neurovegetative ocular and labyrinthic regulation.

27.2 Diagnosis

The clinical examination proposed can be divided into six principal parts:

1. *Static examination of the rachis*, of the head and limbs in an upright position paying visual attention to the anatomic elements concerning modifications of the physiological or pathological curves of the rachis and the position of the head, shoulders and hips.
2. *Dynamic examination of "segment" movements*, to identify limitation of movement, point of pain occurrence during circular movement, abnormalities during harmonious movements and the rigid tracts of the spine or deviations from the movement plan noted during bending and lateral-bending movement.
3. *Examination of mobile vertebral – segments* comprising a series of provocative manoeuvres to provoke pain in the "mobile segment", that is, the intervertebral articulation, in the entire rachis, in a caudal sense from C6 to L5, searching for one or more painful mobile segments:
   - Axial pressure on the spinous processes
   - Lateral pressure on the spinous processes
   - Pressure on the first supraspinous and interspinous segment
   - Search for the paramedian articular pain point
4. *Examination of the cutaneous, subcutaneous, sinuous, periosteal and muscular tissues*, that is, of the "myofascial" pain. R. Maigne described a series of signs visible at the cutaneous, subcutaneous, fasciae, tendons, periosteum and muscular levels which he called "cellulo-periosteo-myalgic syndrome".
5. *Examinations of neurological signs and of the pachymeninx*

   The description of a complete neurological examination is beyond our topic, but it should be systemically carried out in WI and is extremely important for decisions about instrumental exams and therapeutic choices.
6. *Pre-manipulation tests*

   The following are absolutely necessary before proceeding with cervical manipulation:
   - Romberg, sensitized by rotation and extension of the head
   - Localization of the spontaneous and positional nystagmus mainly by rotation and extension of the head

- Rancurel test for haemodynamic vertebral basilar insufficiency
- Positioning and cautious tensioning in cervical rotations assessing the patient's sensations

27.3 Treatment

Modern MM employs various manual techniques including both active and passive mobilization, J. Mennel's joint play, manual traction, transverse and longitudinal muscle stretching and Mitchell's post-isometric techniques as well as "vertebral manipulation" differencing from the aforementioned in the way it is done and the type of sensorial and proprioceptive stimulation, aiming at a major impact and rapidity of action.

Alongside the above methods all the modern antalgic techniques are used in MM, such as articular, vertebral and peridural infiltrations, mini-invasive techniques, instrumental and rehabilitative therapies amongst which the recent spinal stabilization through biofeedback [7, 8] and Natchev's vertebral auto-traction [9].

27.3.1 Manual Therapy

All "soft tissues", skin, subcutaneous, fasciae, periosteum and muscles are obviously an integral part of the movement apparatus, both because they move together with bone segments, that is, by accompanying movement – in the case of muscles they are the engine – and because they are closely connected to the rachis for the metameric distribution of the somatic and sympathetic innervation, and also, even if in a less clear way, they are connected to extra-vertebral articulations.

Thus, for different reasons, but mainly for the achievement of a good clinical result, it is necessary to be able to use these techniques correctly. They are extremely useful both as a gradual preparation for manipulation or as a substitute when manipulation is not possible owing to general or topical causes. These techniques can also be employed to eliminate problems which persist after manipulation and which could impede a quicker functional recovery.

As we have already mentioned, manual techniques can be subdivided into various chapters, but those with more interest for us can be gathered into three groups:

27.3.1.1 Articular Techniques

To perform a mobilization of intervertebral and peripheric articulations.

1. Passive articular mobilization following the direction of active joint movements. These are part of traditional kinesiatrics together with active or active-assisted mobilization.
2. "Joint play" by J. Mennel [10], passive articular mobilization using lateral or sliding movements which the articulation is not able to do actively.
3. Post-isometric relaxation (PIR) by Mitchell [11] or post-isometric release.

   This technique entails guiding the two articular extremities to their maximum excursion, i.e. in tension, in a state of maximum release; then the therapist

asks the patient to move in the opposite direction against a minimum resistance provided by the therapist for a duration of about 10–30 s: the therapist then moves the articulation back to a maximum excursion and repeats this 3–5 times.
4. Inhibition of the antagonist. Requires isometric contraction against a minimum resistance and then passively move the articulation in the same direction.
5. Inhibition of the agonist, who is asked to contract isometrically against a minimum resistance and then move the articulation passively in the opposite direction. These techniques utilize the two laws of Sherrington such as the Kabat method but without using maximum contractions.

27.3.1.2 Muscular Techniques

The aim is to release muscles which are prone to local contractions which may vary in degree. The most efficient techniques are those which utilize stretching through passive articular movement preceded by an agonist or antagonist's contraction according to what is expounded above. These movements must be associated with manual transversal or longitudinal stretching and to techniques to facilitate the neuro-motorial response.

27.3.1.3 Skin and Subcutaneous Techniques

These are of scarce interest for problems of equilibrium, but mobilization of the skin and subcutaneous techniques are useful for diagnosis and treatment of allodynia areas which are generally residues from vertebral treatment and can perpetuate continual pain, sometimes deep and widespread, to the patient.

Other interesting techniques are Dicke's connectival reflexogenic massage, Teirich-Leube massage, Vodder's lymphodrainage and Cyriax's deep massage.

We believe that it is indispensible to know how to use these techniques as they can lead to a good practice of manipulation and in some cases in its substitution.

27.3.2 Vertebral Manipulation

Vertebral manipulation consists of forced passive mobilization which stretches the joint elements beyond their physiologic or pathologic barrier up to the limit of their passive movement. It is called "high speed" or "with impulse". An abrupt movement is used in vertebral movement and causes a high-frequency ascending flux, a rapid proprioceptive re-information to the medulla centres which control the movement of the articulation. This discharge is therefore able to restore the normal fluxes to the centres which had become unaccustomed through movement limitations caused by pain spasms, in our case, after sprain trauma, or owing to balance or postural problems, even if pain free or caused by previous traumas or micro-traumas, or for other causes. Some rules must be followed to obtain these results, such as R. Maigne's "rule of no pain and reverse movement", needing the manipulation to be carried out in the opposite direction to the painful one. The no pain rule must also be respected in manipulative therapy of equilibrium problems.

As has been demonstrated through studies on cadavers using accelerometers and intra-discal pressure gauges [12], the movement of articular heads is slight but extremely rapid, almost explosive.

Manipulation is not only an antalgic treatment but is above all the first and most precise and delicate phase of a rehabilitative treatment.

One of the most interesting aspects of this treatment is the possibility to rapidly modify rachis movement patterns through precise manoeuvres and therefore restore its function as receptor and effector of equilibrium.

It is indeed in an alteration of the rachis motorial patterns, not only at the cervical level but also in the thorax and lumbar zones and in their clinical expression, i.e. DDIM, that we should look for the causes of some equilibrium disorders and chronic post-whiplash pain, above all at the "passage" level, that is, the passage zones between one sector and another of the rachis, also called "transitional zones".

These zones are:

1. The occipit(o)-atlanto-epistrophei passage
2. The cervical-thoracic passage
3. The thoracic-lumbar passage
4. The lumbar-sacral passage
5. The sacral-coccygeus passage which can also be situated between the 1st and the 2nd coccygeus

Teyssandier describes another functional passage in the medio-thoracic segment at level T7–T8 [13].

From a clinical point of view, it is advisable to intervene on these passage areas in order to modify the rachis motorial patterns. R. Maigne has described a "transitional zone syndrome" [14], meaning intervertebral malfunction disorders which can be situated in two or more passages contemporaneously and all on the same side.

Vertebral manipulation is not only performed on the proprioceptive afferents but almost certainly on the vegetative nervous system channels.

Vertebral manipulation may engender vegetative phenomena, such as sweating, and eliminate other phenomena: closed nostrils and unilateral lacrimation in certain cervical cephaleas, cutaneous areas of allodynia which instantly disappear, and therefore they must be related to the vasomotor phenomenons.

In cervical whiplash we find a reduced efficiency both in the dynamic control of head stability and in the strategies of pelvic control of equilibrium, especially in brusque disturbances in walking [15].

It is in fact "hip" strategy (hip strategy by Nashner) which controls a vast range of reactions to destabilizing factors and which appears insufficient in many of the above-mentioned clinical cases.

By "hips" we refer to: the T-L passage, the L-S passage, sacroiliac and pelvis, focusing not only on the joints, but also on the motorial coordination obtained through exact muscular sequences.

This complex sector is also the one which oversees walking, in which, according to a recent theory [16], does not originate in the limbs but in the thoracic-lumbar passage and in the lumbar rachis and is transmitted from here through the sacroiliacs to the lower limbs which provide the kinetic energy necessary.

This movement propagates from the lower area up to the first cervical vertebrae through the anatomic conformation of the cervical joint facets and by the contrasting movement of the humeral-omeric scapular.

The functional synchronization of the phasic muscles of the inferior limbs and the tonic ones of the spine takes place in the lower passages and moves upwards [17].

One must never forget that in the damaging mechanism of "whiplash injury", the first impact is in the inferior dorsal and lumbar region which is nearly always involved in this syndrome.

Therefore, we believe that it is necessary to begin treatment on the inferior passages especially from the lumbar-sacral and then gradually proceed upwards.

The cervical rachis can only be treated after treatments of the inferior levels have not been able to restore the correct vertebral function.

There are a series of reasons why particular precaution must be taken during manipulative treatment of the cervical rachis:

A great part of the errors which occur during vertebral manipulation concerns this zone: such errors are rare but generally serious.

- The major danger has to do with the anatomical situation of the vertebral arteries and possibilities of undiagnosed past pathologies.
- The importance of the neck in the sphere of the Equilibrium System is because of the connection of the cervical roots with the vestibular nuclei and also for the compensation phenomenons which can occur at this level.
- Effective risk-free cervical manipulation calls for great manual and clinical experience, acquired by the operator, through long formative and practical training.

In cases of "whiplash" treatment, it is necessary to begin manipulation from lower vertebral levels, rising gradually, and then treating the neck only if the lesion is contained in the first two stages of the Quebec Task Force classification WAD [18], i.e. cervical pain and stiffness without clinical evidence or only with skeletal-muscle evidence. Even in these cases great caution must be used and manipulation should not be carried out before 1–3 months have passed, and in full respect of the treatment rules, always starting with the above-mentioned manual manipulation, and after having carried out the pre-manipulative tests.

Manipulation techniques should be used to resolve PMID treating the active ones (spontaneously painful) and the inactive (non-spontaneously painful) when localized in specific zones: the most significant inactive PMID in this context is usually located in the "passage area" also called "transition zones" which we have already mentioned.

It is therefore advisable to begin treatment searching for the PMID, even the inactive ones, at the lumbar-sacral and mid-lumbar passage, at L3–L4, thus proceeding with their treatment through mobilization techniques until the correct tension is reached or with vertebral manipulation with impulse.

Subsequently you seek the PMID, also the inactive ones of the thoracic-lumbar segment, and then mid-thoracic (D7–D8), and these are preferably treated by the operator creating an epigastric support extension position.

Then the cervical-thorax segment is treated, also in the absence of PMID, in extension by the operator using a sternum support position, or with the patient in a supine position, and always respecting the treatment limits of the specific patient.

In the case of radicular pain pathologies in any of the spinal segments, one must keep to a "legeartis" treatment, taking all the necessary precautions.

As we have already said, the real cervical treatment must be particularly delicate and we reaffirm that at this level it is absolutely necessary to correlate the vestibular, neurologic and algologic physical diagnosis to the vertebral one.

The "compensatory PMID" should never be treated with impulsive manipulation but only through gentle, superficial stretching. On the contrary, the pathogenic PMID should be resolved with the use of all Manual Medicine techniques, therefore starting with post-isometric release and then proceeding with passive mobilization or "joint play" manoeuvres and if possible concluding with real "high speed" vertebral manipulation.

The atlantooccipital segment is where it is more difficult to distinguish between compensatory "PMID" and pathogenic ones. It is in fact possible, at this level, to have secondary problems to those of occlusion, or either of ocular fusion or of mono lateral auditory ones. It is also a zone with high intrinsic risks of both slight and severe complications. It is therefore advisable to avoid abrupt manipulation and utilize "gentler" techniques, mainly progressive ones such as fibromyolysis to be carried out manually with the patient in a supine or sitting position, or simply through occipit-atlo-epistropheus techniques [19].

One to six sittings twice a week are generally necessary and it is advisable to carry out a single manipulative movement at the beginning and then to evaluate the results and add further manoeuvres at higher levels.

In synthesis, the cervical segment can be treated through abrupt manipulation only in the following cases:

- In the absence of contraindications, especially vascular ones, or of vertebral instability
- In the presence of active PMID
- In 1st and 2nd grade "Whiplash – associated disorders" (WAD) (TAEC)
- In post-acute phases, rarely in subacute ones and never in an initial acute phase
- Respecting the "no pain rule"
- If treatment of the lower levels has resulted ineffective
- By an expert operator

Conclusion

The elements necessary to proceed to manipulative therapy of after effects of whiplash (cervical trauma), both for pain or equilibrium dysfunctions, are:

1. Exact neurologic, algologic and equilibrium diagnoses
2. General medical diagnosis, orthopaedic-physiatric and Manual Medicine diagnosis

3. Competence, ability and experience in Manual Medicine

This procedure could undergo further development through deeper knowledge of the Equilibrium System and of the neuro-motorial control of the rachis.

There are numerous lesions which can pass unobserved in post-traumatic cervical trauma pathology [19]: therefore, manipulation must be carried out with extreme caution.

Clinical and "treatment" diagnosis of Manual Medicine is the key to manage a multi-method therapy in which manipulation has a precise indication.

The Quebec Task Force on WI recommends a special preparation for operators in this difficult field: Manual Medicine, because of its topographic ability in pain diagnosis, and for the direct treatment which can restore the normal neuro-motorial control of the rachis, is the appropriate discipline suitable to teach operators a complete approach to "whiplash" trauma [20–22].

References

1. Teyssandier MJ, Brugnoni G (2000) Quelques aspects de l'osteopathie moderne aux Etats Unis d'Amerique. La Riabilitazione 33(4):141–150
2. Richardson C, Hodges P, Hides J (2004) Therapeutic exercise for lumbopelvic stabilization, 2nd edn. Churchill Livingstone, Edinburgh
3. Maigne R (2006) Douleurs d'origine vertébrale. Elsevier Masson, Issy-les-Moulineaux
4. Maigne J-Y et al (2009) Interexaminer agreement of clinical examination of the neck in manual medicine. Ann Phys Rehabil Med. doi:10.1016/j.rehab.2008.11.001
5. Brugnoni G, Martini S (2008) Reproductibilité inter opérateurs de quatre tests cliniques de Médecine Manuelle dans les cervicalgies communes. Revue de Médecine Manuelle-Ostéopathie 25:4–6
6. Cesarani A, Brugnoni G, Barozzi S (1999) Vertige de la maladie de Ménière Traitement par manipulation vertebrales. Revue de Médicine Orthopedique 59:17–19
7. Kaner T, Ozer AF (2013) Dynamic stabilization for challenging lumbar degenerative diseases of the spine: a review of the literature. Adv Orthop 753470:1–13
8. Canbay S, Aydin AL, Aktas E, Erten SF, Basmaci M, Sasani M, Ozer AF (2013) Posterior dynamic stabilization for the treatment of patients with lumbar degenerative disc disease: long-term clinical and radiological results. Turk Neuro Surg 23(2):188–197
9. Tesio L, Luccarelli G, Fornari M (1989) Natchev's auto-traction for lumbago-sciatica: effectiveness in lumbar disc herniation. Arch Phys Med Rehabil 70(12):831–834
10. Mennel JB (1952) The science and art of manipulation, 2nd edn. Churchill, London
11. Mitchell FL, Mitchell PKG (2002) The muscle energy manual, 2nd edn. MET Press, East Lansing
12. Maigne JY, Guillon F (2000) Highlighting of intervertebral movements and variations of intradiskal pressure during lumbar spine manipulation: a feasibility study. Manipulative Physiol Ther 23(8):531–535
13. Teyssandier MJ (2009) Le syndrome de la charnière médio-thoracique et les deux rachis fonctionnels. Revue de Mèdecine Manuelle-Osteopathie 27:18–24
14. Maigne R (1984) Das syndrom der ubergangszonen der Wirbelsaule. Manuelle Medizin 22:122–124
15. Van Oosterwijck J, Nijs J, Meeus M, Paul L (2013) Evidence for central sensitization in chronic whiplash: a systematic literature review. Eur J Pain 17(3):299–312
16. Gracovetsky S (2002) Le role des membres superieurs dans le control du pelvis et du cou durant la marche. Revue de Medicine Vertebrale 8:4–8

17. Allum JH, Adkin AL (2003) Improvements in trunk sway observed for stance and gait tasks during recovery from an acute unilateral peripheral vestibular deficit. Audiol Neurootol 8(5):286–302
18. Scientific Monograph on Whiplash-Associated Disorders (1995) Redefining "whiplash" and its management. Spine 20(Suppl 8):1S–73S
19. Jonsson HJ Jr, Bring G, Rauschning W, Sahlstedt B (1997) Hidden cervical spine injuries in traffic accident. La Revue de Medicine Orthopédique 50:3–12
20. Falla D, Dall'Alba P, Rainoldi A, Merletti R, Jull G (2002) Location of innervation zones of sternocleidomastoid and scalene muscles – a basis for clinical and research. Electromyography applications. Clin Neurophysiol 113:57–63
21. Jull GA (2000) Deep cervical neck flexor dysfunction in whiplash. J Musculoskelet Pain 8(1/2):143–154
22. Sterling M (2011) Whiplash-associated disorder: musculoskeletal pain and related clinical findings. J Man ManipulativeTher 19(4):194–200

Rehabilitation Strategy According to the Quebec Classification

28

S. Negrini, P. Sibilla, S. Atanasio, and G. Brugnoni

28.1 Introduction

Whiplash injuries entail lesions in the cervical spine. There may be elongations of ligaments, smaller or more serious vertebrae fractures, disc compressions, prolapses or dislocations of the vertebrae.

The treatment strategy depends upon the type and degree of cervical lesion. Stabilizing surgery may be indicated in severe cases. Psychological approaches are a necessity. Simultaneous damage to the brain, brainstem, inner ear, back, pelvis or lower extremities has to be taken into consideration when planning treatment. Physiotherapy in whiplash injuries has a central role.

In order to assess the lesions, case history, clinical investigation and imaging with radiology and MRI are mandatory. This should be performed before the patient is seen by the physiotherapist.

The manual examination sometimes has to be postponed due to the cervical pain. The degree of active movement is of importance to notice. Pain may contraindicate some parts of the examination and physiotherapy, especially in the acute stage.

S. Negrini (✉)
Department of Clinical and Experimental Sciences, University of Brescia, Viale Europa 11, 25123, Brescia, Italy
e-mail: stefano.negrini@med.unibs.it

P. Sibilla
Scoliosis Center, IRCCS "Don Carlo Gnocchi" Foundation, via capecelatro 66, Milan, Italy

S. Atanasio
Istituto Italiano Colonna – ISICO, via Crivelli 5, Milan, Italy
e-mail: salvatore.atanasio@isico.it

G. Brugnoni
Italian Academy of Manual Medicine,
Italian Institute for Auxology, Milan, Italy
e-mail: guido.brugnoni@libero.it

D.C. Alpini et al. (eds.), *Whiplash Injuries*,
DOI 10.1007/978-88-470-5486-8_28, © Springer-Verlag Italia 2014

Neck hyperextension and dislocation should be noticed and may contraindicate most physiotherapeutic manoeuvres. One must proceed with caution in implementing neck therapy if the assessment is not performed in an adequate way by the responsible physician and in some parts completed by the physiotherapist. Cervical lesions may be worsened by too brisk examinations.

The Bone and Joint Task Force on Neck Pain and Its Associated Disorders [1] conducted a critical review of the literature on assessment tools and screening protocols for traumatic and non-traumatic neck pain. According to the Task Force, in the absence of serious pathology, clinical physical examinations are more predictive at excluding than confirming structural lesions causing neurologic compression, that to say the physiotherapist could be, at the same time, the more appropriate health professional to diagnose and treat a WAD patient.

As usual in the rehabilitation field, attention has been recently more and more drawn to the biopsychosocial aspects and to the changes in the quality of the lives of patients who have suffered neck trauma. The strategies of behavioural medicine intervention are particularly useful, meaning an individual approach with the therapist, with a group or through telematics monitoring. The patient follows a standard exercise programme at home and therefore should be able to monitor himself and recognize the changes in his health during daily activities.

To describe the most determinant clinical symptoms, the Quebec Task Force (QTF) developed in 1995 [2] a classification system which allows a good assessment of the severity of the injury. In cases of QTF I and II whiplash injuries, the posttraumatic treatment is a domain of conservative therapy. Therapeutic measures have been exhaustively studied and compared. Physical therapy has been assessed predominantly with respect to its effects on pain intensity and improving patients' range of motion. It seems that its efficacy is limited to a certain degree of improvement of these parameters in the acute stage of convalescence. We would like to emphasize the importance of a multidisciplinary approach within which the psychological and behavioural aspects are of considerable significance to the rehabilitation of the patient with WAD (whiplash-associated disorders). Furthermore, we suggest the distribution of informative pamphlets and the training of the patient by experts in the emergency departments during the early stages of the post-trauma period. Early recognition of the patients' emotional state could be a useful instrument in shortening the necessary recovery time, reduce eventual unsatisfactory results and lower the total costs of treatment.

For handling patients with whiplash injuries, a team of specialists is necessary. The members of different professions need special expertise concerning orthopaedics, neurology, neck physiology and neuro-otology. The legal questions can best be answered by a physician in the whiplash team. The physiotherapist must have a profound knowledge of neck physiology and treatment, balance problems and vertigo. Education and information of physicians and physiotherapists are necessary to increase the awareness of the whiplash phenomenon, thereby preventing harmful delay in treatment and referral.

Table 28.1 Clinical classification on whiplash-associated disorders proposed by the Quebec Task Force (1995)

Grade	Clinical presentation
0	No complaint about neck pain No physical signs
I	Neck complaint of pain, stiffness or tenderness No physical signs
II	Neck complaint Musculoskeletal signs including: Decreased range of movement Point tenderness
III	Neck complaint Musculoskeletal signs Neurological signs including: Decreased or absent deep tendon reflexes Muscle weakness Sensory deficits
IV	Neck complaint and fracture or dislocation

Table 28.2 Clinical spectrum of whiplash-associated disorders as proposed by the Quebec Task Force (1995) [2]

Grade	Presumed pathology	Clinical presentation
I	Microscopic or multimicroscopic lesion Lesion is not serious enough to cause muscle spasm	Usually presents to a doctor more than 24 h after trauma
II	Neck sprain and bleeding around soft tissue (articular capsules, ligaments, tendons and muscles) Muscle spasm secondary to soft tissue injury	Usually presents to a doctor in the first 24 h after trauma Nonspecific radiation to the head, face, occipital region, shoulder and arm form soft tissues injuries Neck pain with limited range of motion due to muscle spasm
III	Injuries to neurologic system by mechanical injury or by irritation secondary to bleeding or inflammation	Presents to a doctor usually within hours after the trauma Limited range of motion combined with neurologic symptoms and signs

28.2 WAD Classification

In the literature there has been a great heterogeneity of classifications. The Quebec Task Force on Whiplash-Associated Disorders proposal represents a milestone for both clinicians and researchers.

This classification is summarized in Table 28.1. To better compare this classification with the one we have proposed, we present, in Table 28.2, other clinical and pathological specifications proposed by the Quebec Task Force on Whiplash-Associated Disorders and, in Table 28.3, a summary of our classification.

Table 28.3 Summary of our classification

Degree	Lesion	Treatment
1st	Simple strain	Soft collar, 20 days
2nd	Strain	Soft collar with a good containment, 20 days
3rd	Serious strain	Hard collar, 25/30 days
4th	Compromising of mechanical stability	Minerva in Articast, 30/40 days
5th	Articular dislocation and/or bony fractures	Surgery

It must be said that we proposed our classification during the S. Margherita Meeting in January 28, 1995, before the appearance in the literature of the Quebec Task Force classification. The two are surprisingly similar, but ours is more pertinent to our way of treatment and is derived from a more practical, clinical point of view. The Quebec Task Force classification is designed to better compare the literature results about different types of patients.

28.3 Whiplash Rehab According to Quebec Task Force Classification

In this chapter we will discuss the rehabilitative treatment of whiplash, identifying five clinical degrees of pathology and proposing specific rehab therapeutic approaches based on clinical evaluation of patient. The rehabilitative tool is particularly focused on the restoration of neck functioning [3–7].

28.4 First-Degree Whiplash

28.4.1 Anatomical Pathology

First-degree whiplash is a simple strain of the cervical spine ligaments. The zygapophyseal joints do not show severe lesions although they have been stressed in distraction and compression according to the mechanism of injury. In the outer part of the discs, tears can appear that can justify tardy painful syndromes due to disc protrusions. The muscles are stretched, usually without lesions of their bodies and/or their tendons. An involvement of the sympathetic plexus or nerve roots is seldom [8, 9].

28.4.2 History

The pain is not very accentuated, and is usually local, but sometimes there are irradiations to the head and/or shoulders. If trigger points appear, there can be irradiation to the upper extremities, but these are not due to nerve root involvement.

Symptoms usually are increased by active movements and by prolonged periods of standing and/or sitting. Sympathetic symptoms are rare, but sometimes difficult to treat.

28.4.3 Clinical Examination

If there has been a lateral impact and/or the head of the patient was rotated when the accident occurred, there can be a torticollis, usually with the head away from the pain.

28.4.4 Range of Movement

Usually the cervical spine is relatively mobile. Movements are painful in any direction at the last degrees of the range of movement, and the most involved are extension and particularly retraction; many times flexion is free. If there is a lateral component, rotation and lateral flexion are more painful on one side than the other. It's important here to remember that rotation tests better assess the upper cervical spine (occiput-C2), while lateral flexion assesses the medial and inferior segments.

Testing each articular level it is usually possible to find some joints that are more involved. This evaluation is fully compatible with the mechanism of the injury: upper spine if protrusion was prevalent, C5-C6 if flexion-extension was more important, symmetry if only sagittal movements occurred and asymmetry sometimes with differences between the lower and upper cervical spine if a lateral component was present.

It is possible to verify RoM also in the supine position, where there are not many differences apart from a trivial increase in the RoM.

28.4.5 Palpation

Muscles are not very painful. A light contracture is present, sometimes only in a few fibres; occasionally trigger points are detectable. Examining the zygapophyseal joints, it is possible to "feel" their involvement as shown by the RoM segmental evaluation. Also the lateral apophysis can be painful [5].

28.4.6 Neurologic Examination

It is usually normal.

28.4.7 Diagnosis

There is not real boundary between first- and second-degree whiplash: they describe a continuum in which the first degree represents the less important clinical lesion and the second degree represents an important clinical picture, with little movement, significant contracture and frequent irradiation of pain.

28.4.8 Treatment

A soft collar must be prescribed for 10/20 days, because it is necessary to let the ligaments heal. This happens in 18 days normally [10, 11]. The soft collar permits a little protected motion inside. It is not possible to move the cervical spine more than at the beginning of the RoM, but this motion is not only allowable, it is also advisable. In fact it is known that the ligaments heal along the force lines of the movement, if this is permitted, if it is not, the ligamentous tissue repairs in a perturbed fashion.

Rehabilitation can begin after the collar is no longer needed [12, 13].

28.5 Second Degree

28.5.1 Anatomical Pathology

Second-degree whiplash is a real strain of the ligaments and capsules of the zygapophyseal joints. These do not show dislocations: the capsular involvement depends on their distraction, sometimes internal derangement can be demonstrated. Disc lesions can be protrusions or bulging. The muscles are overstretched, sometimes without lesions of the body: these are more likely to involve tendons at their insertions. There is usually an involvement of the sympathetic plexus. The medulla can be slightly stretched, and sometimes nerve roots are involved too.

28.5.2 History

Pain is local with irradiations to head and/or shoulders. Irradiation to upper extremities is common, rarely due to nerve root lesions. Active movements are sometimes impossible, in most cases they are possible only to a minor degree. Vertigo, dizziness, nausea, vomiting, scotoma and photophobia are common. Sometimes drop attacks can appear too.

28.5.3 Clinical Examination

Usually patients present with a fixed position, fully compatible with the mechanism of injury, including both impact and head position.

28.5.4 Range of Movement

The cervical spine is relatively blocked. Movements ar0e painful in any direction at the very beginning of the RoM: many times the flexion is less involved and the most involved are rotations. The more blocked movements permit one to understand how the accident happened.

To test the more blocked articular levels is usually not useful nor possible, because all of the cervical spine is involved. The RoM in the supine position is usually a little bit less obstructed.

28.5.5 Palpation

Muscles are painful, usually more at their insertions. An important muscular contracture is present, usually in trapezium, sternocleidomastoid and elevator scapulae. Trigger points in the same muscles are usually detectable.

Examining the zygapophyseal joints, it is possible to "feel" their involvement which, at this stage, is normally very important and bilateral, depending on the mechanics of injury. The lateral apophyses are usually painful.

28.5.6 Neurologic Examination

There can be weakness, sensory impairment and/or reflex alterations. These have to be monolateral and monoradicular; otherwise it is necessary to evaluate more thoroughly the lower extremities and the other neurologic functions to investigate a possible medullar or central involvement (rare in second-degree whiplash).

28.5.7 Imaging

Reduction of cervical lordosis, localized inversion of the curve or rigidity of a few segments is more likely in this case.

28.5.8 Diagnosis

As was described above, between second- and third-degree whiplash, the differences are only clinical: in third degree usually movements are completely blocked due to the pain, which is more intense and irradiated compared to a second-degree lesion. Also sympathetic symptoms are more pronounced.

28.5.9 Treatment

A soft collar with good containment (this means that it allows less movement), or a hard collar must be prescribed for 20 days. It is necessary to pay particular attention to sustaining the cervical spine without distracting/elongating it. It is also very important not to keep the cervical spine in an incorrect position: usually patients with these collars are followed by a technician and not by a physician and this is a mistake. It is important not to hold the patient in protrusion, because this can be exactly the position in which the lesion occurred, but to restrain movements keeping a correct position. If the head is maintained in a protracted position, as long as the patient is sustained he feels well, but when the collar is removed his symptoms return, often worsened exactly by the collar. Rehabilitation must begin after removing the collar. The process must be gradual and determined by the physiotherapist (according to the physician's prescription) on the basis of the gradual training of muscles [14–17].

28.6 Third Degree

28.6.1 Anatomical Pathology

Third-degree whiplash is a serious strain of the ligaments that are partially split. Zygapophyseal joints in this case too do not show dislocations: there is only capsular distraction and sometimes internal derangements can be demonstrated. Disc lesions can reach real herniation. Muscles are overstretched, sometimes without lesions of the body but always of tendons at their insertions. There is an important involvement of sympathetic plexus. The medulla can be stretched, and nerve roots usually are involved too [18].

28.6.2 History

Pain is always irradiated to the head and/or shoulders and many times to the upper extremities due to nerve root lesions. Active movements are impossible and when the patient is asked to move the neck, he only moves his eyes. Vertigo, dizziness, nausea, vomiting, scotomata, photophobia and drop attacks are present in most patients. Sometimes there is tachycardia, pins and needles to both upper and lower extremities (one or both sides), strength or sensory deficits, eye alterations and sweating to one upper extremity, revealing significant lesions to nervous structures.

28.6.3 Clinical Examination

The patient presents in a fixed position that in this case too is normally a clue to the mechanism of the injury.

28.6.4 Range of Movement

The cervical spine is completely blocked. Active and passive movements are impossible in any direction, although sometimes a little bit of motion appears offering a clue as to how the accident happened. It is important to be very cautious when testing RoM in the supine position in these patients.

28.6.5 Palpation

Muscles are painful and very contracted, but palpation at this stage is not very useful, due to the obvious clinical picture [19, 20].

28.6.6 Neurologic Examination

This exam is very important at this stage, and central signs must be very thoroughly examined, because as reported in the literature there may also be encephalic involvements. Nerve root signs are not rare.

28.6.7 Diagnosis

Between third- and fourth-degree whiplash there is a definite boundary: a radiographically evident lesion with sub-dislocation of zygapophyseal joints.

28.6.8 Treatment

A hard collar must be prescribed for 25–30 days. In these cases it is important to offer a support to both chin and occiput. Many times it is also necessary to extend anteriorly to the sternum, blocking in this way the possibility of moving the head anteriorly or maintaining an incorrect position. Obviously not distracting/elongating the cervical spine nor keeping an incorrect position is crucial here. Rehabilitation must begin after removing the collar and must be very gradual. The collar must be removed gradually over 15–30 days, always determined by the physiotherapist according to the physician's prescription and closely monitoring training of the muscles [21–24].

28.7 Fourth Degree

28.7.1 Anatomical Pathology

Fourth-degree whiplash is a condition in which the mechanical stability of the cervical spine has been compromised. There is a capsular disruption of zygapophyseal joints combined with a ligamentous strain that allows pathological movements between vertebral bodies. In this case too disc lesions such as definite herniation are common. Neurological lesions can include all of what has been described above together with a possible direct compression of nerve structures. A medullar damage can be suspected, but sometimes it appears only later rather than immediately after the injury occurred.

28.7.2 History

Pain is particularly important and does not respond to treatments. Active movements are impossible. All neurological symptoms mentioned above can be presented by the patient.

28.7.3 Clinical Examination

There are not important differences from what has been mentioned regarding third-degree whiplash.

28.7.4 Diagnosis

Between fourth- and fifth-degree whiplash, there is another definite boundary: a complete articular dislocation [25–27].

28.7.5 Treatment

A Minerva collar in Articast (less heavy than one in simple cast) has to be prescribed for as long as 30–40 days, assuring in this way a complete blockage for a period long enough to permit stabilization. If this does not occur, it is necessary to stabilize the cervical spine surgically. The rehabilitation process must be as presented above [28–31].

28.8 Fifth Degree

This lesion is not completely pertinent to our work. It is very rare, it has a dramatic clinical picture and it is characterized by dislocation of one or more articular processes or by bony fractures.

The risks are very high and it is necessary to act surgically to reduce the lesion with an anterior or posterior fusion.

28.9 To Immobilize or Not to Immobilize: That Is the Question

We discuss this issue because our proposal is somewhat different from what can be found in the recent literature. One of the biggest problems that we have to face nowadays regarding harmless spinal pathologies is if rest or early mobilization is the best treatment. In some ways, low back pain and whiplash injury are similar because the general consensus of treatment by rest (should it be bed rest or collars) has shifted to a less general, but still common, consensus in promoting mobility as early as possible.

The Quebec Task Force on Whiplash-Associated Disorders stated: "Based on limited evidence and reasoning by analogy, it is the Task Force consensus that the use of non steroid anti-inflammatory and analgesics, short-term manipulation and mobilization by trained persons, and active exercises are useful in Grade II and III WAD, but prolonged use of soft collars, rest or inactivity probably prolongs disability in WAD".

In any case, this consensus does not mean that it is proven that mobilizing is the correct answer to the problem, particularly in the case of a whiplash-injured patient.

We have to remember that:

- All the studies addressing the problem have evaluated short-term disability, but we know that long-term results should be the most important for this type of patients.
- Soft collars do not immobilize the neck, but only restrict wide-range movements.
- Mobilization must be in any case a step in the treatment that we proposed, but this does not mean that must it be the first one.
- Many times the inadequate results of patients that have used a collar are due to the lack of a good rehabilitative process after removing the collar.
- Doctors must not abdicate their role of making the diagnosis and choosing treatments according to the level of pathology: research results say only what is better for most (statistical significance), not for all.

Bearing in mind these points, we think that it is not sound to propose, as many do, that mobilization should be prescribed until it has been shown that immobilization is superior to mobilizing interventions.

Whiplash is presumably a form of distortion of the cervical spine. This pathogenic mechanism acts on a composed structure made up of many articulations, a large quantity of muscles with a very fine regulation and large bands with a stabilizing, not a blocking, function.

A general rule is that ligamentous or capsular stretchings require immobilization as a means of repair. This must be prolonged to at least 18 days to be effective. Immobilization can be partial or total according to the severity of pathology; it is also possible to prolong the immobilization time according to necessity.

The real goal of treatment is to avoid over time pain and development of a possible instability at a distance. Our experience over the years has taught us that a cervical, whiplash-injured spine that did not remain immobilized sufficiently can more frequently cause problems and that these problems last for a longer time.

Therefore, mobilization is possible only if the trauma is so minor that there has not been a real lesion of ligamentous structures, but only a lengthening. If there is an involvement of capsules, ligaments or tendons, it will be necessary to immobilize [32–36].

We think that only when mobilization proves more effective than immobilization will it be possible not to observe these cautious rules.

References

1. The Bone and Joint Decade 2000–2010 Task Force on Neck Pain and Its Associated Disorders, Nordin M, Carragee EJ, Hogg-Johnson S, Weiner SS, Hurwitz EL, Peloso PM, Guzman J, van der Velde G, Carroll LJ, Holm LW, Côté P, Cassidy JD, Haldeman S (2009) Assessment of neck pain and its associated disorders: results of the bone and joint decade 2000–2010 task force on neck pain and its associated disorders. J Manipulative Physiol Ther 32(Suppl 2):S117–S140
2. Spitzer WO, Skovron ML, Salmi LR, Cassidy ID, Duranceau J, Suissa S, Zeiss E (1995) Scientific monograph of the Quebec task force on whiplash-associated disorders. Redefining "whiplash" and its management. Spine 20(8):1S–73S2
3. Verhagen AP, Scholten-Peeters GG, de Bie RA, Bierma-Zeinstra SM (2007) Conservative treatments for whiplash. Cochrane Database Syst Rev 2007(2):CD003338
4. Allen ME, Weir Jones I, Motiuk DR, Flewin KR, Goring RD, Kobetitch R, Broadhurst A (1994) Acceleration perturbations of daily living. A comparison to "whiplash". Spine 19(11):1285–1290
5. Barnsley L, Lord S, Bogduk N (1993) Comparative local anaesthetic blocks in the diagnosis of cervical zygapophysial joint pain. Pain 55(1):99–106
6. Carette S (1994) Whiplash injury and chronic neck pain. N Engl J Med 330(15):1083–1084
7. Maimaris C (1989) Neck sprains after car accidents. BMJ 299(6691):123–131
8. Simons DG (1989) Myofascial trigger points and the whiplash syndrome. Clin J Pain 5(3):279–282
9. Dehner C, Kraus M, Schöll H, Schneider F, Richter P, Kramer M (2012) Therapy recommendation "act as usual" in patients with whiplash injuries QTF I°. Glob J Health Sci 4(6):36–42
10. Fisher SV, Bowar JF, Awad EA, Gullikson G (1977) Cervical orthoses effect on cervical spine motion: roentgenographic and goniometric method of study. Arch Phys Med Rehabil 58:109–115
11. Johnson RM, Hart DL, Simmons EF, Ramsby GR, Southwick WO (1977) Cervical orthoses. A study comparing their effectiveness in restricting cervical motion in normal subjects. J Bone Joint Surg Am 59:332–339
12. Foley Nolan D, Barry C, Coughlan R, O'Comnor P (1990) Pulsed high frequency (27 Mhz) electromagnetic therapy for persistent neck pain. A double blind placebo controlled study of 20 patients. Orthopedics 13:445–451
13. McKinney LA (1989) Early mobilisation and outcome in acute sprains of the neck. BMJ 299:1006–1008
14. Foley Nolan D, Moore K, Codd M, Barry C, O'Connor P, Coughlan RJ (1992) Low energy high frequency pulsed electromagnetic therapy for acute whiplash injuries. A double blind randomized controlled study. Scand J Rehabil Med 24(1):51–59
15. McKinney LA, Doman JO, Ryan M (1989) The role of physiotherapy in the management of acute neck sprains following road traffic accidents. Arch Emerg Med 6(1):27–33
16. Mealy K, Brennan H, Fenelon GC (1986) Early mobilisation of acute whiplash injuries. BMJ 292:656–657
17. Dehner C, Elbel M, Strobel P, Scheich M, Schneider F, Krischak G, Kramer M (2009) Grade II whiplash injuries to the neck: what is the benefit for patients treated by different physical therapy modalities? Patient Saf Surg 3:2
18. Pato U, Di Stefano G, Fravi N, Arnold M, Curatolo M, Radanov BP, Ballinari P, Sturzenegger M (2010) Comparison of randomized treatments for late whiplash. Neurology 74(15):1223–1230
19. Cecchi F, Negrini S, Pasquini G, Paperini A, Conti AA, Chiti M, Zaina F, Macchi C, Molino-Lova R (2012) Predictors of functional outcome in patients with chronic low back pain undergoing back school, individual physiotherapy or spinal manipulation. Eur J Phys Rehabil Med 48(3):371–378

20. Vismara L, Cimolin V, Menegoni F, Zaina F, Galli M, Negrini S, Villa V, Capodaglio P (2012) Osteopathic manipulative treatment in obese patients with chronic low back pain: a pilot study. Man Ther 17(5):451–455
21. Casale R, Negrini S, Franceschini M, Michail X (2012) Chronic disabling pain: a scotoma in the eye of both pain medicine and rehabilitation in Europe. Am J Phys Med Rehabil 91(12):1097–1100
22. Negrini S, Zaina F (2013) The chimera of low back pain etiology: a clinical rehabilitation perspective. Am J Phys Med Rehabil 92(1):93–97
23. Negrini S (2006) Usefulness of disability to sub-classify chronic low back pain and the crucial role of rehabilitation. Eura Medicophys 42(3):173–175
24. Negrini S (2007) The neck is not the back: obvious, but the research gap should be reduced. Eura Medicophys 43(1):75–77
25. Newman PK (1990) Whiplash injury. BMJ 301(6749):395–396
26. Pearce JM (1989) Whiplash injury: a reappraisal. J Neurol Neurosurg Psychiatry 52(12): 1329–1331
27. Pearce JM (1990) Whiplash injury. BMJ 301(6752):610
28. Pearce JM (1993) Subtle cerebral lesions in "chronic whiplash syndrome"? J Neurol Neurosurg Psychiatry 56(12):1328–1329
29. Pearce JM (1993) Polemics of chronic whiplash injury. Neurology 44(11):1993–1997
30. Pennie B, Agambar L (1991) Patterns of injury and recovery in whiplash. Injury 22(1):57–59
31. Pennie BH, Agambar LJ (1990) Whiplash injuries. A trial of early management. J Bone Joint Surg Br 72(2):277–279
32. Radanov BP, Sturzenegger M, De Stefano G, Schnidrig A (1994) Relationship between early somatic, radiological. Cognitive and psychosocial findings and outcome during a one year follow up in 117 patients suffering from common whiplash. Br J Rheumatol 33(5): 442–448
33. Redmond AD (1992) Prognostic factors in soft tissue injuries of the cervical spine. Injury 23(4):285
34. Gebhard JS, Donaldson DH, Brown CW (1994). Soft-tissue injuries of the cervical spine. Orthop Rev Suppl:9-17. Review. PubMed PMID: 8090555
35. Luo ZP, Goldsmith W (1991) Reaction of a human head/neck/torso system to shock. J Biomech 24(7):499–510
36. Radanov BP, Schnidrig A, Di Stefano G, Sturzenegger M (1992) Illness behaviour after common whiplash. Lancet 339(8795):749–750

Whiplash-Associated Equilibrium Disturbances (WAED) Rehabilitation: Vestibular Re-education and Vestibular Rehabilitation

29

D.C. Alpini, A. Cesarani, and F. Di Berardino

29.1 Introduction

The human equilibrium system derives much of its strength and plasticity from the fact that the specific neuronal and growing software is moulded in childhood during the maturation phase, under the influence of permanent information from the world we live in. The software overlying the structural, sensorial and central nervous hardware creates the so-called space concept within the brain. Post-whiplash failures of the sensory inputs as well as of the central equilibrium regulation may lead to vertigo, blurred vision, static and/or dynamic head and body instability. The system has many inborn possibilities for internal stabilization and compensation; in fact after injuries there are different neurophysiological phenomena involved in the restoration of the equilibrium function [1, 2].

Rehabilitation specifically acts activating one or more of these phenomena [3]. They are:

Restitution can be defined as a complete reparation after a temporarily limited lesion.

Adaptation means that the human equilibrium system can adapt itself to physiologically, as well as to pathologically, altered conditions. The central regulatory system can reweigh sensitivity of the vestibular, retinal and other receptors used to

D.C. Alpini (✉)
ENT-Otoneurology Service, IRCCS "Don Carlo C. Gnocchi" Foundation, Milan, Italy
e-mail: dalpini@dongnocchi.it

A. Cesarani • F. Di Berardino
Department of Clinical Sciences and Community Health, University of Milan, Milan, Italy

Audiology Unit, IRCCS "Ca' Granda" Ospedale Maggiore Policlinico, Milan, Italy
e-mail: antonio.cesarani@unimi.it; federica.diberardino@unimi.it

D.C. Alpini et al. (eds.), *Whiplash Injuries*,
DOI 10.1007/978-88-470-5486-8_29, © Springer-Verlag Italia 2014

regulate equilibrium. It comprises all phenomena which ensure that a patient with a persisting peripheral dysfunctional state reattains a normal – or near normal – behaviour in relation to his space orientation and balance in rest as well as when executing movements. He again maintains his erect standing position and has no more "odd" feeling categorized as vertigo or dizziness. The messages sent by the sense organs into the brainstem are more and more suppressed and prevented from reaching the higher centres the longer the steady state in the surrounding world persists. The subject has adapted itself to conditions imposed by the outer world. Yet the slightest change in stimulatory conditions not pertaining to the steady state will alarm.

Habituation is defined by the reduction of the intensity and duration of the subjective vestibular reactions, for example, vertigo and nausea in the case of seasickness. Habituation is a term used in the sense that repeated exposure to a "mismatched" sensory situation (e.g. during caloric testing, postural vertigo, motion sickness conditions) induces such changes in the central processing as to annihilate the undesirable effects and to do so with a prolonged effect. It has been based upon the development of conditioned compensatory reactions to oppose inappropriate responses associated with visuo-vestibular conflicts and exposure to unusual motion environments.

Compensation describes another type of central nervous counter-regulation as a result of functional deterioration due to a vestibular or other equilibrium lesion. It utilizes supplementary functions which are added so that an overlay of additionally activated functions covers the underlying equilibrium lesions by mean of its neuronal plasticity. However, primary lesion continues to exist and can, in the case of a special conflict, manifest itself in the clinical phenomenology. It is a goal-directed process induced by some recognized "error" in the system and directed to its elimination. Thus compensation may be defined as an error-controlled goal-directed learning process.

These phenomena lead to different levels of recovery. Recovery is essentially due to the integration of different level of substitution:

Sensorial substitution, in which the movement of the subject is identical to the one before the lesion but the subject uses different set of sensory receptors for triggering and control

Functional substitution, in which the neuronal mechanisms subtending the movement have been changed but still belong to the subsystems normally used by the subject

Behavioural substitution, by which the nervous system calls for new motor behaviours not belonging to its normal repertoire

Under another point of view, the evolution of a lesion can be interpreted into three stages of damage:

- The primary damage: the lesion that induces the onset of symptomatology
- The secondary damage: the pathological modification of the compensatory systems
- The tertiary damage: chronicization of pathological adaptive phenomena

Treatment had to be pointed to limit primary damage (usually by means of pharmacotherapy), to reduce secondary damage and to avoid tertiary damage.

29.2 Vertigo

Benign paroxysmal positional vertigo (BPPV) is due to displacement of otoconia as a consequence of the head concussion during whiplash, and BBPV is the most common cause of vertigo caused by vestibular pathology; it is very frequent after head trauma but this is not the case after whiplash. Anyway, it has to be taken into account also in whiplash-associated equilibrium disturbances (WAED) patients: whiplash-associated BBPV (WA-BPPV).

The characteristic presentation of this disorder involves repeated episodes of the transient illusion of spinning, triggered by head motion in the plane of the involved semicircular canal (SCC). Cupulolithiasis and canalolithiasis [4] have both been proposed as pathophysiologic mechanisms underlying BPPV. Canalolithiasis, involving free-floating otolithic particles moving within the affected SCC, is responsible for the majority of WA-BPPV cases. Of the three SCCs, the posterior SCC is most commonly affected because of its anatomical location inferior to the utricle.

Most cases of WA-BPPV can be treated using physical therapy, with the Epley's [5] canalith-repositioning procedure (CRP) in the case of canalolithiasis and Semont's [6] liberatory manoeuvre in the case of cupulolithiasis, both acting through *restitution* phenomenon. In this sense these kinds of procedures have to be considered in vestibular re-education.

Although both manoeuvres have been shown to have therapeutic benefits, they require sequential procedures involving moving the patient's head and body into unnatural positions, making them sometime unsuitable for WAED patients with cervical or back disorders, especially for older patients.

In WAED patients, it is thus better to use more conservative procedures like the supine to prolonged lateral position (SPLP) [7] or the rolling-over manoeuvre (ROM) [8].

SPLP contained two steps. First, the patient was instructed to start in an upright sitting position and then lie down supinely on the bed and maintain this position for 3 min. During this step, it was proposed that the trapped otolithic particles would move away from the ampulla (ampullofugal), drift towards the common crus by crossing the horizontal SCC plane and stay in the superior arm of the posterior SCC. In the second step, the patient was asked to sleep on their healthy side by turning their head and body from the previous supine position towards the healthy side laterally. This process allowed the particles to slip through the common crus into the utricle. To facilitate their movement back into the utricle and to prevent any floating particles in the utricle from being trapped in the posterior SCC again, a prolonged side lateral position (minimum duration 30 min) was suggested at bedtime, with or without a pillow support.

ROM involves moving the patient from supine to nose-up position to a right ear-down position and maintaining this position for 10 s, before subsequently returning the head to a nose-up position, which is maintained for further 10 s. The patient is then moved to the left ear-down head position which is maintained for 10 s. Patient repeats these manoeuvres 10 times in a set and two sets in day, before getting up in the morning and before sleeping in the night.

ROM can be performed either by neck rotation or by whole-body movements without any cervical torsion. This is very suitable for whiplash patients, especially in the early phases of trauma.

29.3 Dizziness and Disequilibrium

Dizziness and disequilibrium following whiplash may be recovered by means of *vestibular rehabilitation*, which is a special rehabilitation of motion intolerance and imbalance problems. Although it has only recently gained wide attention, the concept of head, body and coordinated eye exercises as a treatment for vestibular disorders is actually over 50 years. As far back as the mid-1940s, an English otolaryngologist Sir Cawthorne [9] observed that some patients who experienced dizziness did better or recovered sooner when performing rapid head movements. In cooperation with a physiotherapist, Cooksey, he developed a regimen of exercises which, with some modifications, are frequently still used today. Cawthorne-Cooksey [10] protocol is based on the concepts of habituation and sensory substitution (Table 29.1).

Vertigo and dizziness are conscious symptoms and the disturbances are not disequilibrium or nystagmus but the *consciousness* of disequilibrium and nystagmus. Thus physical rehabilitation must not only be pointed to resolution of objective disorder but it must be aimed to resolution of subjective consciousness of the disorder itself. Such a particular kind of treatment needs a particular theoretical basis. This is the reason why we structured our method of rehabilitation on a particular model of the vestibular system: the *MCS* method [11–13]. *MCS* is the acronym of mechanic, cybernetics and synergetics [14].

Table 29.1 Cawthorne-Cooksey Protocol

Exercises
In Bed 1. Eye movements, at first slow, then more quickly: (a) Up and down. (b) From side to side. (c) Focusing on fingers moving from 3 feet to 1 foot away from head. 2. Head movements, at first slow, then quick. Later with eyes closed. (a) Bending forwards and backwards. (b) Turning from side to side.
Sitting 1. Eye movements as above. 2. Head movements as above. 3. Shoulder shrugging and circling. 4. Bending forwards and picking up objects from the floor.
Standing 1. A-1 & A-2 & B-3 as above. 2. Changing from sitting to standing position with eyes open and with eyes shut.

3. Throwing a small ball from hand to hand, above eye level.
4. Throwing ball from hand to hand, under knee.
5. Change from sitting to standing and turning around in between.

Dynamic
1. Circle around the centre person who will throw a large ball and to whom it will be returned.
2. Walk across room with eyes open and then eyes closed.
3. Walk up and down slope with eyes open and then closed.
4. Walk up and down steps with eyes open and then closed.
5. Any games involving stooping and stretching such as frisbee, catch or basketball.

Under a *mechanic* point of view, we can consider the equilibrium function as the result of the *sum* of vestibular reflexes, the contemporary but distinct activation of some or all of these reflexes, according to the need: gaze, standing and walking.

Under a *cybernetics* [15] point view, all the structures, peripheral and central, that contribute to the balance ocular reflexes (BOR) and balance spinal reflexes (BSR) [16] constitute a system, that to say, a network of different structures *interconnected* and *interacting* to reach a common goal. In this case the goal is human balance.

Under a *synergetic* point of view, equilibrium *is* the result of integration different functional levels, orientation and coordination [17].

On the basis of *MCS* model of equilibrium system, different protocols for the different vestibular impairments have been prepared, including WAED patients. Protocols combine physical and instrumental exercises and they are subdivided into a part to be executed with the physiotherapist in the gymnasium and in self-administrated exercise, at home.

From an MCS point of view, WAEDs are caused by distortion and desynchronization of the proprioceptive chain:

- Modification of the proprioceptive cervical inputs to the vestibular nuclei and reticular formation
- Desynchronization between vestibular cues and general cervical inputs regarding head position and movement
- Modification of the cervico-spinal reflexes
- Head-to-trunk dynamic stabilization

Treatment is pointed to:

1. Restore cervico-dorsal mobility
2. Restore dorsolumbar mobility
3. Reorganize proprioceptive informations from the neck and the pelvis
4. Avoid secondary damage characterized by reduction of the movement of the body along the neck with involvement of the thoracolumbar segment and the pelvis
5. Restore head-neck coordination
6. Restore the control of head stabilization during gait
7. Reorganize self-perception of posture

Because whiplash injuries cause different and variable damage and symptoms, the following protocol is only a general guide about what action we think is useful in patients after such a trauma. In every patient suffering vertigo and balance disorders, but especially in WAED cases, treatment closely tailored to the patient is necessary.

Rehabilitation may be combined also with pharmacotherapy (see Chap. 19) like decontracturings or myorelaxants (*Diazepam*) or *L-sulpiride* (at low doses). If cognitive functions are compromised, *nicergoline or citicoline* may be useful. If cervical proprioceptors are hyperactive, *cinnarizine* or *flunarizine* may be used at low doses for a short period.

Physical exercises are reported in Tables 29.2 and 29.3, while instrument-assisted treatment is described in the specific following chapters.

Table 29.2 MCS Physical Exercises

I Week: Mechanics Phase

Goals:

- Enforcement of extensor antigravity muscles
- Mobilization of ankle and pelvis joints

Exercises:

The patient takes his two knees to the chest, contemporary, helping and softly, with the hands

With the flexed legs and the feet on the bed, the patient rotates his pelvis rightwards and leftwards keeping his knees flexed and your legs united

The patient lifts his pelvis taking contemporary his arms extended over his head. Then he retakes his arms along the body lowering his pelvis

In quadrupedal position the patient extends contemporary the right arm and the left leg. Then he repeats with the left arm and the right leg

In prone position the patient lifts his left arm and the right leg maintaining his forehead over the bed. Then he repeats with the right arm and the left leg

The patient repeats as above but lifting contemporary also the head

The patient inhales. Exhaling, he bends forwards taking his head on the right knee. He waits 10 s. Inhaling he returns in sitting position. Exhaling, he bends forwards taking his head on the left knee. He waits 10 s and then inhaling he returns seated

II Week: Cybernetics Phase

Goals:

- To improve interaction between ocular and spinal performances

Exercies:

The patient fixates a target on the ceiling and slowly moves his head rightwards and leftwards

The patient looks for two equidistant targets on the ceiling, and then he fixates them alternatively first moving only the eyes and then moving only the head

The patient from supine position passes to the sitting position fixating a point straight in front of him

From the supine position, the patient passes to the sitting position fixating a point sited on his right

From the supine position, the patient passes to the sitting position fixating a point sited on his left

The patient goes up and down a step, fixating a target according the following sequence:

Right foot up	Left foot up	Right foot down
Left foot down	Left foot up	Right foot up
Left foot down	Right foot down	

Then he repeats with eyes closed

III Week: Synergetics Phase

Goals:

- Integration of cognitive and motor performances

Exercises:

The patient extends his right arm and lifts his thumb. Then he moves slowly his arm to and fro before along a horizontal direction and then along a vertical direction. The patients is instructed to pursue his thumb with eyes only, first slowly and then increasing progressively the velocity of thumb displacement.

After that, he has to perform the exercise as above but moving contemporary also the head trying to maintain the eyes still.

The patient opens a book in front of him. Then he sends it away from him extending his arms reading it. Then he brings it near to him slowly, trying to read it. Then he sends it away again and he repeats some times to and fro.

Table 29.3 Home Protocol

Exercises have been subdivided according to different phases of equilibrium, from supine to standing to moving. In each phase, there is a progression from mechanic to synergetics exercises

Home exercises cannot ever substitute the therapeutic programmes showed in the previous chapter performed with the therapist. Home exercises complete the therapeutic period and maintain the obtained results.

Supine

1. Take your two knees to the chest, contemporary, helping and softly, with the hands
2. Put a pill under your leg. Bound a 2 kg weight on your ankle with the flexed knee; then extend it alternating the right and left legs
3. With the flexed legs and the feet on the bed, rotate your pelvis rightwards and leftwards keeping your knees flexed and your legs united
4. Lift your pelvis taking contemporary your arms extended over your head. Then retake your arms along the body lowering your pelvis
5. Fixate a target on the ceiling and slowly move your head rightwards and leftwards
6. Look for two equidistant targets on the ceiling and then fixate them alternatively, first moving only the eyes and then moving only the head

(continued)

7. In the quadrupedal position, inhale and arch your back (hyperkyphosis) taking your head between your arms. Then exhale bending your head and rotating the pelvis in hyperlordosis
8. From supine position pass to the sitting position fixating a target straight in front of you
9. In quadrupedal position extend contemporary the right arm and the left leg. Then repeat with the left arm and the right leg
10. In prone position lift your left arm and the right leg lifting contemporary also the head. Then repeat with the right arm and the left leg

Sitting

11. Extend your right arm and lift your thumb. Move slowly your arm to and fro before along a horizontal direction and then along a vertical direction. Pursue your thumb with eyes only, first slowly and then increasing progressively the velocity of thumb displacement
12. As in the previous exercise but moving contemporary also the head trying to maintain the eyes still
13. Move your head first slowly and then faster in all directions fixating a target straight in front of you
14. Inhale. Exhaling, bend forwards taking your head on the right knee. Wait 10 s. Inhaling return in sitting position. Exhaling, bend forwards taking your head on the left knee. Wait 10 s and then inhale and return seated
15. Inhale. Exhaling bend forwards to keep an object on the floor. Inhale and take it up over your head and then fixate it for 10 s. Inhale. Exhaling bend forwards and take the object on the floor
16. Open a book in front of you. Read it moving, contemporary, the book right and left and then to and fro

Standing

17. Fixate yourself in a mirror. Align correctly your position. Maintain equilibrium for 1 min and then close your eyes looking your correct position in your mind and remain in this position for at least 1 min
18. Repeat the same, standing on a soft mattress
19. Fixate yourself in a mirror; then, keeping your feet still, bend your trunk to and fro and right and left with eyes closed standing on a soft mattress
20. Keep a little object and lift it over your head. Fixate it. Inhale. Then exhale and bend yourself forwards taking the object on the floor. Wait 10 s and then inhaling lift again the object over your head
21. Standing on soft mattress, keep a little object and lift it over your head. Fixate it. Lift it over your head and then, with your straight arms, move the object drawing circles and, bending contemporary your trunk and your knees, after that take it on the floor

Moving

22. Stepping with eyes closed, moving the head to and fro
23. Stepping, reading a book
24. Stepping on a soft mattress, reading a book
25. Go up and down a step, moving to and fro your head, according the following sequence:

Right foot up	Left foot up	Right foot down
Left foot down	Left foot up	Right foot up
Left foot down	Right foot down	

References

1. Bronstein AM, Brandt T, Woollacott MH (eds) (1996) Clinical disorders of balance, posture and gait. Arnold, London
2. George FH (1962) The brain as a computer. Pergamon Press, Oxford
3. Claussen CF (1994) Vestibular compensation. Acta Otolaryngol (Stockh) 513(Suppl):33–36
4. Rajguru SM, Ifediba MA, Rabbitt RD (2005) Biomechanics of horizontal canal benign paroxysmal positional vertigo. J Vestib Res 15(4):203–214
5. Epley J (1992) The canalith reposition procedure: for the treatment of benign paroxysmal vertigo. Otolaryngol Head Neck Surg 107:399–404
6. Semont A, Sterkers JM (1980) Reeducation vestibulaires. Les Cahiers D'Orl 15:305
7. Shih CP, Wang CH (2013) Supine to prolonged lateral position: a novel therapeutic maneuver for posterior canal benign paroxysmal positional vertigo. J Neurol 260(5):1375–1381. doi:10.1007/s00415-012-6807-9
8. Sugita-Kitajima A, Sato S, Mikami K, Mukaide M, Koizuka I (2010) Does vertigo disappear only by rolling over? Rehabilitation for benign paroxysmal positional vertigo. Acta Otolaryngol 130(1):84–88
9. Cawthorne T (1944) The physiological basis of head exercises. J Chart Soc Physiother 30:106
10. Dix DR (1974) Treatment of vertigo. Physiotherapy 60:380
11. Cesarani A, Alpini D (1991) New trends in rehabilitation treatment of vertigo and dizziness. In: Akyildiz N, Portmann M (eds) Vertigo and its treatment. Proceedings of international symposium for Prof. G. Portmann's Centenary, Ankara, 16–18 May 1990, Ankara, pp 90–104
12. Cesarani A, Alpini D (eds) (1994) Equilibrium disorders. Brainstem and cerebellar pathology. Springer, Milano
13. Cesarani A, Alpini D (1999) Vertigo and dizziness rehabilitation. Springer, Milan
14. Gluck MA, Rumelhart DE (eds) (1990) Neuroscience and connectionist theory. Lawrence Erlbaum Associates Publishers, Hillsdale
15. Ashby WR (1956) An introduction to cybernetics. Chapman & Hall, London
16. Norrè ME (1990) Posture in otoneurolog. Acta Otorhinolaryngol Belg 44(2–3):55–364
17. Haken H (2006) Synergetics of brain function. Int J Psychophysiol 60(2):110–124

Vestibular Electrical Stimulation 30

A. Cesarani, D.C. Alpini, and E. Filipponi

30.1 Introduction

Peripheral proprioceptors of the muscles and the joints have a feedback control on the vestibular nuclei through the spino-vestibular pathways. Neuromuscular spindles and Golgi receptors are dynamometers and they are particularly sensitive to variations in muscle length and tension. Joint receptors, Ruffini and Golgi bodies, give information regarding the position of a joint and its movement. The portion of the neck including the first three vertebrae is particularly involved during the major part of everyday head movements [1, 2].

The paravertebral muscles of this region are very rich in proprioceptors. They are especially concentrated in the splenius capitis, the rectus capitis major, the longissimus capitis, and the semispinalis capitis. These muscles comprise the deep plane of the nuchal muscles. The splenius is more superficial. The muscles act in the extension of homolateral bending and rotation of the head. During head movements they discharge to the vestibular nuclei [3, 4].

A. Cesarani
Department of Clinical Sciences and Community Health,
University of Milan, Milan, Italy

Audiology Unit, IRCCS "Ca' Granda" Ospedale Maggiore Policlinico, Milan, Italy
e-mail: antonio.cesarani@unimi.it

D.C. Alpini (✉)
ENT-Otoneurology Service, IRCCS "Don Carlo C. Gnocchi" Foundation, Milan, Italy
e-mail: dalpini@dongnocchi.it

E. Filipponi
S.I.T.R.A. (Rehabilitation) - Audiology Unit,
IRCCS "Ca' Granda" Ospedale Maggiore Policlinico, Milan, Italy

D.C. Alpini et al. (eds.), *Whiplash Injuries*,
DOI 10.1007/978-88-470-5486-8_30, © Springer-Verlag Italia 2014

It is known that vibration of muscles or muscle tendons alters proprioceptive input and produces kinesthetic illusions in human subjects. A lot of clinical and experimental evidence exist regarding the effects of vibration of the paravertebral muscles on posture control and head-trunk coordination. Generally the effects are based on the activation of the cervico-spinal reflexes (CSRs): bending the neck and turning the head relative to the body evokes reflexes in the limb muscles either in decerebrate cats [4] or in human beings [5].

It is possible [6–8], in the absence of any actual movement, to induce kinesthetic illusions and associated motor responses in humans when mechanical vibrations are applied either to the distal tendon of a limb muscle or to the neck. Illusory movements and/or motor responses can be extended to the whole body when vibrations are applied to muscles involved in postural stance, such as neck muscles.

Vibration therefore constitutes an efficient means of obtaining true copies of actual sensory messages and thus eliciting "at will" illusory movements, the direction, speed, and duration of which can be preselected.

Vibration of the posterior muscles of the neck has been shown to induce illusions of changed position and of motion of a visual target when the target is presented with no visual background [9].

Cervical muscle proprioceptors are sensible to superficial electrical stimulation (SES), too. SES is a noninvasive technique that provides nerve and/or muscle stimulation by means of surface electrodes. The characteristics, the size, and the site of application of the electrodes and the characteristics of the electrical waves play a fundamental role in the neurophysiological effects of the SES. Our previous experimental experiences [10–16] showed that vibration of the paravertebral muscles can be substituted by SES. Usually, handheld antalgic electrostimulators are called TENS stimulators, which means transcutaneous electrical nerve stimulations [17]. The excitation of the peripheral motor nerves and the associated muscle activation is caused by the application of an electric current to the skin, which usually corresponds to the motor points. This kind of stimulation induces depolarization of the motor nerves either in the centrifugal or in the centripetal sense. Furthermore this kind of stimulation induces an activation of the sensitive nerves of the skin. Thus it is difficult to divide the motor and the sensitive effects of the SES.

Lackner [7] remarked that the vestibular nuclei are really polysensorial relays and that they are not only labyrinth correlated. The author underlined that it is not possible under natural circumstances to activate the vestibular receptors without implicating other force-sensitive receptor systems that convey information relevant to spatial orientation.

On the basis of this extensive, but physiologically justified, point of view of the vestibular system, we refer to superficial paravertebral electrical stimulation as vestibular electrostimulation (VES).

It was shown that neurophysiological effects of VES are strictly dependent on the characteristics of the electrical wave. Thus the definition of VES pertains only to those waves able to induce measurable neurophysiological cervico-spinal effects.

Fig. 30.1 The device

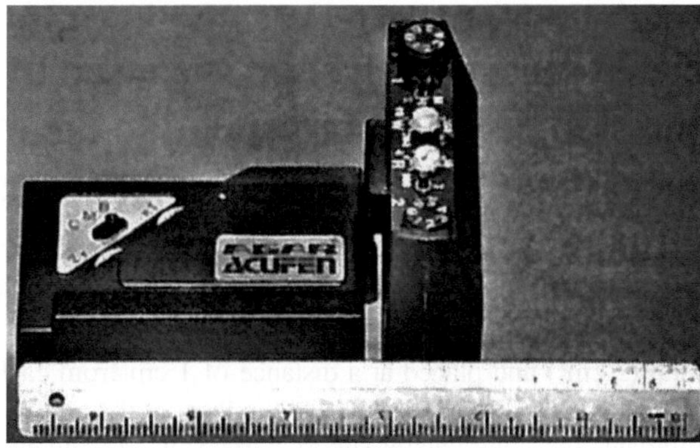

30.2 The Device

Either for experimentations or for clinical application, we used an electrostimulator, agar. It is a small (25×36×91 mm) and light (88 g) portable device prepared at Hadassah University Hospital of Jerusalem (Israel) and approved by the US Food and Drug Administration.

The mean currency intensity is 0.9 pAlmm^2 and the impulse currency intensity is 30 CLA/rnm^2, the maximum impulse power is 5 W, the maximum impulse charge is 22 p C, and the mean impulse charge is 0.55 C.

The device is able to produce different stimulation modes (Fig. 30.1).

Burst. This consists of short pulse series at a high frequency repeated at slow frequency. This stimulation mode is used for pain relief. The stimulation should be so strong that muscle contractions can be seen. Usually the electrode is placed on a large muscle near the aching spot. Burst is not useful for vestibular stimulation.

30.2.1 TENS

It consists of short electric impulses and is used for pain relief.

The stimulation must never be so strong that muscle contractions are found.

The electrodes are normally placed on nerve paths leading away from the aching spot. Sometimes this wave can be varied as regards both pulse width and stimulation currency. The variations are random but pulse width multiplied by stimulation current is constant (i.t. = constant charge). This stimulation mode prevents tolerance to a set pulse width.

Muscle Stimulation Used for Rehabilitation of Muscles. The stimulation should be so strong that the muscles contract. The stimulation consists of stimulation (on time) with a slow rise (rise time) and a pause (off time). This sequence is repeated and makes the muscle slowly contract and be tight for some time. It is often used on weak muscles (rehabi1itation); the stimulation frequency is kept low (20–30 Hz) to avoid tiring out the muscle. For sports training higher frequencies are used. This wave is not useful for vestibular stimulation.

30.2.2 VES

This is an electric stimulation of cervico-dorsal muscles by using a biphasic asymmetrical modulated square wave. The modulation program randomly modifies the duration of each wave. The mean duration is 100 ps while the frequency is 80 Hz. Electrodes are small (2 cm^2) and placed at a distance of 1 cm from each other. A pair of electrodes stimulates paravertebral muscles at the level of the second cervical vertebra, and a pair stimulates the contralateral superior trapezius. The intensity of VES is never able to induce muscle contractions. The frequency used is in the muscle spindle range of vibratory activation (80 Hz). Thus, it is likely that VES activates the same spinal pathways of the CSRs. VES modulates the lower limbs postural reflexes in the same way.

Vibratory stimulation of muscle in a range between 1 and 100 Hz is able to activate muscle spindles. The vibratory stimulation of the neck muscles produces proprioceptive inputs to the brainstem. These afferent volleys are able to evoke postural reflexes from the muscle of the lower limbs: CSRs. By means of the same mechanism, vibration is also able to evoke alterations of the perceptual representation of the shape and orientation of the whole body and/or body parts.

The experimental results obtained by VES show that this kind of stimulation clearly influences the excitability of the motor neurons of the lower limbs. This influence resembled the action of CSRs on the extensor lower muscles (see Chap. 31 by Osio et al.).

Alteration of proprioceptive input from the neck by VES led to changed perception of head position. The manipulated proprioceptive input is incorporated in the head position signal with any other input contributing to head and body position control [18, 19].

30.3 Indications

After whiplash injuries, two conditions are especially indicated for VES treatment:

1. Paroxysmal positional vertigo
2. Unsteadiness and dizziness with VOR (vestibuloocular reflex) and/or VSR (vestibulospinal reflex) asymmetry

Posttraumatic positional vertigo is, generally, atypical: it is often bilateral, not resolved by Semont maneuver. Nystagmus has no latency or it does not decrease by repeating the movements.

Usually we treat the patient with one or two Semont maneuvers. When they are uneffective we employ VES. The electrodes are placed on the cervical paravertebral muscles ipsilateral to the fast phase of positioning nystagmus (that is usually concording with the vertiginous position) and on the contralateral trapezius. Each stimulation lasts 30 min. During stimulation the patient walks or performs simple and provocative rehabilitative exercises such as Cawthorne-Cooksey protocol. According to intensity of the symptoms, the patient is treated once a day for 5 days a week for 2 weeks or once a day every 2 days for 2 weeks.

When paroxysmal positional vertigo is bilateral, cervical electrodes are placed on the most intense side if there are no important VOR and/or VSR asymmetries.

When unsteadiness is associated with asymmetrical vestibular reflexes, the cervical electrodes are placed on the opposite side of the VOR hyporeflexia and/or Romberg deviation and/or stepping deviation. In some cases VOR hyporeflexia is not accompanied by ipsilateral stepping and/or Romberg deviation. This can be generally due either to the modification of the postural dynamic caused by the trauma or to pre-trauma postural conditions.

In these cases it is sometimes difficult to interpret if VOR prevalence compensates VSR deficit or if postural asymmetries compensate VOR hyporeflexia or if previous musculoskeletal conditions induce unexpected VSRs.

In these cases the sites of stimulation cannot be standardized but have to be chosen on the basis of a complete postural evaluation and a complete neuro-otological examination with special regard to smooth pursuit, optokinetic nystagmus, and VVOR (visuo-vestibuloocular reflex).

The general rule is that cervical electrodes are placed on the prevalent site and the trapezius electrodes are placed on the deficit site.

The treatment protocol lasts 2 weeks (a stimulation once a day) or 3 weeks (a stimulation every 2 days).

VES is frequently used to prepare the patient for rehabilitative treatment when vertigo and dizziness provoked by head/body is intense. There is no contraindication in the combination OWES and some early orthopedic treatment such as the collar. Obviously, in these cases VES is performed without the collar.

VES is particularly indicated starting "equilibrium rehabilitation", in the early phases of the trauma, and to treat also "low compliance" patients.

Some simple tasks during VES improve the effects of the treatment and the best results have been obtained combining VES and some cognitive involved rehabilitation procedures such as center of gravity visual feedback reeducation.

References

1. Berthoz A, Llinas R (1974) Afferent neck projection to the cat cerebellar cortex. Exp Brain Res 20:385–401
2. Boyle R, Pompeiano O (1981) Convergence and interaction of neck and macular vestibular inputs on vestibulospinal neurons. J Neurophysiol 45:852–866; Biguer B, Donaldson IML, Hein A, Jannerod M (1988) Neck muscle vibration modifies the representation of visual motion and direction in man. Brain 11(1):1405–1424
3. Ghez C (1991) Posture. In: Kandel ER, Schwartz JH, Jessel TM (eds) Principles of neural science, 3rd edn. Elsevier, New York, pp 596–607
4. Brink EE, Suzuki I, Timerick SJB, Wilson VJ (1985) Tonic neck reflex of the decerebrate cat: a role for propriospinal neurons. J Neurophysiol 54:978–987

5. Dumas G, Lion A, Gauchard GC, Herpin G, Magnusson M, Perrin PP (2013) Clinical interest of postural and vestibulo-ocular reflex changes induced by cervical muscles and skull vibration in compensated unilateral vestibular lesion patients. J Vestib Res 23(1):41–49
6. Kobayashi Y, Yagi T, Kamio T (1988) The role of cervical inputs in compensation for unilateral labyrinthectomized patients. Adv Otorhinolaryngol 42:185–189
7. Lackner JR (1988) Some proprioceptive influences on the perceptual representation of body shape and orientation. Brain 111:281–297
8. Lackner JR (1992) Multimodal and motor influences on orientation: implications for adapting to weightless and virtual environments. J Vestib Res 2:307–322
9. Wang Y, Rahmatalla S (2013) Human head-neck models in whole-body vibration: effect of posture. J Biomech 46(4):702–710
10. Cesarani A, Alpini D, Barozzi S (1990) Electrical stimulation in the treatment of acute vertigo. In: Sacristan T, Alvarez-Vincent JJ, Bartual J, Antoli-Candela F (eds) Otorhinolaryngology, head & neck surgery. Proceedings of the XIV World Congress of Otorhinolaryngology, Madrid, 1989. Kugler & Ghedini Publ, Amsterdam/Berkeley/Milano
11. Cesarani A, Alpini D, Barozzi S (1990) Neck electrical stimulation in the treatment of labyrinth acute vertigo. Riv Ital EEG Neurof Clin 13(1):55–61
12. Cesarani A, Pertoni T, Alpini D (1988) L'electrostimulation cervicale posteriore dans la rehabilitation des handicaps vestibulaires. XXII Reunion de la Societe d'otoneurologie de Langue Francaise, Toulose, May 1988
13. Cesarani A, Alpini D, Barozzi S (1989) L'electrostimulation electrique dans la reeducation vestibulaire: indications, limites, perspectives. XXIII Reunion de la Societe d'Otoneurologie de Langue Francaise, Modena, June 1989
14. Cesarani A, Alpini D (1991) New trends in rehabilitation treatment of vertigo and dizziness. In: Akyildiz N, Portmann M (eds) Vertigo and its treatment. Proceedings of international symposium for Prof G Portmann's Centenary, Ankara, 16–18 Maggio 1990, pp 90–104
15. Cesarani A, Alpini D, Barozzi S (1992) Superficial paravertebral electrical stimulation. A conservative treatment of vertigo and dizziness. In: Claussen CF, Kirtane MV, Schneider D (eds) Conservative versus surgical treatment of sensorineural hearing loss, tinnitus, vertigo and nausea. Proceedings of the XVIII NES Congress, Dr Werner Rudat & Co, Nach. edi, m + p, Hamburg
16. Cesarani A, Alpini D, Barozzi S, Osio M (1993) Superficial paravertebral electrical stimulation (SPES) in the treatment of vertigo and disequilibrium disturbances. In: Dufour A (ed) Proceedings XXVII symposium Societe d'Oto-Neurologie de Langue Francaise Sanremo, p 47
17. Cesarani A (1994) The cervical electrostimulation. Neurootol Newslett 1(1):67–72
18. Alpini D, Cesarani A, Barozzi S (1992) Non pharmacological treatment of acute vertigo. In: Claussen CF, Kirtane MV, Schneider D (eds) Diagnostic procedures and imaging techniques used in neurotology. Proceedings of the XVI NES Congress, Dr Werner Rudat & Co, Nachf ed, m + p, Hamburg, pp 337–34018
19. Tseng CC, Wang SJ, Young YH (2013) Comparison of head elevation versus rotation methods for eliciting cervical vestibular-evoked myogenic potentials via bone-conducted vibration. Int J Audiol 52(3):200–206

The Neurophysiological Basis of Vestibular Electrical Stimulation

31

M. Osio, L. Brunati, G. Abello, and A. Mangoni

31.1 Introduction

Bending the neck and turning the head respecting to the body cause the stimulation of the cervical proprioceptors. This kind of receptors activates a pathway projecting to the vestibular nuclei.

The impulses are reflected through the nucleo-reticular formation and then to the spinal cord. Such activation allows movements of the neck to influence the postural set and to modify the activation of the antigravity muscles of the lower limbs.

This pattern of muscular activation is hypnotized on the basis of the so-called neck-postural reflexes, or better named cervico-spinal reflex [1]. During the contraction of the paravertebral muscles of the neck, there is a response characterized by inhibition of ipsilateral soleus in respect to the side of neck stimulation and facilitation of the contralateral muscles [2, 3]. During the superficial electrical stimulation (SES), the paraspinal muscles are also activated and there are previous studies that show that SES is able to reduce vertigo and dizziness [4]. This kind of stimulation is also able to evoke changes in activity of the muscles of the legs. We used a neurophysiological test named H-reflex to control this modification. It holds special interest because it can attest the activation of the vestibular-spinal way during the stimulation of the paraspinal muscles through the modification of excitability of the motoneuron. Under appropriate conditions, a single electrical shock to the tibial nerve will evoke two discrete motor action potentials in the calf muscles. The

M. Osio (✉) • A. Mangoni
Department of Neurology, Neurophysiology "Sacco" Hospital,
Via G.B. Grassi, 74, 20157, Milano, Italy
e-mail: osio.maurizio@hsacco.it

L. Brunati
"Pro Juventute" Foundation, IRCCS "Don Carlo Gnocchi" Foundation,
Via Capecelatro 66, 2100, Milan, Italy

G. Abello
Bioengineering Department, Politecnico di Milano, Via C. Golgi, 39, 20133, Milano, Italy

D.C. Alpini et al. (eds.), *Whiplash Injuries*,
DOI 10.1007/978-88-470-5486-8_31, © Springer-Verlag Italia 2014

first potential, the M-wave, results from direct stimulation of motor nerve fibers. The second potential, the H-wave, is the expression of a monosynaptic reflex, which runs in afferent fibers (I1 a) from the neuromuscular spindles and back again through motor afferents. Since no interneurons are involved, the size of the second action potential will provide a measure of motoneuron excitability under a variety of experimental conditions [5, 6].

31.2 Material and Methods

Eight normal subjects (5 females and 3 males), aged between 20 and 33 years old, were admitted to the study. Subject did all sit in a comfortable armchair, with cervical spine at rest position with non-flexion, extension, or lateral bending and head support and not rotated with respect to the trunk.

Legs were at rest and supported, the hips were flexed at 90°, the knees were flexed at 120°, and the ankles were flexed at 90°. Patients were in a quiet room and were awake and relaxed with eyes closed.

Recording of the H-reflex was obtained with pregelled surface electrodes. Active electrode was fixed on the distal on the belly of soleus muscle, while reference electrode was fixed 30 mm below. Stimulation of the tibial nerve was performed with surface electrodes at the popliteal fossa. Interelectrodes distance was 25 mm. Stimulus duration was 1 ms. All this is in accordance with the indication of the literature [5]. Stimulus intensity was between 5 and 21 mA at the intensity needed to evoke the maximum amplitude of the H-reflex (H Max) for each subject.

H Max from soleus muscle right and left legs was recorded every 5 min before, during, and after the stimulation of the muscles. In particular superficial electrical stimulation (SES) of neck paravertebral muscles and contemporary contralateral upper part of the trapezius was applied. SES of the neck muscles was applied with pulse rate of 80 Hz and a pulse width randomly modulated between 100 and 200 ps of duration (so-called vestibular electrical stimulation – VES – see Chap. 30). First VES application was performed for 15 min contemporaneously on the right paravertebral muscles of the neck and on the left upper part of trapezius muscle. After 30 min VES was applied to the contralateral paravertebral of the neck and trapezius muscle for a duration of 15 min. The recordings of the H Max were obtained by left and right leg. We calculated mean (M) and standard deviation (SD) of the five consecutive H Max responses, and obtained values were tabulated. Measures of H Max value were done every 5 min. For each subject were recorded one H Max basal value before application VES, 3 H Max were obtained every 5 min during VES applied to the right paravertebral and left trapezius muscle; 3–6 H Max during to recovery phase, 1 H Max basal, 3 H Max values during VES applied to the left paravertebral muscle and right trapezius muscle, and 3–6 H Max values obtained during a second recovery phase. Statistical analysis was performed with the Student's *t*-test comparing H Max recorded before, during, and after each VES application.

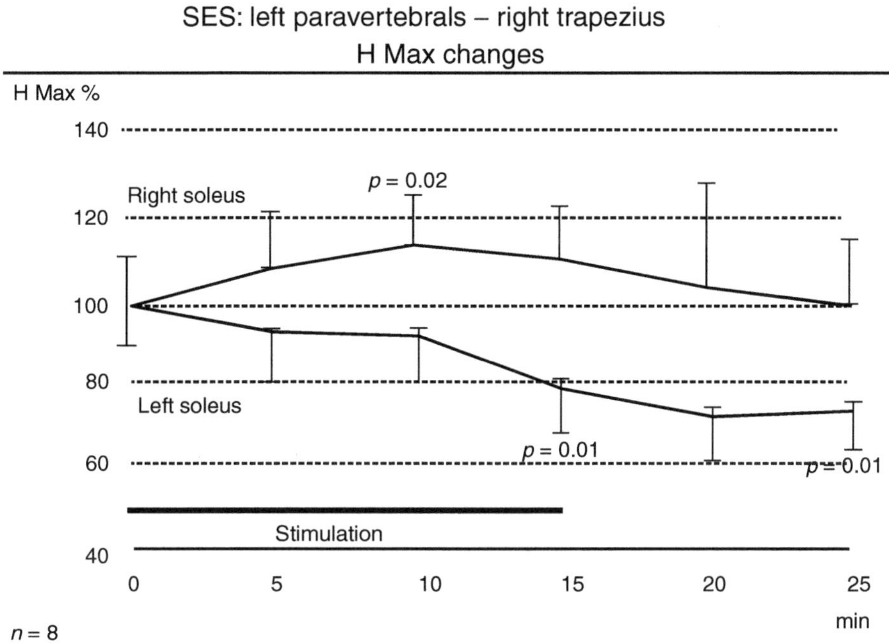

Fig. 31.1 Effects of electrical stimulation on H-reflexes

31.3 Results

They were homogeneous in all subjects both for the stimulation patterns. The contemporary VES of the left paravertebral cervical muscles and of the right trapezius was enhanced in all subjects after 10 min, H Max amplitude (14 % of the maximum amplitude; $p=0.02$) of the right soleus muscle, and reduced after 15 min, H Max amplitude (–20 %; $p=0.001$) of the soleus muscles. H Max amplitude returned to the basal values 10 min after the end of the stimulation on the right soleus and was still reduced (–36 %; $p=0.001$) 10 min after the end of SES on the left soleus. In some subjects H Max values lasted less than normal for 30 min after the end of VES. Recording from the right soleus showed that 10 min after the end of VES amplitude was still decreased (27 %; $p=0.001$) in some subject inhibition of the H-reflex that lasted over 30 min (Fig. 31.1).

The stimulation by VES of the right paravertebral cervical muscles and left trapezius induced, after 5 min, an increase of the left side values (20 %; $p=0.001$) and reduced, after 15 min, the amplitude of the right values (–32 %; $p=0.001$). In a short time after the end of the SES, left H-reflex returns to basal values. When a paradoxal second phase begins, H-reflex decreases slowly but progressively reaching a new “basal” value that is significantly ($p=0.001$) lower. Right H-reflex remains reduced at least 10 min after the end of SES (–27 %; $p=0.001$) (Fig. 31.2).

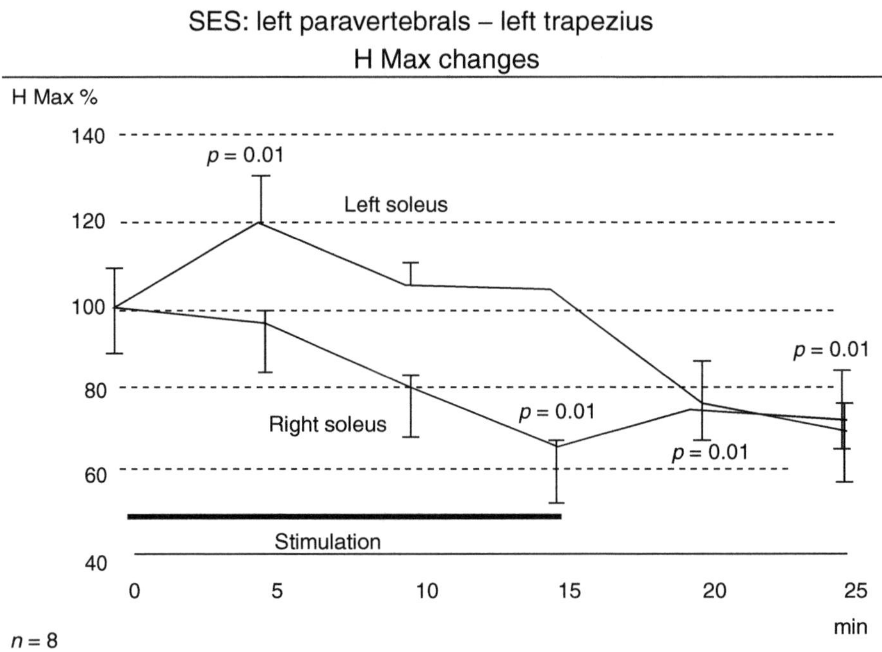

Fig. 31.2 Effects of electrical stimulation on H-reflexes

Conclusions

The results of the present study showed that VES of the neck muscles clearly influenced the excitability of the motor neurons of the lower limbs.

It is important to underline that VES at the intensity to which was applied never evoked muscles contraction. On the contrary VES was applied in the same frequency range (80 Hz) which is able to activate muscles spindles by vibratory stimulation. Thus, it is likely that VES activate the same spinal pathways activated from the cervico-spinal reflexes, modulating in the same way the postural reflexes of the lower limbs. This action is probably mediated from proprioceptive input originated in the spindles of the neck muscles [7]. Otherwise we cannot exclude the action of skin receptors mediating the vibratory sense.

Proprioceptive afferent input evoked from VES of the neck muscles could reach also contralateral Deiters vestibular nuclei and cortex, probably by mean of reticular pathways. In such way SES may influence the equilibrium system. It is known [8] that if vestibular apparatus is damaged, the reflexes of the neck, limb, and eyes muscles become prominent. Therefore it is possible that VES action in treatment of vertigo and dizziness is based on the modulation of the proprioceptive input from neck muscles.

At last there is the observation that inhibitory effect is more pronounced and long lasting than the excitatory one. Supraspinal pathway activation [9] may give account of this phenomenon, but further investigations are needed to verify such hypothesis.

References

1. Ghez C (1991) Posture. In: Kaendel ER, Schwartz JH, Jessell TM (eds) Principles of neural sciences, 3rd edn. Elsevier, New York/Amsterdam/London/Tokyo, pp 596–607
2. Angel RW, Hofmann WW (1963) The H reflex in normal, spastic and rigid subjects. Arch Neurol 8:591–596
3. YaM K (1979) The organization of voluntary movement. Neurophysiological mechanisms, vol II. Plenum Press, New York/London, pp 27–503
4. Alpini D, Cesarani A, Barozzi S (1992) Non pharmacological treatment of acute vertigo. In: Claussen CF, Kirtane MV, Schneider D (eds) Diagnostic procedures and imagining techniques used in neurotology. Proceedings of the XVI NES Congress. Werner Rudat & Co, Nachf ed m+p, Hamburg, pp 337–340
5. Thompson AK, Chen XY, Wolpaw JR (2013) Soleus H-reflex operant conditioning changes the H-reflex recruitment curve. Muscle Nerve 47(4):539–544
6. Oliveira MI, Machado AR, Chagas VG, Granado TC, Pereira AA, Andrade AO (2012) On the use of evoked potentials for quantification of pain. Conf Proc IEEE Eng Med Biol Soc 2012:1578–1581
7. Shields RK, Dudley-Javoroski S (2013) Fatigue modulates synchronous but not asynchronous soleus activation during stimulation of paralyzed muscle. Clin Neurophysiol 11:S1388-2457(13)00278-2
8. Okuma Y, Bergquist AJ, Hong M, Chan KM, Collins DF (2013) Electrical stimulation site influences the spatial distribution of motor units recruited in tibialis anterior. Clin Neurophysiol 18: S1388-2457(13)00315-5
9. Lagerquist O, Mang CS, Collins DF (2012) Changes in spinal but not cortical excitability following combined electrical stimulation of the tibial nerve and voluntary plantar-flexion. Exp Brain Res 222(1–2):41–53

Ski Trainer Oscillating Platform: Proprioceptive Reeducation

32

M. Savini, D.C. Alpini, and A. Cesarani

32.1 Introduction

Reeducation of the proprioceptive reflexes is especially indicated in posttraumatic disequilibrium. This method uses the theoretical premises of the method known as "proprioceptive neuromuscular facilitation" by (1) the use of nervous information of surface origin (tactile data) and (2) coordination of the information of deep origin (joint place, stretching of tendons, and capsuloligamentous complexes).

This peripheral information stimulates the nervous system, which triggers the muscle. In this way the patient may relearn to balance on his foot or knee via recoordination of the reflexes in unstable positions. He thus learns progressively to admit and understand the unstableness after an accident and is guided to fight against this residual unstableness through an improved muscular interplay [1, 2].

Skitter is a ski trainer platform comprised of an oscillating plate on which two foot pads are placed. Each foot pad is able to move anteroposteriorly (toes up and toes down) and lateral senses also allow torsional movement of each foot. The plate on which the two foot pads are placed is able to surf on an oscillating small table (Fig. 32.1a).

The oscillations of the table are slowed by elastic cords that regulate the resistance with which the device opposes the patient's movements. These movements of

M. Savini
Istituto Clinico Città Studi, via Jommelli 17, Milan, Italy

D.C. Alpini (✉)
ENT-Otoneurology Service, IRCCS "Don Carlo C. Gnocchi" Foundation, Milano, Italy
e-mail: dalpini@dongnocchi.it

A. Cesarani
Department of Clinical Sciences and Community Health,
University of Milan, Milano, Italy

Audiology Unit, IRCCS "Ca' Granda" Ospedale Maggiore Policlinico, Milano, Italy
e-mail: antonio.cesarani@unimi.it

D.C. Alpini et al. (eds.), *Whiplash Injuries*,
DOI 10.1007/978-88-470-5486-8_32, © Springer-Verlag Italia 2014

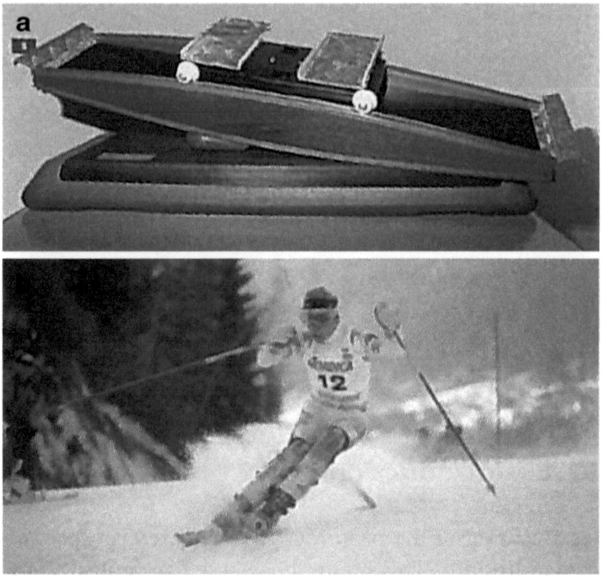

Fig. 32.1 Skitter (**a**) and skier (**b**)

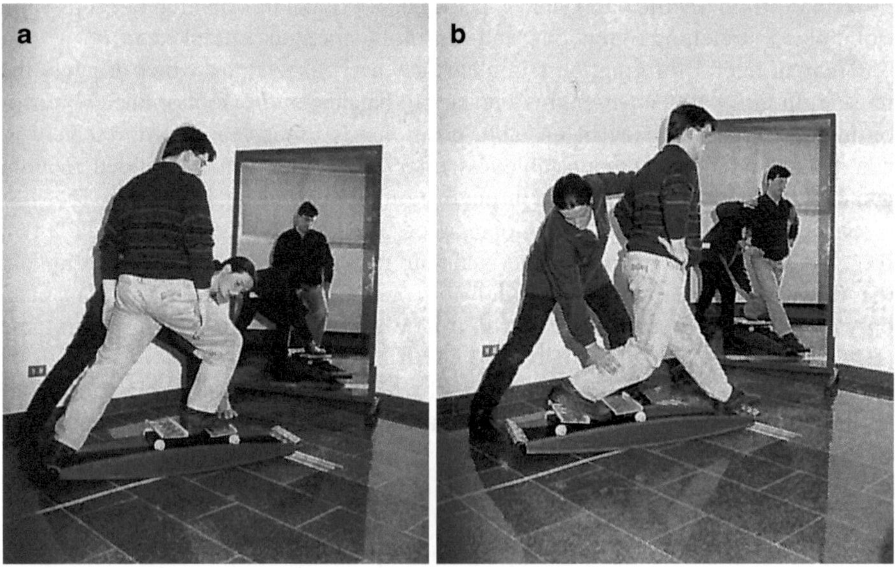

Fig. 32.2 Forward (**a**) and backward (**b**) leg extensions

the feet and, especially, surfing and oscillating of the body simulate the movements performed during skiing (Fig. 32.1b).

We usually employed Skitter for proprioceptive reeducation of posttraumatic unsteadiness and dizziness because it allows the use of cognitively involved exercises and improvement of sensorial coordination when visual feedback is

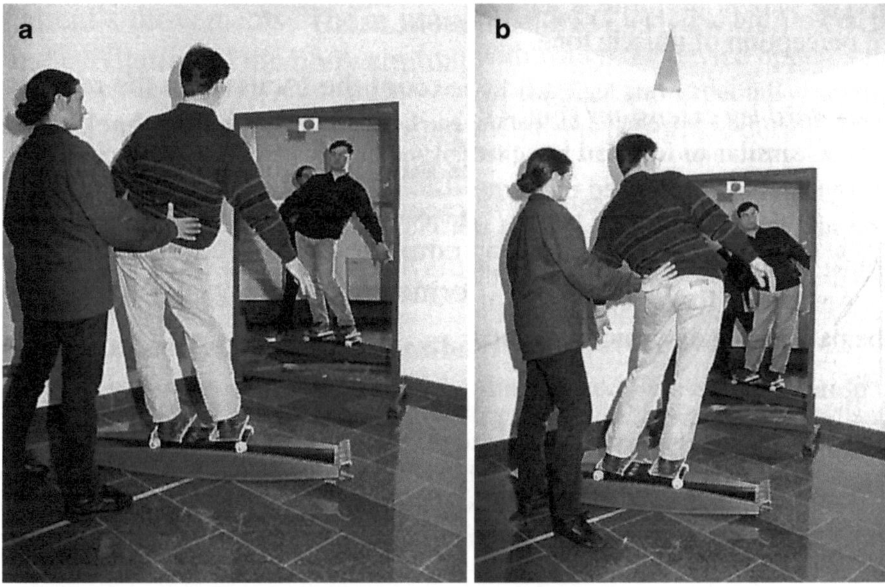

Fig. 32.3 Ankle-hip lateral strategies (**a**) and with oscillations (**b**)

associated in order to improve head-to-trunk dynamic stabilization [3]. To successfully reeducate reflexes by this method, active cooperation of the subject is needed. The careful activity of a reeducator or of a physiotherapist offers better chances of success [4].

In whiplash patients we standardized a protocol that has been used in patients ranging from 18 to 45 years of age. According to the obvious limits of age, Skitter can be employed (with the constant help of the reeducator) also in older subjects, but usually it is not possible to perform the entire protocol. To achieve a good result, it is crucial that the articulations of ankle, knee, and hip are complete and that the muscular tone, especially of the thigh, is good. Sometimes previous tonification of the muscles is in fact necessary before starting reeducation of the proprioceptive reflexes.

32.1.1 Forward Leg Extensions (Fig. 32.2a)

1. With one foot on the end cap and the other across the foot pad, the patient keeps his weight forward and extends the front leg in a controlled manner, then he returns slowly and repeats. It improves quads and trunk muscles and stabilizes ankles and knees.
2. The patient maintains the leg extension position, and the therapist destabilizes him by moving the platform during visual fixation of a point.
3. The patient performs a leg extension with closed eyes to improve self-perception of muscle tone.

32.1.2 **Backward Leg Extensions** (Fig. 32.2b)

This is similar to forward leg extensions except the focus is on the rear leg. With a stable, controlled movement, the patient extends the leg back to the end and repeats on both legs. It improves gluts and quads, hamstrings, and *trunk* muscles, and stabilizes ankles and knees.

According to the neuro-otologic and equilibriometric characteristics of the patient, leg extensions should be performed for both legs or only for one leg.

32.1.3 **Ankle-Hip Strategies** (Fig. 32.3a)

The patient steps on the foot pads with feet centrally positioned. Then he concentrates on proper posture using a mirror to see his reflection and transfers his weight from one foot to the other with a smooth flowing motion.

During this smooth and rhythmic weight transfer, the therapist induces body movements according to ankle or hip strategies.

32.1.4 **Visual Feedback**

The patient is comfortably stable on the foot pads. With his thumbs and extended limbs, he tries to touch some visual targets placed in different positions on a mirror in front of him.

32.1.5 **Oscillations** (Fig. 32.3b)

The patient steps on foot pads with feet centrally positioned. Then he concentrates on proper posture using a mirror to see his reflection. With eyes closed he transfers his weight from one foot to the other with a smooth flowing motion. During this smooth and rhythmic weight transfer, the therapist pushes the bumpers at one end of the Skitter inducing a sudden and unpredictable inclination of the device.

32.1.6 **One Leg**

The patient maintains equilibrium on one leg with the other extended (Fig. 32.4a) or flexed (Fig. 32.4b) or with one leg lateral (Fig. 32.5). The therapist helps the patient either to maintain equilibrium or to correct his posture. A mirror facilitates postural equilibrium strategies correction.

32.1.7 **Slalom** (Fig. 32.6)

The patient steps on the foot pads with feet centrally positioned. Then he concentrates on proper posture using a mirror to see his reflection and begins to transfer his weight from one foot to the other with a smooth flowing motion. As his rhythms

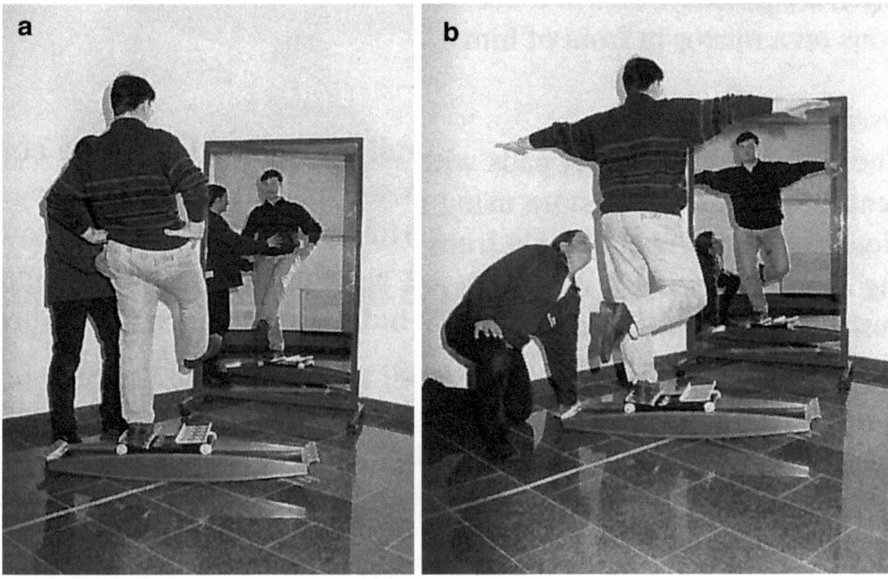

Fig. 32.4 Extended (**a**) or flexed (**b**) exercises with one leg

Fig. 32.5 One-leg exercise

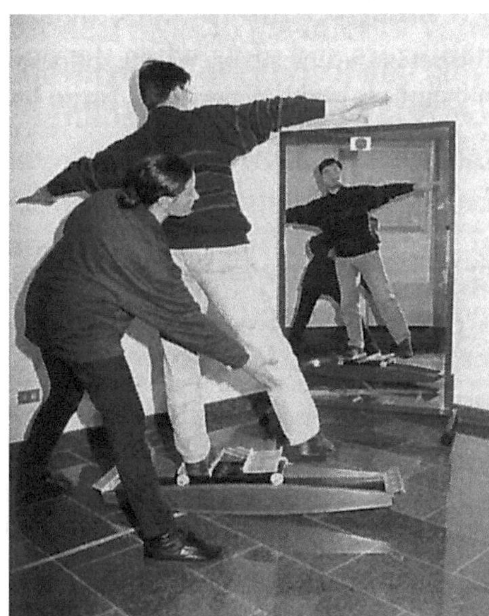

increase he will get closer to the bumpers at each end, always maintaining good upright posture with eyes focused in the mirror and paying attention to his balance. If the exercise is performed with limited upper body movement (such as in slalom), it improves hip rotators, quads, and calves, while it stimulates abdominal stabilizers and gluts when the patient includes upper body motion (such as in giant slalom). Exercises have to be performed concentrating on proper edge setting techniques.

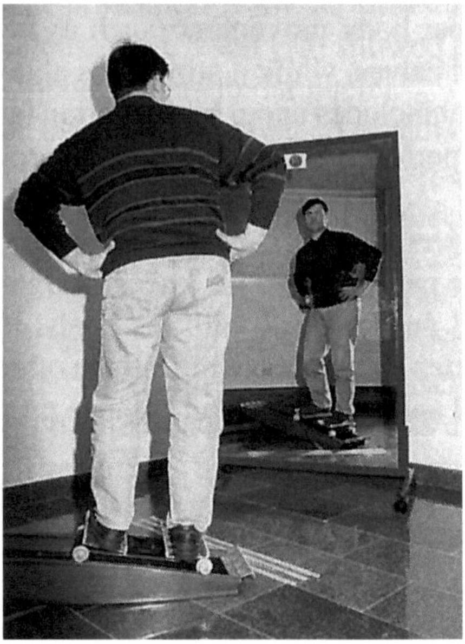

Fig. 32.6 Slalom exercise

32.1.8 Ankles Stability

The patient keeps his knees straight pushing the skate forward with his toes and pulling back with his heels. He has to concentrate on using only the ankles and calves, while all the other muscles are relaxed. It improves calves and ankle stability and balance proprioception.

References

1. Corna S, Nardone A, Prestinari A, Galante M, Grasso M, Schieppati M (2003) Comparison of Cawthorne-Cooksey exercises and sinusoidal support surface translations to improve balance in patients with unilateral vestibular deficit. Arch Phys Med Rehabil 84(8):1173–1184
2. Nardone A, Godi M, Artuso A, Schieppati M (2010) Balance rehabilitation by moving platform and exercises in patients with neuropathy or vestibular deficit. Arch Phys Med Rehabil 91(12):1869–1877
3. De Nunzio AM, Nardone A, Schieppati M (2005) Head stabilization on a continuously oscillating platform: the effect of a proprioceptive disturbance on the balancing strategy. Exp Brain Res 165(2):261–272
4. Fairburn PS, Palmer R, Whybrow J, Fielden S, Jones S (2000) A prototype system for testing force platform dynamic performance. Gait Posture 12(1):25–33

Visual Feedback Postural Control Re-education

33

D.C. Alpini, A. Cesarani, M. De Bellis, R. Kohen-Raz, and D. Riva

33.1 Introduction

Maintaining postural stability is a complex process [1] involving the coordinated actions of biomechanical, sensory, motor, and central nervous system components. A relatively simple biomechanical definition for postural stability can be formulated in terms of the position of the body center of gravity relative to the base of support. The body movements used to maintain postural stability, however, are complex because of the number of joint systems and muscles involved. The center of gravity (CoG) is the point at which the whole weight of a body may be considered to act. In humans who are standing quietly and vertically erect, the CoG is located at the level of the hips and slightly forward of the ankle joints. CoG height is 0.5527 of total height. CoG and center of mass (CoM) are equivalent points in space when the gravitational field is uniform and gravity is the only force under consideration.

Shumway-Cook et al. [2] conducted the first study that used objective visual feedback (VFB), based on symmetry of postural sway (movement of the CoG), for training purposes.

D.C. Alpini (✉)
ENT-Otoneurology Service, IRCCS "Don Carlo C. Gnocchi" Foundation, Milan, Italy
e-mail: dalpini@dongnocchi.it

A. Cesarani
Department of Clinical Sciences and Community Health, University of Milan, Milan, Italy

Audiology Unit, IRCCS "Ca' Granda" Ospedale Maggiore Policlinico, Milan, Italy
e-mail: antonio.cesarani@unimi.it

M. De Bellis
ENT Department, Desio Hospital (Mi), Milan, Italy

R. Kohen-Raz
The school of Education, The Hebrew University of Jerusalem, Har ha-Tsofim, Jerusalem, Israel

D. Riva
International Society of Proprioception and Posture, via Valgioie 87, 10146 Torino, Italy

D.C. Alpini et al. (eds.), *Whiplash Injuries*,
DOI 10.1007/978-88-470-5486-8_33, © Springer-Verlag Italia 2014

Nowadays, a lot of different posturographic equipments are available and VFB is frequently used to improve postural stability control.

For the scope of the chapter, even if nowadays for postural visual feedback rehabilitation [3–5], examples are based on the Balance Master System (Neurocom, Clackamas, OR, USA, http://resourceonbalance.com), Tetrax FB System (Tel Aviv Israel, www.tetraxfb.com), and the Delos System (Turin, Italy, www.delos-international.com).

Balance Master is an equipment that allows, by means of a dual footplate, a visual feedback of CoG position, projected on a computer screen facing the patient standing on the platform [6–8] (see also Chap. 15).

Tetrax system is based on recording of separate CoG of the anterior and posterior part of the 2 ft [9–16] (see also Chap. 15).

Delos System is an equipment constituted by a unstable and oscillating platform and two accelerometers, one on the trunk [17] and one on the head (see also Chap. 16). In this way the visual feedback projected on the screen may regard the movements of the table or the trunk or the head or a combination of the three.

33.2 Balance Master

When normal subjects maintain a vertically erect position, the CoG is located directly over the area of the feet support, slightly forward of the ankle joints. This position can be maintained without stepping or reaching for support if sway does not exceed the subject's limits of stability (Fig. 33.1).

Functional stability limits (limits of stability, LoS) have been calculated to be 6.25″ anteriorly and 4.45″ posteriorly for the average adult subject. The angular limits of stability are very nearly the same for all adults regardless of height. The biomechanical properties that determine the LoS are similar for standing in place, walking, and sitting without trunk support. For these reasons reeducation of the limits of stability in standing in place can be used to rehabilitate the patient to regain normal LoS during walking, too.

LoS test and exercise require the subject to be able to actively move his/her CoG away from the center toward a visual target and maintain that position for the required time. The correct execution of the LoS test requires normal combined and integrated ankle-hip strategies (Fig. 33.2).

LoS parameters to be considered are:

Movement time, how many seconds the patient takes to reach the desired target (including the reaction time).

Path sway, that refers percentage of path length.

Target sway, percentage of maximum CoG area maintained on the target.

Patient position, value given in polar coordinates that represents the average position of the COG during the period of target sway assessment. If the target was not reached, the patient position score reflects the point of closest approach to the target.

Distance error, difference between the patient's average position and the center of target. This parameter allows one to see how far away from the center the patient is willing and able to move in a given direction.

Fig. 33.1 Balance Master equipment

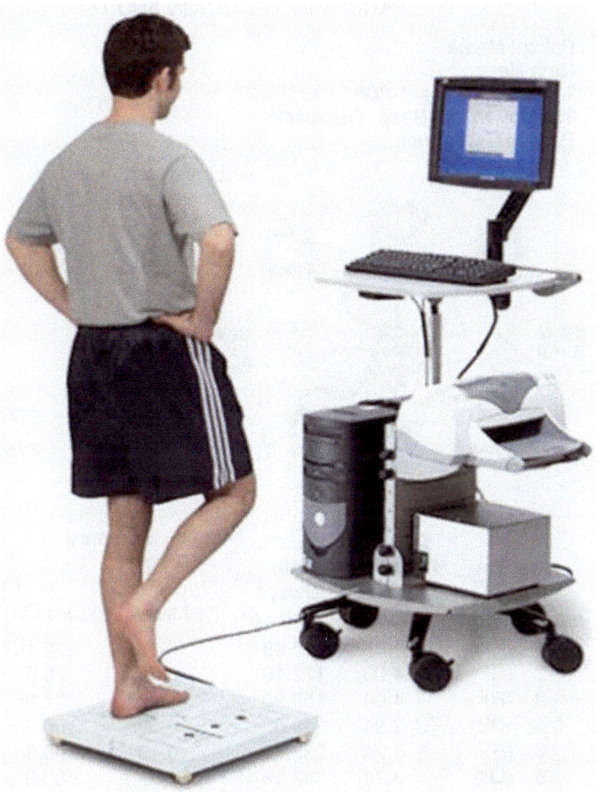

LoS misperception is common findings in whiplash patients. In these cases training aimed at teaching the appropriate conditions for using ankle movements can have a positive impact. In contrast, weakness of ankle joint muscles, loss of ankle sensation, reduced mobility about the ankles, or combinations of these factors prevent the patient from generating effective ankle movements and might be an abnormal adaptation used by a dizzy patient to minimize head movements and associated stimulation of the neck and vestibular system.

By means of the Balance Master it is possible to treat patients ranging from 76 to 203 cm in height and from 18 to 138 kg in weight. Each treatment session can be performed according to the LoS, ranging from 25 to 100 % of the predictable LoS, in 5 % increments. The target pacing is 1, 3, 5, 7, 10, 15, and 20 s. If trying to promote faster movement, then low pacing settings (1, 2, 5 s) are appropriate. If stability at points in space is desired, then higher pacing settings (10 s or higher) are appropriate so that the patient must "hold" a position (Fig. 33.3).

The duration of each session treatment is 20 min. The frequency generally varies from twice a week to every day treatment. The frequency of training sessions is dependent on a combination of other rehabilitative treatments such as physical therapy and vestibular electrical stimulation.

PATIENT INFORMATION AND TEST SETTINGS

Patient Name:	Age: 30	Test Date. 02/16/95
Data file	Ht.: 172 cm	Order #: 6
Target/prot. Type: SP06	LOS: 75 %	Pacing Speed: 10 sec
Therapy Mode: Beep, Feedback		
Post-Test Comment:		

Limits of stability

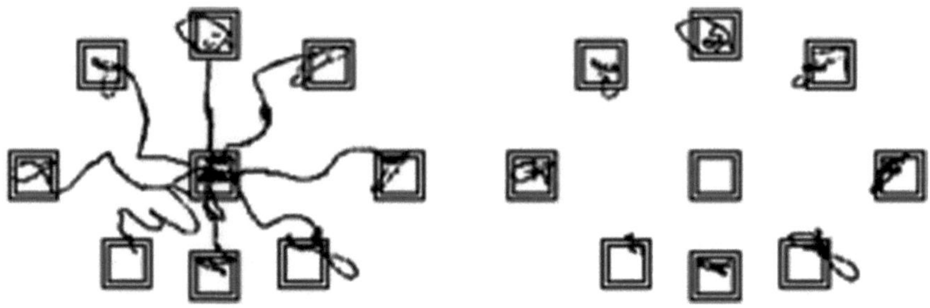

Numeric Summary

Transition	Mvt Time (sec)	Path Sway (% Path Len)	Target Sway (% Max Area)	Patient Position (% LOS)	Patient Position (deg)	Distance Error (% LOS)	Direction Error (deg)
1 (F)	4.28	127.68	N/S	<72.1>	<359.2>	<–2.9>	<–0.8>
2 (RF)	4.00	172.16	0.41	70.8	42.7	–4.2	–2.3
3 (R)	4.04	157.96	N/S	<71.8>	<87.8>	<–3.2>	<–2.2>
4 (RB)	2.94	169.83	0.58	68.6	124.8	–6.4	–10.2
5 (B)	3.74	237.19	0.13	66.8	176.6	–8.2	–3.4
6 (LB)	6.72	347.19	N/S	<60.6>	<230.8>	<–14.4>	<–5.8>
7 (L)	4.50	188.06	N/S	<73.4>	<271.9>	<–1.6>	<1.9>
8 (LF)	3.70	158.90	0.20	70.1	314.2	–4.9	–0.8

Fig. 33.2 Example of LoS, a not completely statistical representation

33.2.1 Tetrax FB

Tetrax FB works within the principles of Simplexity [18], which state that a human body's balance in space is based on the cooperation and interaction of a multiplicity and complexity of many subsystems which are under the control of efficient neurophysiological mechanisms. It consists of four independent mobile force plates, two for each foot. Each plate contains a strain-gauge force transducer, which is sensitive to vertical force. Tetrax provides independent output from the four balance plates. Subjects are requested to stand quietly on the platforms and control CoG displacements using both feet, toes, and heels in a synchronized and coordinated way. "Tetra CoG" have to be moved along visual presented pathways (e.g., a labyrinth, Fig. 33.3) as correctly as possible (Fig. 33.4).

The pressure fluctuations produced by the heels and toes of a subject standing with different positions of the trunk or the head may be visually balanced through the feedback presented on the screen.

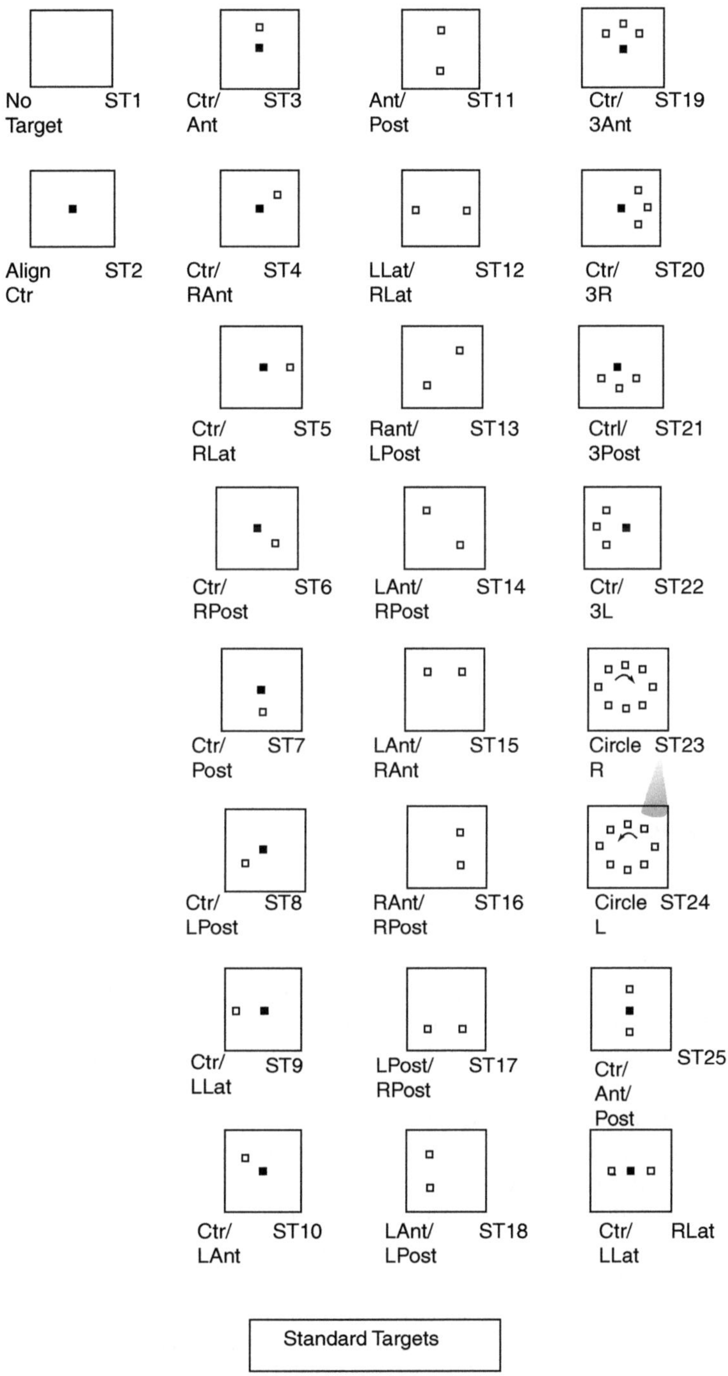

Fig. 33.3 Standard targets available for treatment

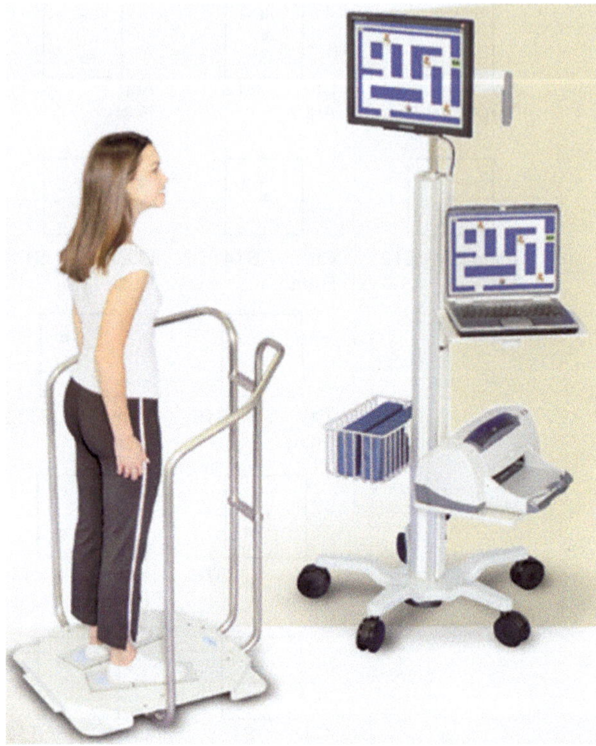

Fig. 33.4 Tetrax FB equipment

33.2.2 Delos

It is based on an electronic rocking board, with "a degree of freedom" and visual tracking of the micro-rolling of the point of support. Its exclusive rocking movement, combined with the subcortical visual tracking in real time, creates conditions of instability capable of activating high-frequency proprioceptive flows both in standing (Fig. 33.5) and sitting position (Fig. 33.6).

The rolling surfaces with variable radius permit the proposal of different levels of instability and the selective activation of the postural strategies. The postural reader measures the subject's levels of stability in static and dynamic, monopodalic, bipodalic, and seated conditions. It records and visualizes in real time the movements on the frontal and sagittal planes in relation to the vertical axis. The system may use also a wireless electronic rocking board with "3 degrees of freedom" with visualization in real time of the movements on the *x*-, *y*-, and *z*-axis. Tridimensional view of the trials represents the completion of DEB2 proposal, widening the number of biomechanical and postural situations to be managed. The rolling surfaces with variable radius permit the proposal of increasing levels of instability.

Figs. 33.5 and 33.6 Delos DEB 2 equipment comprising the electronic rocking board and the two accelerometers on the head and the trunk

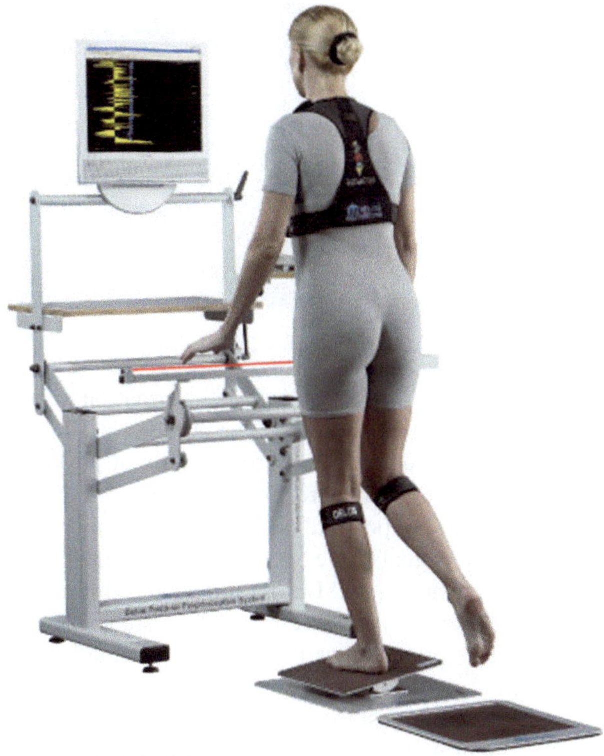

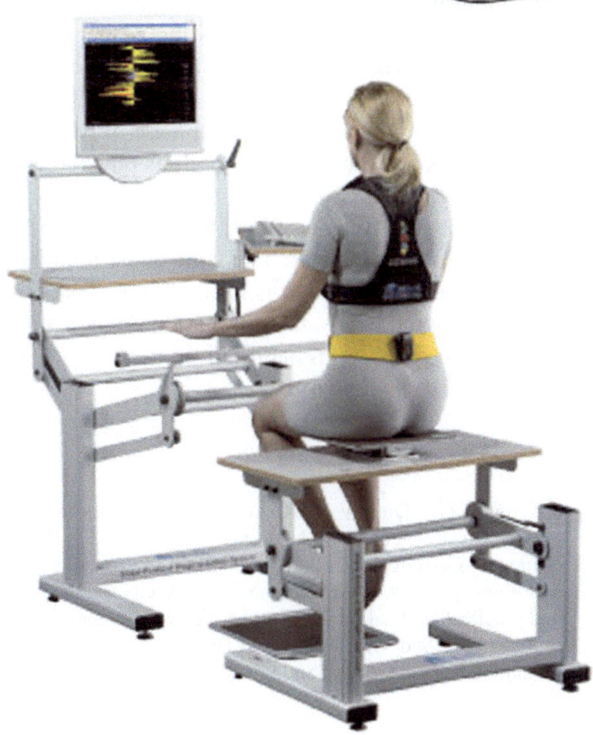

Figs. 33.5 and 33.6 (continued)

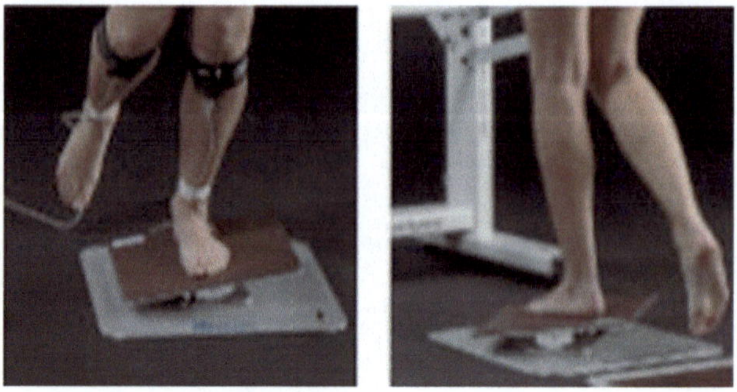

Conclusions

VFB provides a ready source of information about postural instability for both the patient and the therapist. The purpose of VFB is to detect and make available to the patient objective information about physiological function or movement that is not ordinarily perceived by the patient (e.g., Balance Master).

In the case of postural instability caused by whiplash injuries, visual and auditory (beep) signals have been used to give the patient information about head and trunk orientation (e.g., Delos) and about symmetry of weight bearing through the lower extremities (e.g., Tetrax). The assumption is that the patient can use visual or auditory cues better than he or she could use somatosensory or vestibular inputs.

For the therapist the VFB facilitates the design of custom treatments, and for the patient it enhances motivation through real-time visual feedback, links perception to movement, internalizes the appropriate alignment or movement pattern, improves volitional control, and builds confidence to perform activities of daily living.

Recently it has been proposed the use of Nintendo Wii, a popular virtual reality (VR) video gaming system, both as physiotherapist-assisted [19] and home-based [20] exercises.

Nintendo Wii Balance Board is cost-effective and user-friendly [21] and has been proposed as an alternative to other popular frequently used systems in elderly patients [22], but it is limited in its customizability to accommodate different functional levels, thus in our experience, professional equipments have to be preferred for WAD rehabilitation.

References

1. Horstmann GA, Dietz V (1990) A basic control mechanism: the stabilization of the center of gravity. Electroenceph Clin Neurophysiol 76:165–176
2. Shumway-Cook A, McCollum G (1991) Assessment and treatment of balance deficits in the neurologic patients. In: Montgomery P, Connelly B (eds) Motor control. Theoretical framework and practical application, & physical therapy. Chattanooga Corp, Chattanooga, pp 123–138
3. Di Fabio RP, Andersen JH (1993) Effect of sway-referenced visual and somatosensory inputs on human head movement and postural patterns during stance. J Vest Res 3:409–417

4. Hamann KF, Krausen C (1990) Clinical application of posturography. Body tracking and biofeedback training. In: Brandt T, Paulus W, Bles W (eds) Disorders of posture and gait. Thieme, Stuttgart, pp 295–298
5. Lee DN, Lishrnan JR (1975) Visual proprioceptive control of stance. J Hum Mov Stud 1:87; Moore S, Wollacott MH (1993) The use of biofeedback devices to improve postural stability. Phys Ther Pract 2(2):1–19
6. Nashner L (1994) Evaluation of postural stability, movement, and control. In: Hasson SM (ed) Clinical exercise physiology. Mosby, St Louis, p 57
7. Neurocom International Inc. (1989) Balance master operator's manual. Neurocom, Portland
8. Daleiden S (1990) Weight shifting as a treatment for balance deficits. A literature review. Physiother Can 48:81–87
9. Alpini D, Cesarani A, Pugnetti L, Cardini R, Hahn A, Sambataro G (2000) Project to prevent mobility related accidents in elderly and disabled. Proceedings of the 3rd international conference on disability, virtual reality and ass. Tech., Alghero, Italy, pp 249–254
10. Himmelfarb R, Kohen-Raz R, Rapaport J, Bloom A (1992) The application of posturography in the assessment of vertiginous disorders caused by head and neck injuries. Proceedings of he international meeting on whiplash injuries. University of Wales, Wales
11. Kohen-Raz R, Gentaz R (1993) Posturographic characteristics of patients with lower back pain. Cahiers de Posturologie, Paris
12. Kohen-Raz R (1986) Learning disabilities and postural control. Freund Publishing House, Tel Aviv
13. Kohen-Raz R, Roth V (1998) Posturographic characteristics of Whiplash patients. Proceedings of the XII regular meeting of the Barany Society, Wuerzburg, Germany. In: Claus CF, Claus-Toni H, Hoffenberth B (eds) Equilibrium research, Clinical equilibriometry and modern treatment. Elsevier, Amsterdam, 2000
14. Roth V, Perlson Y (1997) The contribution of an interactive balance recording system (IBS) to the diagnosis, treatment and follow up of Foot and Ankle Injuries. Proceedings of the international congress on foot and ankle injuries, Jerusalem, January 1997
15. Turner D (1998) Evaluation of the tetrax interactive balance system and equitest using normal subjects. MSc thesis, University of Southampton
16. Lee KG, Chun MH, Kang SH, Kim BR (2008) The evaluation of effect after biofeedback training using interactive balance system in sub-acute stroke patients. Asan Medical Center Korea, XVII. European stroke conference Nice, France. Poster Session: Recovery and rehabilitation, May 2008
17. Sjostrom H, Allum JH, Carpenter MG, Adkin AL, Honegger F, Ettlin T (2003) Trunk sway measures of postural stability during clinical balance tests in patients with chronic whiplash injury symptoms. Spine 28(15):1725–1734
18. Berthoz A (2012) Simplexity. Yale University Press, London
19. Levac DE, Miller PA (2013) Integrating virtual reality video games into practice: clinicians' experiences. Physiother Theory Pract;29(7):504–512
20. Prosperini L, Fortuna D, Giannì C, Leonardi L, Marchetti MR, Pozzilli C (2013) Home-based balance training using the wii balance board: a randomized, crossover pilot study in multiple sclerosis. Neurorehabil Neural Repair 27(6):516–525
21. Sparrer I, Duong Dinh TA, Ilgner J, Westhofen M (2013) Vestibular rehabilitation using the Nintendo® Wii Balance Board – a user-friendly alternative for central nervous compensation. Acta Otolaryngol 133(3):239–245
22. Taylor MJ, Shawis T, Impson R, Ewins K, McCormick D, Griffin M (2012) Nintendo Wii as a training tool in falls prevention rehabilitation: case studies. J Am Geriatr Soc 60(9):1781–1783

34 Neurorehabilitation of Ataxia

M. Forni

34.1 Introduction

The meaning of ataxia is failure of coordination. Ataxic patients are not able to define the width, velocity, and rhythms of muscle contractions and cannot coordinate more muscle groups which are synchronously activated. The ataxia can be determined by (1) injury of the proprioceptive afferences, (2) labyrinthic injury, and (3) injury of cerebellum or its connections which are reciprocally connected to the cerebral cortex (neocerebellum), the spinal cord (paleocerebellum), and the vestibular system (archeocerebellum).

Post-whiplash ataxia is not frequent and it attains to polytrauma patients. The walking ataxia – often generically considered as walking balance disease – can also be generated by an injury of the pyramidal paths causing a heavy recruitment deficit of the lower limb proximal areas. We use the word "ataxia" with the meaning of coordination and motor control alteration due to the inability of the antagonistic muscle couples to synergistically operate. It can occur as postural instability of one or more body segments or as dyssynergia when holding a posture during the execution of a complex motion [1, 2]. Ataxia can be often found in whiplash-type injuries and sometimes in the acute phase shows reversibility, probably because it is supported by a simple neuro-apraxia of the corresponding nervous paths. In cases in which the ataxia is present with instability, it is usually supported by injuries of the direct or indirect proprioceptive paths or the cerebellospinal paths flowing to the cervical spinal cord. From the functional point of view, ataxia can be defined as a specific difficulty in controlling the center of gravity of the whole body or of single articulated segments. In fact, it magically disappears when the patient is immersed into water [3].

M. Forni
Rehabilitation Unit, IRCCS "Don Carlo Gnocchi" Foundation,
Marina di Massa (MS), Italy
e-mail: mforni@dongnocchi.it

D.C. Alpini et al. (eds.), *Whiplash Injuries*,
DOI 10.1007/978-88-470-5486-8_34, © Springer-Verlag Italia 2014

34.1.1 Treatment Outlines

If considered on the plane of a system which can be influenced by therapeutic exercise, that is, on the interface between environment and spinal segmentary systems (receptor level and muscle effector level), ataxia can be defined as the inability to couple suitably coactivation and reciprocal activation, the latter the pathologically prevalent characteristic. From the spinal cord point of view, in fact, hypotonia could be considered as the cause of the ataxia. In fact, if we consider ataxia as increase of the stretching reflex threshold due to decreasing of the fusi basal discharge, we can formulate the hypothesis that the motion desynchronization is supported by a decreasing of the tonic "brake," due to perceptive distortions connected to the proprioceptor-altered operation. Further, we could consider ataxia as the extreme pole of a continuous path with variable prevalence grades between coactivation and reciprocal activation, in which the opposite is spasticity. In fact, correct motion requires a rigidity entity which is able to withstand stimuli or a flexibility that is the ability to follow stimuli. Ataxia can be considered as an excessive flexibility. The posturogram of a normal person is known to often show variability in the center of gravity displacement, which is the expression of physiological flexibility. The motion pre-patterns, that is, the anticipatory muscle activation of an intentional motion being carried out, are one of the physiological examples of the control of this CNS variability. The therapeutic approach to ataxia cannot be separated from such considerations [4]. The most important problem in the spontaneous adaptation to the symptom in the atactic patient is normally that the spontaneous reaction increases the symptom.

The "body's intelligence" reacts against the instability by increasing the rigidity, that is, the cocontraction, which is the real mechanism altered by the pathology. This condition activates the paradoxical happening so that the instability increases with the increasing of attempts aimed to limit it. Some preliminary therapeutical results can be obtained simply by disconnecting this vicious circle by means of relaxation techniques (which could be claimed as not suitable with regard to muscle tone assessment), also of the psychomotor type. Taking into consideration that often the whole spontaneous attempt of stopping the symptom accentuates it, the proposal of "balance exercises" for the ataxic patient seems to be not justifiable. In fact, these exercises are based on quick changes of the center of gravity, as imposed by the rehabilitator, and are also based on the idea that after some stress of this type, an adaptation should occur. It is my opinion that this adaptation – based on the idea that the repetition is one of the mechanisms starting the process of learning – makes the ataxia problem not solvable from the rehabilitation point of view.

An exercise plan for the ataxic patient should be based on a functional assessment, recognizing the motion-specific characteristics as well as the necessary changes needed to modify it. For example, we can examine whether the ataxic motion is sensitive to inertial changes applied to the end of the considered segment (weights), or to intentional changes (automatic-voluntary dissociation), or even whether it uses any, and if so which, privileged afferent channels. Furthermore, the description of the altered motion should include the planes on which the alteration

Table 34.1 Correlations between lesions and symptoms

Lesion topography	Functions	Postural reactions	First-order lesion associations	Second-order lesion associations
Efferent motor paths	Pyramidal	Inhibited		
Posterior cord afferent paths	Kinesthetic and proprioceptive (deep sensory)	Uncompleted, delayed	With synergically reduced reactions	
Cerebrocerebellar paths	Neocerebellar	Sequentially altered		With dissociated reactions
Spinocerebellar paths	Paleocerebellar	Increased intensity	With reactions uninhibited in direction and intensity	
Vestibulocerebellar paths	Archeo-cerebellar	Dynamically displaced with distal prevalence		
Vestibulospinal paths	Vestibular	Statistically distorted with proximal prevalence		

is mainly evident as well as the articular angles and motion velocity at which the motion is mainly compromised. Furthermore, we should examine whether the motion is dynamically or statically altered.

The most interesting classification from the rehabilitation point of view is still P. Gasco's one [5], relevant to rehabilitation of motion in patients suffering from multiple sclerosis in its different expressions (Table 34.1).

Therefore we propose a descriptive assessment protocol to be associated, when possible, with instrumental evaluations [1, 5]:

1. Assessment of ataxia "migration" in different body areas, with reference to posture; in fact, often the oscillation of one segment is complementary to and compensates the adjacent segment oscillation and does not represent the injury site from the topological point of view. The patient is evaluated in different postures taking into consideration the syndrome's acuteness: for example, in the erect position (possibly also the monopodalic position), both with extended and flexed knees, in a quadruped position, in crouched position, sitting down to exactly examine the planes at which the motion is more compromised, and the postural conditions in which the instability is evidenced in each body area. In the most difficult cases, the patient can also be evaluated in a supine position thanks to suitable supports, able to allow the cingulum to move with one or more degrees of freedom.
2. Evaluation of synergies most stressed by the ataxia in the same body area [6]. Various modes of execution of the same action are evaluated (e.g., reaching to a point in the space with one limb end or with the head or tracking of a trajectory

with one limb or the eyes, grasping of objects, reaching possible positions). In this phase, the performance success or the execution correctness is not evaluated, but the chosen "strategy," above all on the basis of the degrees of freedom or constraints imposed on the various segments implied or possible to be implied in the motion.
3. Evaluation of the maximal voluntary cocontraction effects on the symptoms: the patient is asked to *try* to actively stop the tremor or the postural instability by stiffening as much as possible the involved segment and the adjacent segments. Under the same other conditions, we note cases in which this operation is successful and cases in which this operation causes instability or increasing incoordination.
4. Evaluation of differences in the symptoms with respect to the voluntariness or automatism of the motion; for example, in exercises with multiple conditions in which an upper limb is laid on a moving plane and executes automatic support functions, while the other limb executes an intentional job referred to a target imposed by the examiner, then the operation of the examined limbs is inverted. We note instability conditions which tend to occur more intentionally, than automatically, and vice versa (considering the required cautions due to the kinesiologic differences between the two tasks).
5. Evaluation of differences in the symptoms [7] subsequent to segmentary motions which are freely chosen by the patient, or segmentary motions imposed by the examiner, but without perceptive guide, or motions with perceptive guide, such as reaching a target or executing a trajectory following paths imposed by the examiner.
6. Evaluation of the effect of suppression, increase, or distortion of one or more perceptive channels (acoustic, visual, or proprioceptive) on the posture or motion. The above six factors allow a functional assessment of the ataxia which is more suitable than the traditional one used to plan therapy. In this way, the therapeutic approach can be oriented to correction of the most specific aspects which determine the incoordination or balance deficiency.

Naturally, this approach should be widened and validated, if possible, with instrumental analysis able to control both the assessment correctness and the efficiency of the therapeutic approach.

34.1.2 Treatment

Research evidence of activity-dependent central nervous system (CNS) plasticity and the requisite motor learning principles can be used to construct an efficacious motor recovery intervention. Brain plasticity after trauma refers to the regeneration of brain neuronal structures and/or reorganization of the function of neurons. Not only can CNS structure and function change in response to injury, but also the changes may be modified by "activity." For gait training or upper limb functional training for stroke survivors, the "activity" is motor behavior, including coordination and strengthening exercise and functional training that comprise motor learning. Critical principles of motor learning required for CNS activity-dependent plasticity include close-to-normal movements, muscle activation driving practice of movement, focused attention, repetition of desired movements, and training specificity.

The ultimate goal of rehabilitation is to restore function so that a satisfying quality of life can be experienced.

Accurate measurement of dysfunction and its underlying impairments are critical to the development of accurately targeted interventions that are sufficiently robust to produce gains not only in function but also in quality of life.

When it is not possible to adopt sophisticated instrumental evaluations, we think it is very useful to monitor the condition with videotapes, which can be associated with a functional assessment and allow one to have a relatively accurate idea about the efficiency of the treatment. [7]

The International Classification of Functioning, Disability, and Health (ICF) model of disablement, put forth by the World Health Organization, can provide not only some guidance in measurement level selection but also can serve as a guide to incorporate function and quality of life enhancement as the ultimate goals of rehabilitation interventions. Based on the evidence and principles of activity-dependent plasticity and motor learning, we developed gait training and upper limb functional training protocols.

An interesting perspective in ataxia therapy has been offered by the application of "perceptive conflict" exercises for treatment of feedback control deficiency. This approach, which can even use sophisticated methods such as virtual reality, is based on the importance given in the determination of ataxia to the perceptive aspect and to the possibility to restructure the balance system in the peripheral environment through induced perceptive alterations.

Another interesting attempt is the use of an EMG-acoustic device able to monitor muscular recruitment sequences in ballistic movements for treatment of preprogramming level. In addition, the technique known as kinematic muscle shortening with traction stress has also been successfully used. This method, based on motor action organization theories – the best known of which is A. Feldman's "equilibrium point" – is based on the possibility of recalling not present motion components, shortening a muscle when contemporarily a vibration is applied to the muscle itself (traction stress). In ataxia this exercise cannot be applied to all muscle groups; in fact, the associated hypotonia implies that the strengthening reaction is recalled at higher muscle lengths than the normal ones; sometime these lengths can exceed the articular limits of the considered segment. The muscles on which the exercise can be usually executed are short, generally phasic, muscle such as the posterior neck muscles, to which the head is suspended in the vertical posture. This exercise allowed us to obtain preliminary interesting results in head tremor control.

Other otoneurological techniques, almost of all which involve reflexologic imprinting, are exhaustively described in other reports.

In many serious cases, it is possible to use technology to enable people with ataxia to perform intended tasks such as feeding themselves. There are three ways of reducing the effects of ataxia: (1) isolation from direct control, (2) modification of feedback, and (3) mechanical loading for increasing inertia by adding a spring with a definite stiffness, by adding mass, and by viscous damping. Many damped orthoses have been created for many activities of daily living.

The ICF model suggests that we intervene at multiple lower levels (e.g., pathology and impairment) in order to improve the higher levels of function and life role participation. With the ICF model proffering the challenge of restoring life role participation, it then becomes important to design and test interventions that result in impairment gains sufficiently robust to be reflected in functional activities and further in life role participation. Fortunately, CNS plasticity and associated motor learning principles can serve well as the basis for generating such interventions. These principles are useful in generating both efficacious gait training and efficacious upper limb functional training interventions. These principles also supported incorporation of functional task practice and the demand of attention to task practice within the intervention. The ICF model provided the challenge to restore function and life role participation. The means to that end was provided by principles of CNS plasticity and motor learning.

Despite multimodal intervention, persistence of tandem gait abnormality [8] is particularly common.

Treadmill may be a useful tool to improve gait control in ataxic patients [9] with possible gains in walking speed, Timed Up and Go, step length and balance, and Rivermead Visual Gait Assessment. Freund and Stetts [10] to improve trunk stabilization proposed a training and locomotor training (LT) using body-weight [11] support on a treadmill (BWST). They reported improvement in movement, transverse abdominis thickness, and isometric trunk [12] endurance tests after 10 weeks of intervention.

Trunk control improvement has to be one of the main goal of posttraumatic ataxia rehabilitation. In this way conventional [13] Bobath approach, also in its "modern" reconceptualization [14, 15], seems to be still nowadays the best approach to regain the ability to move selectively and the ability to produce coordinated sequences of movement and vary movement patterns to fit a task, on the basis of sensory input in motor behavior and learning.

Contemporary practice in the Bobath concept utilizes a problem-solving approach to the individual's clinical presentation and personal goals [16]. Treatment is focused towards remediation, where possible, and guiding the individual towards efficient movement strategies for task performance [17].

References

1. Dietz HC et al (1992) The coordination of posture and voluntary movement in patients with cerebellar dysfunction. Mov Disord 7(1):14–22
2. Marsden CD (1975) The physiological basis of ataxia. Physiotherapy 61(11):326–328
3. Solari A, Filippini G, Gasco P, Colla L, Salmaggi A, La Mantia L, Farinotti M, Eoli M, Mendozzi L (1999) Physical rehabilitation has a positive effect on disability in multiple sclerosis patients. Neurology 52(1):57–62

4. Grimaldi L et al (1986) Evocazione di componenti motorie assenti nelle lesioni del sistema nervoso centrale. 11. Criteri di organizzazione degli atti motori. Giardini, Pisa
5. Gasco P (1994) La terapia riabilitativa dei pazienti con sclerosi multipla. In: Cazzullo CL et al (eds) Sclerosi Multipla. Masson, Milano
6. Morgan MH et al (1975) Intention tremor-a method of measurement. J Neurol Neurosurg Psychiatry 38:253–258
7. Sanes JN et al. (1988) Visual and mechanical control of postural and kinetic tremor in cerebellar system disorders. J Neurol Neurosurg Psychiat 51:934–9438; Daly JJ, Ruff RL (2007) Construction of efficacious gait and upper limb functional interventions based on brain plasticity evidence and model-based measures for stroke patients. Sci World J 7:2031–2345. doi: 10.1100/tsw.2007.299
8. Walker WC, Pickett TC (2007) Motor impairment after severe traumatic brain injury: A longitudinal multicenter study. J Rehabil Res Dev 44(7):975–982
9. Vaz DV, Schettino Rde C, Rolla de Castro TR, Teixeira VR, Cavalcanti Furtado SR, de Mello Figueiredo E (2008) Treadmill training for ataxic patients: a single-subject experimental design. Clin Rehabil 22(3):234–241
10. Freund JE, Stetts DM (2010) Use of trunk stabilization and locomotor training in an adult with cerebellar ataxia: a single system design. Physiother Theory Pract 26(7):447–458
11. Hewer RL et al (1972) An investigation into the value of treating intention tremor by weighting the affected limb. Brain 95579–590
12. Michaelis J (1993) Mechanical methods of controlling ataxia. In: Bailliere's (ed) Clinical neurology. Bailliere's Clinical Neurology 2(1): 121–139
13. Graham JV, Eustace C, Brock K, Swain E, Irwin-Carruthers S (2009) The Bobath concept in contemporary clinical practice. Top Stroke Rehabil 16(1):57–68
14. Keser I, Kirdi N, Meric A, Kurne AT, Karabudak R (2013) Comparing routine neurorehabilitation program with trunk exercises based on Bobath concept in multiple sclerosis: pilot study. J Rehabil Res Dev 50(1):133–140
15. Karthikbabu S, Nayak A, Vijayakumar K, Misri Z, Suresh B, Ganesan S, Joshua AM (2011) Comparison of physio ball and plinth trunk exercises regimens on trunk control and functional balance in patients with acute stroke: a pilot randomized controlled trial. Clin Rehabil 25(8):709–719
16. Brock K, Haase G, Rothacher G, Cotton S (2011) Does physiotherapy based on the Bobath concept, in conjunction with a task practice, achieve greater improvement in walking ability in people with stroke compared to physiotherapy focused on structured task practice alone?: a pilot randomized controlled trial. Clin Rehabil 25(10):903–912
17. Serrao M, Mari S, Conte C, Ranavolo A, Casali C, Draicchio F, Di Fabio R, Bartolo M, Monamì S, Padua L, Pierelli F (2013) Strategies adopted by cerebellar ataxia patients to perform U-turns. Cerebellum 12(4):460–468

Rehabilitation in Polytrauma

35

E. Spadini

Perceptive surface (SUPER) represents a new therapeutic system based on interaction between the body surface of the patient and a perceptive support through small latex hemispheres. Hemispheres consist of materials varying in height and elasticity and are applied to the bed. Patient is laid up on the bed, stimulating cutaneous and proprioceptive receptors and allowing an antalgic reflex and a relaxing action.

35.1 SUPER in the Proprioceptive Rehabilitation of Polytraumatized Patients

In our case series, we present four cases of high-energy fractures and internal injuries in polytraumatized patients. Prolonged immobilization, the long wait for a complete healing of internal injuries, and a precarious stabilization of the fractures prevented carrying out other rehabilitative treatments.

Our sample is composed of four patients, three males and one female between 25 and 42 years old, coming into our department from the Emergency Room. All patients had multiple fractures and internal injuries (liver, lung, spleen, kidney, bladder).

Generally, treatment was articulated in 6 sessions of 1 h per week for a month and then three weekly sessions of 45 min. Duration of stay in the hospital was from 45 days to 3 months.

SUPER hemispheres were composed of latex applied to a bed, positioned next to the body surface of the patient. Hemispheres vary in height, from 4 to 8 cm, and elasticity, being composed by materials of different characteristics that can resume as soon as possible the original form.

E. Spadini
Neuromotor Rehabilitation Unit, "San Filippo Neri" Hospital, Rome, Italy
e-mail: e.spadini@sanfilipponeri.roma.it

D.C. Alpini et al. (eds.), *Whiplash Injuries*,
DOI 10.1007/978-88-470-5486-8_35, © Springer-Verlag Italia 2014

There are three types, corresponding to different colors: yellow, a soft surface; pink, hard surfaces; and blue, harder surfaces. Altogether, hemispheres create a perceptive support that interacts with patient's body surface. Different degrees of elasticity, different heights, and their location are determined by the operator.

The first session was for sensory-motor evaluation: it was to keep confidence with the tool, using the average modulus (pink) as a reference midline and the remaining neutral (yellow). Essential conditions for the therapeutic effectiveness were mastoid reference alignment for anatomical median line, the comfort of patient, the contact surface with the body surface, and the guidance of the therapist. After a few minutes of adaptation and relaxation, the perception of the patient was assessed qualitatively (recognition of stocks) and quantitatively. The patient was asked to describe the sense of body position in general and then in particular the symmetry of loading and the symmetry of the trunk; the curves of the spine; any torsions, translations, and rotations; the support of the foot; and the presence of minor or plus areas of support. After about 30 min, skin signs, left by hemispheres, were evaluated.

Further processing is divided into a perception stage, a perceptual-motor stage, and an active phase, which imply different moments and whose aims are, respectively, recovery of ability to gather information from surfaces of the trunk and the trunk capacity of fragmented elements significant for the task.

35.2 Case Description

Male patient, 42 years old, was admitted to our department for neuromotor rehabilitation, with a diagnosis of polytrauma, left acetabular fracture, diastasis (6 cm) of the symphysis pubis, liver laceration, large open abdominal injuries, ablation of the spleen, and bladder trauma. The prospect of prolonged immobilization, the long wait for a complete healing of internal injuries, a poor stabilization of the pelvis, and a new intervention for the implementation of fixing, in which the pieces could not be subject to the risk of a septic state, have prevented from carrying out other rehabilitative treatment (Fig. 35.1).

SUPER rehabilitation program was carried out in daily sessions for 1 month (1 h) and then three weekly sessions of 45 min (Fig. 35.2).

At the end of rehabilitation, we observed an acceptable realignment of bone heads in all cases and a complete recovery of deambulation, pain reduction as demonstrated by VAS, a good postural control with a full consciousness of the anatomical median line and the body surface, and, finally, a good motor functional outcome. SUPER showed a useful alternative treatment where we cannot resort to other therapeutic means. More studies should be conducted to analyze SUPER.

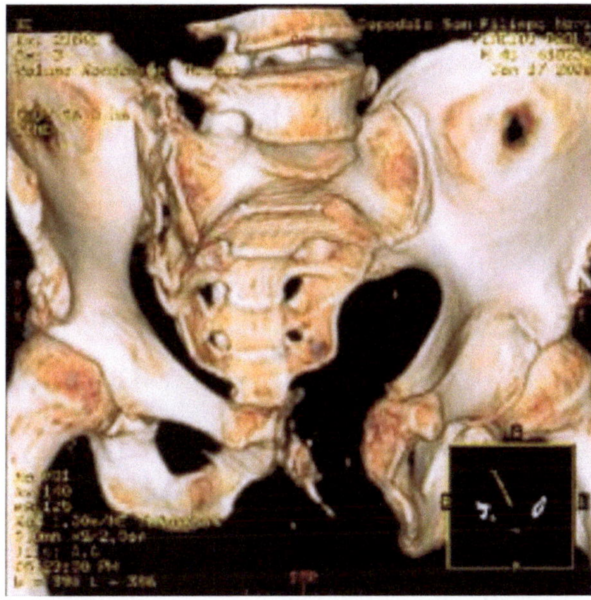

Fig. 35.1 MS CT scan of the described patient

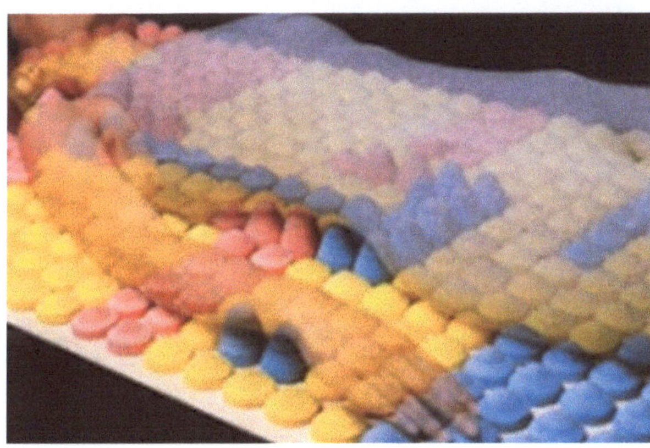

Fig. 35.2 The bed for perceptive surface

Acupuncture and Chinese Medicine: Cervical Disorders and Chronic Pain

36

G. Garozzo

36.1 Introduction

Regarding Chinese medicine, there is always a little bit of prejudice by traditional medical doctors and it is often proposed asthe last chance of therapy, whenever other tretments have failed to cure.

Studying acupuncture with my great Master and Professor, Nguyen Van Ngh, I could observe similarities between the traditional Western medicine and the Chinese one rather than highlight differences [1].

When we talk about medicine, we speak about man, as such, but more as a part of this universe. And it is this, or rather the laws that govern our universe, that make the two medicines (Western and Eastern) the same. The two medicine should never be regarded as conflicting with each other but rather agreeing on the pursuit of health for man.

Prof. Dr. Nguyen Van Nghi has spent all his life in the quest for integration between the two schools of medicine, and he did so through his 10-year study, being able to match part of the famous Rosetta Stone that would allow us to translate a language (such as the synthetic Oriental Medicine) into the analytic of our Western culture.

This integration should not be seen reductively in an explanation of the effects of acupuncture (considering the possible outcomes of Oriental Medicine) as the result of a reflex system. In literature, it has been reported from many years that acupuncture act at a spinal level, modulating the transmition of nociceptive information to the central nervous system and these concepts have been written. However, stimulating acupuncture points with needles, hands or anything else is not only "evoking a reflex", but include a more complex emotional individual response. In the same

G. Garozzo
Acupuncture and Traditional Chinese Medicine,
Artemedica via privata Angera 3, 20125 Milano, Italy
e-mail: gaudenzio62@msn.com

D.C. Alpini et al. (eds.), *Whiplash Injuries*,
DOI 10.1007/978-88-470-5486-8_36, © Springer-Verlag Italia 2014

manner, smiling "after receiving a caress" or "meeting someone you love" is not only a reflex.

Firstly, we want to focus that Traditional Chinese Medicine is one of the oldest Schools of Medicine. The concepts with which it deals with Traditional Chinese Medicine starts considering that man is indivisible, and that there is an intersection between the soma and the spirit; therefore, physiological, chemical and pathological rules are based on this concept of energy, called "qi". Disruptions of the flow of energy thorugh the body are believed to be responsible for disease. It is a genuinely fascinating medicine, its diagnostic approach which takes into account the uniqueness of Man is very advanced considering unsuspected relationships still to be proved by western medicine.

For example, in Oriental Medicine we speak of the *heart* as the center of the whole human being and as emperor (using the way they speak) of a universe related to it. Saying so, it explains the functions and relationships, and one of them is its ability to be the element of "fire" of the entire body (the one that heats and burns). Well, myocardial cells produce two hormones, ANP and BNP, that are able to stimulate lipolysis and thermogenesis, two processes known to consume fats (ANP was discovered in 1981 by a group of experts in Kingston, Canada, led by Adolfo J. de Bold, after noting that the injection of extracts of atrial tissue [but not ventricular] in laboratory mice caused abundant natriuresis [release of sodium in the urine]).

The ANP is involved in the homeostatic control of water, sodium, potassium and fat that is present in the organism. It is released in response to an excessive increase in blood volume (high blood pressure) by particular myocytes, in the auricola of the right atrium of the heart. The ANP acts on the kidneys, to reduce the water, sodium and adipose loads in the circulatory system, thereby lowering blood pressure.

BNP (brain natriuretic peptide) is a vasoactive hormone secreted by the heart – to be exact, by the ventricles – in response to excessive dilation or increased wall stress.

So the two medicines speak the same language but must be analyzed by a tool that can be the equivalent of the Rosetta Stone.

Starting from this premise, it is therefore imperative in order to understand the explanation of pathological mechanisms, to know a bit about the organization of our bodies according to the Eastern point of view.

From an anatomical point of view, provided with the understanding of the anatomical and physiological common acquisitions, Chinese medicine tells us about other structures of different types of energy. Briefly, we can say that in addition to muscles, tendons, blood vessels, tissues, and others, Chinese medicine tells us about the energetic pathways that give us the opportunity to communicate and distribute the set of all the energies in our bodies.

These are called meridians, or as they are called in Chinese "jing luo." In fact, Chinese medicine does no more than clarify the effect and function of substances such as hormones, whose qualities and functions we know, but we believe then that they can only move through traditional anatomical pathways.

So to exemplify all, we say that there are different locations and functions of this pathway, enabling us to divide them as follows:

1. Main meridians or jing mai (12)
2. Secondary meridians are the following:
   (a) jing jin or tendino-muscular meridians (associated in group of three and divided into yin and yang meridians);
   (b) jing bie or divergent meridians (associated in pairs respecting Internal-External the rule, or "biao-li" in Chinese);
   (c) connecting meridians at the Luo points: the 12 regular meridians, externally-internally related in pairs, are linked together by the Luo (connecting) points e related connenting meridians (16 for the former and 12 for the scondary in order to correlate each yin primary meridian with its yang primary meridian); and
   (d) qi jing ba mai or 8 extraordinary vessel (in number of eight associated in pairs).

The different energies can instead be divided into several groups, but for the sake of simplicity, just remember:

(a) Ying Qi – also called Nutritive Energy
(b) Wei Qi – also called Defense Energy
(c) Jing Qi – also called Acquired Energy
(d) Shen Qi – also known as Mental Energy
(e) Yuan Qi – also called Ancestral Energy
(f) Tian Qi – also called Respiratory Energy
(g) Gu Qi – also called Food Energy
(h) Zong Qi – also called Pectoral Energy

36.2 The Tendon-Muscular Meridians (TMM)

The TMM are large vessels that:

1. Start from jing distal points
2. Affect the tendons and muscles
3. Do not penetrate the organs and viscera,
4. Their paths go from bottom to top
5. Play a significant role in the disease known as "external factor"
6. Are not subject to the laws of Yin/Yang alternation.

The three yang meridians of the foot correspond to spring, which are the first, second and third months of the lunar year:

- TMM Stomach is the first month
- TMM Bladder is the second month
- TMM Gall bladder is the third month.

The three yin meridians of the foot correspond to autumn, i.e., on the seventh, eighth and ninth months of the lunar year:

- TMM Spleen/Pancreas is the seventh month
- TMM Kidney is the eighth month
- TMM Liver is the ninth month

The three yang meridians of the hand correspond to summer, i.e., the fourth, fifth and sixth months of the lunar year:

- TMM Intestine is the fourth month
- TMM Small intestine is the spring month.
- TMM San Jiao (also commonly and incorrectly called Triple Burner) is the sixth month

The three yin meridians of the hand correspond to winter, i.e., the tenth, eleventh and twelfth months of the lunar year:

- TMM Pericardium is the tenth month
- TMM Lung is the eleventh month
- TMM Heart is the twelfth month

36.2.1 Bladder

Disorders of the TMM of the bladder (Fig. 36.1) are popliteal muscle contractures, the feeling of a broken spine, contracture of the tendons and muscles of the neck, inability to raise the arm, stabbing pain in the axilla and the supraclavicular fossa, headache, and facial neuralgia.

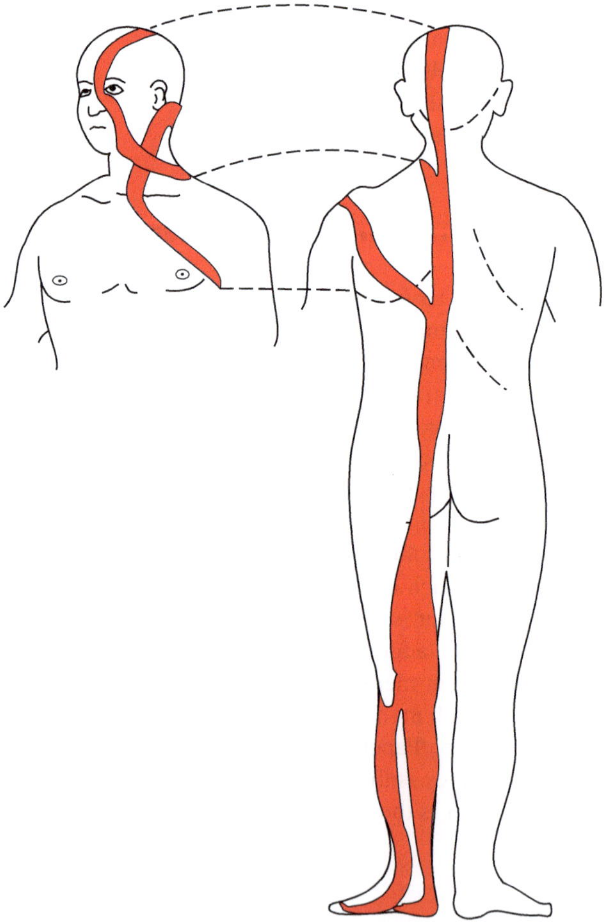

Fig. 36.1 Start at the external corner of the nail of the 5th finger (B67) up to the lateral aspect of the knee (B39), from here: a vessel goes down to the heel, back to the popliteal fossa (B40); a vessel up to the buttock, the medial part of the back and reaches the neck (B10), reaches the base of the tongue, a vessel reaches the skull down to the m around the eye (B2), cheekbone; a vessel reaches the armpit, St12 and reaches the mastoid

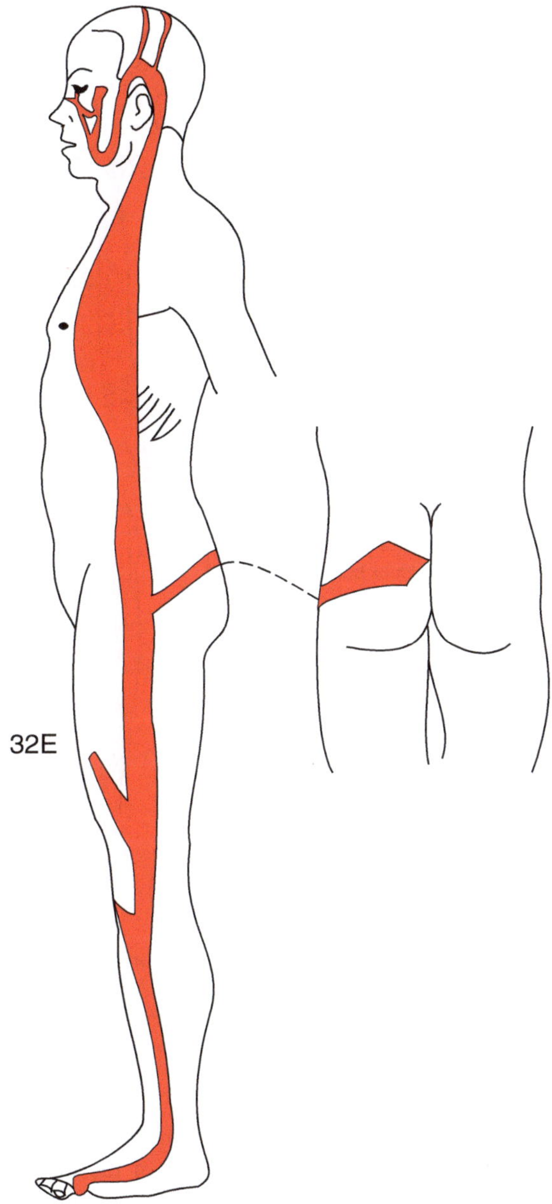

Fig. 36.2 Starts at the external nail of the 4th toe (GB44), climbs the outside face of the legs, inserted on the knee, penetrates to the area of "rabbit crouching" (St32), reaches the thigh and the hip, where a vessel surrounds the buttock, and arrives at the coccyx (DU1). The main vessel climbs to the false ribs, divides into two branches, one arriving at the breast to the supraclavicular fossa St12, the other goes to St8, rises to Baihui, comes back down to the chin and cheekbone SI18, and enters the bone in the external commissure of the eye

36.2.2 Gall Bladder

Disorders of the TMM of the gall bladder (Fig. 36.2) are the inability to stretch and flex the knee associated with pain in the popliteal fossa, pain in the antero-external part of the thigh to the hip, pains in the side up to the ribs, side, chest, breast, supraclavicular region, contracture and pain in the leg up to the lateral malleolus, and contracture of the 4th toe.

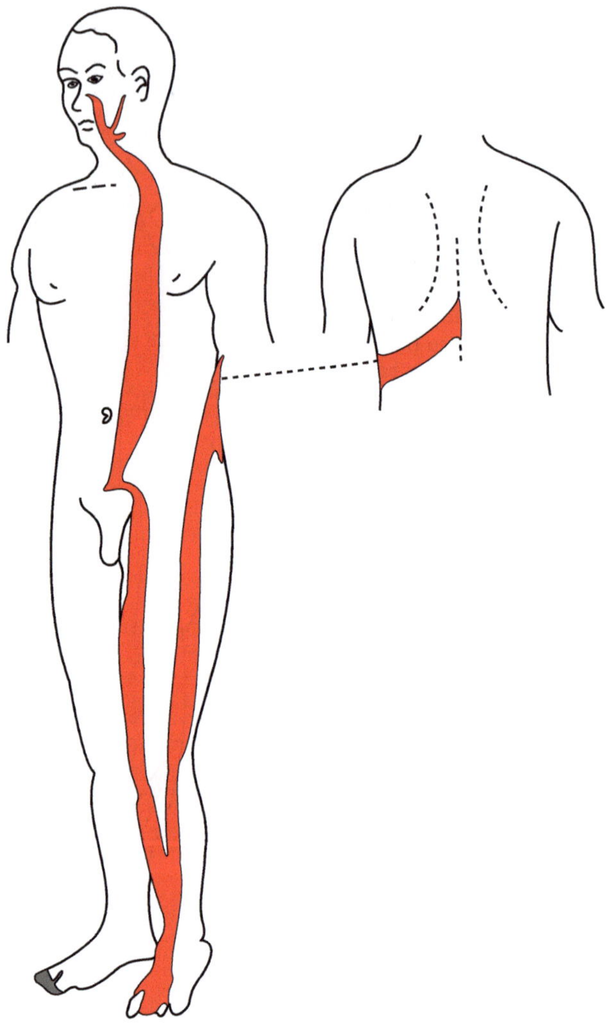

Fig. 36.3 Starts from the external side of the nail of the 2nd, 3rd and 4th toe, rises to the instep and is divided into two branches. The external branch goes up to the Huan Tiao hip point (GB30), goes to the false ribs and is inserted on the spine (DU9). The internal branch goes from the dorsum of the foot, climbs to below the patella and joins the regular meridian of GB; The vertical section runs through the area of the "rabbit crouching" (St32), arrives at Scarpa's triangle, up to RM2 and goes to the m. rectus abdominis, rising up to St12 to the cheekbone (SI18) and to the nose, then to the regular meridian of bladder

36.2.3 Stomach

Disturbances of TMM of the stomach (Fig. 36.3) are swelling below the groin, orchitis, contracture and stiffening of the dorsum of the foot, contracture of the thigh area known as "rabbit crouching," contracture and tightening of the abdominal muscles, sudden deformation of the mouth, pain radiating to the supraclavicular fossa and cheek, contracture of the 2nd toe and leg.

36.2.4 Spleen/Pancreas

Disturbances of TMM of the spleen (Fig. 36.4) are pain in the tibia and knee, pain in the medial side of the thigh, up to the groin, shooting pains in the external

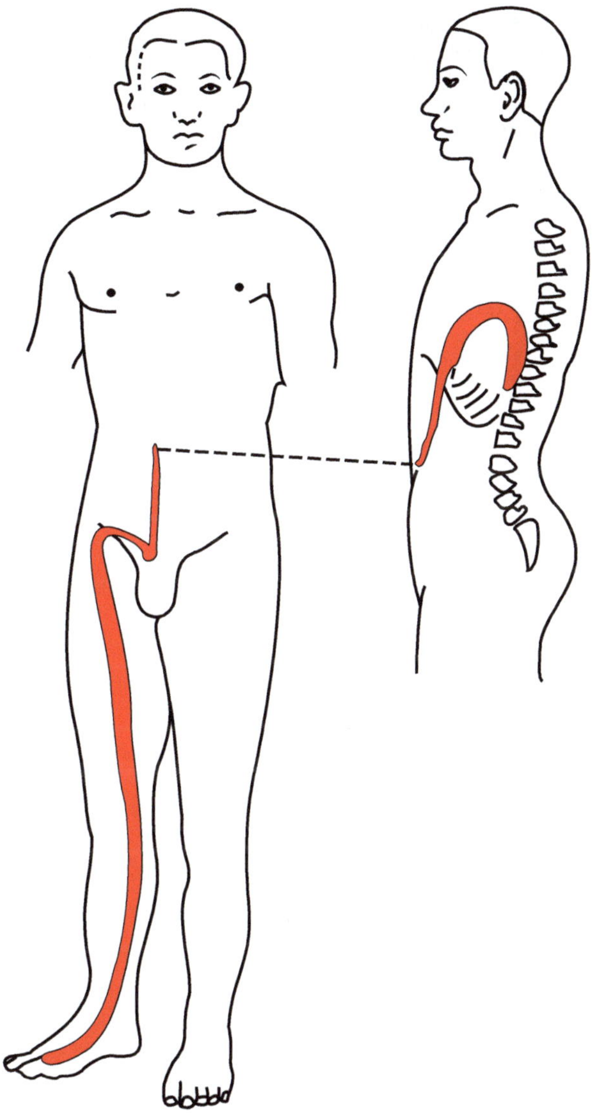

Fig. 36.4 Starts at the medial corner nail of the big toe, goes to the internal malleolus, ascends along the medial aspect of the thigh, reaches Scarpa's triangle, converges towards the external genitalia, penetrates the abdomen, reaches the navel, and then the ribs and the internal part of the thorax. A vessel, from the external genitalia, arrives at the spine

genitals, pain in the navel and hips, widespread pain in the chest and spine, contractures and cramps in the big toe and the internal malleolus.

36.2.5 Liver

Disturbances of TMM of the liver (Fig. 36.5) are contractures and pain in the medial thigh muscle, pain to the tibia tuberosity and medial side of the knee, pain in the big toe up to the internal malleolus, and genital disorders with impotence.

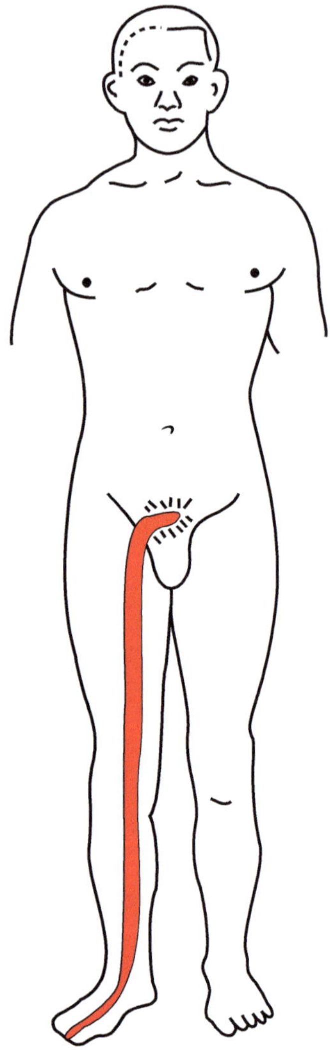

Fig. 36.5 Starts at the big toe, climbs in front of the internal malleolus, passes forward to the spleen jing jin, following the tibia right below the internal tuberosity, up to the groin, converges to the external genitalia to get together with other MTM in the suprapubic region to RM3

36.2.6 Kidneys

Disturbances of TMM of the kidney (Fig. 36.6) are contractures and pain along the entire path, contractures of the plantar muscles, abdominal contracture with the sensation of an anterior weight on the body associated with limiting the ability to bend backwards, abdominal contracture to the external side with a sensation of weight lumbar associated with a limitation to bend forward.

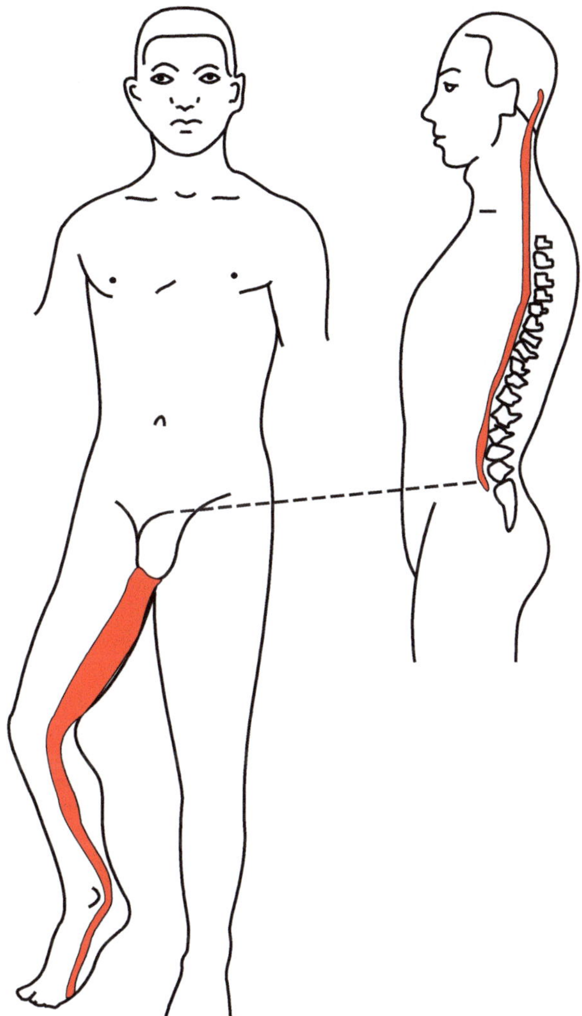

Fig. 36.6 Starts below the 5th toe, reaches Ki1 and follows the TMM of the spleen up to the internal malleolus. Reaches the heel, ascends along the medial aspect of the leg to the internal tuberosity of the tibia, then up to the groin. Converges in the genital region, penetrates the abdomen (RM3) and following the anterior aspect of the spine, a vessel starts to the genital area, passes through the buttock of the opposite side, follows the lateral aspect of the spine, up to the occiput and joins with the TMM of the bladder to B10

36.2.7 Small Intestine

Disturbances of TMM of the small intestine (Fig. 36.7) are pains in the back side of the shoulder to the neck, hearing loss, pains in the ear and chin, eyes closing a moment before looking, muscular contracture of the neck (torticollis), possible pain throughout the path of TMM, internal side pain of the arm from the armpit to the little finger.

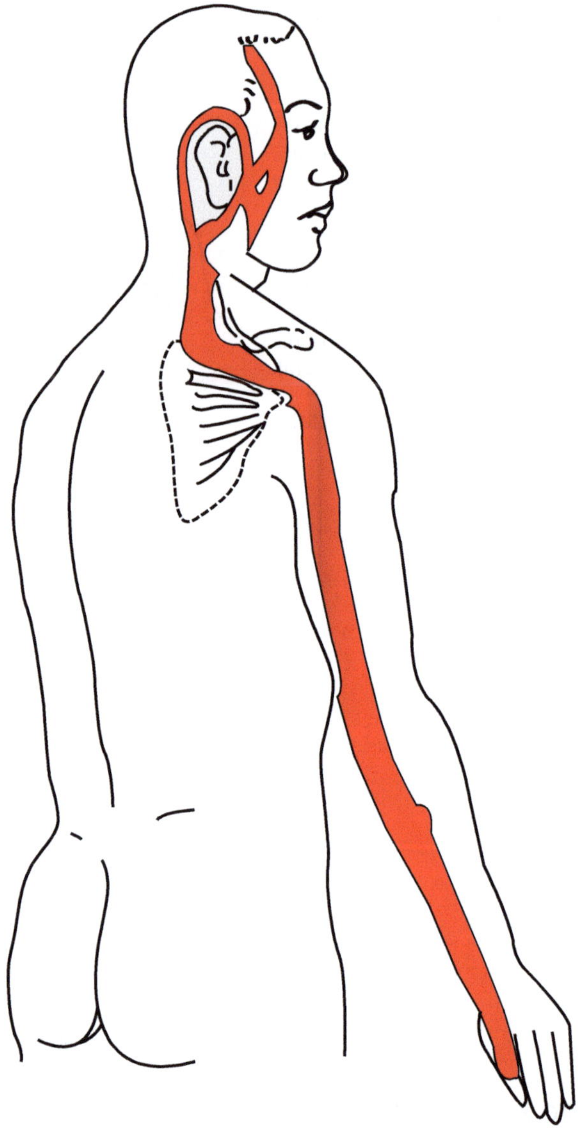

Fig. 36.7 Starts at the external side of the little toenail, goes to the medial epicondyle, reaches the armpit, goes around it, goes to the back side of the shoulder, then up to the neck where it divides into two branches: the secondary branch goes to the mastoid, goes around the ear, then to the jaw and up to the outer canthus of the eye. The main branch goes on the corner of the jaw, St6, passes in front of the tragus, up to the outer corner of the eye and ends at the fronto-parietal region

36.2.8 San Jiao

Disturbances of TMM of san jiao (Fig. 36.8) are contracture and cramping of the entire path, contracture and retraction of the tongue.

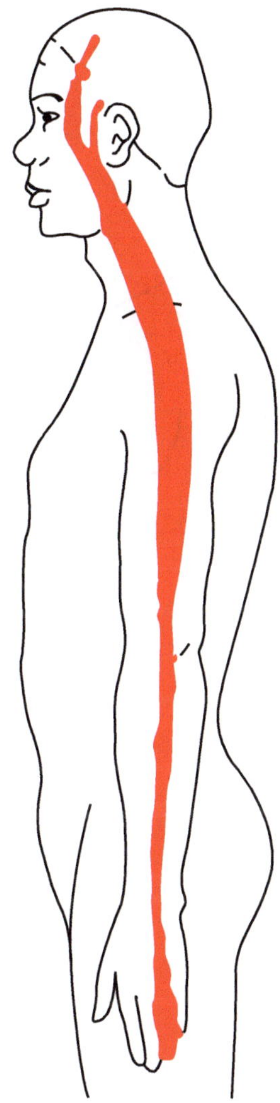

Fig. 36.8 Starts at the external corner of the nail of the 4th finger, goes to the wrist, follows the medial part of the forearm, inserted the olecranon, and climbs up to the shoulder and neck, joins the regular meridian, arrives at the corner jaw (SI17) and is divided into two branches: a vessel enters the throat, reaches the base of the tongue; a vessel from the corner jaw goes to St6, passes in front of the ear, comes to the outer corner of the eye, and fits on the front of the St8

36.2.9 Large Intestine

Disturbances of the TMM large intestine (Fig. 36.9) are "helmet headache," inability to raise the arm, inability to turn the neck, pain, contracture and cramping on the path.

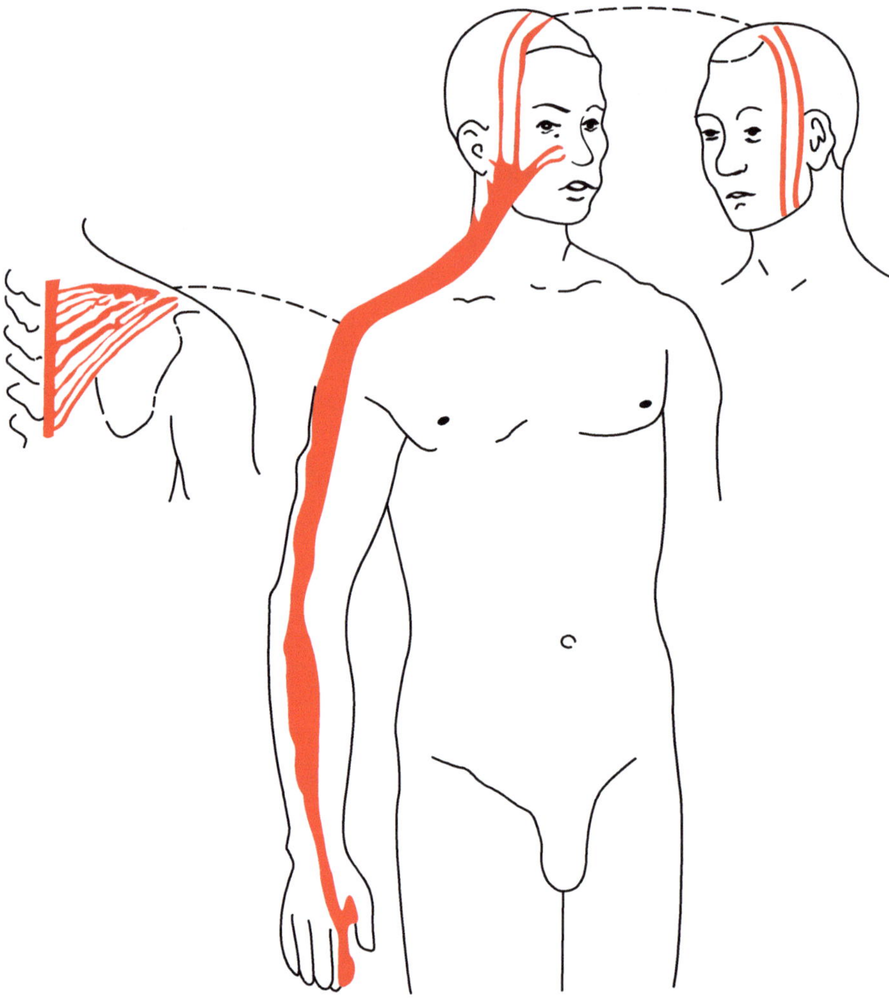

Fig. 36.9 It starts at the external corner of the index fingenr's nail, climbs along the outer edge of the arm (LI11), reaches the jianyu point (LI15) on the shoulder and is split: a branch goes around the shoulder and goes to DU14.The main branch rises to St6, and is divided into two branches, one in the jaw and the other in the cheekbone, one on the forehead at PC 9 up to the corner jaw on the opposite side

36.2.10 Lung

Disturbances of TMM of the lung (Fig. 36.10) are a sore shoulder that cannot be lifted, hypocondralgia, and sometimes haematemesis. The pain, very sharp, causes anxiety and oppression. The muscles on the course of the meridian are contracted or sore.

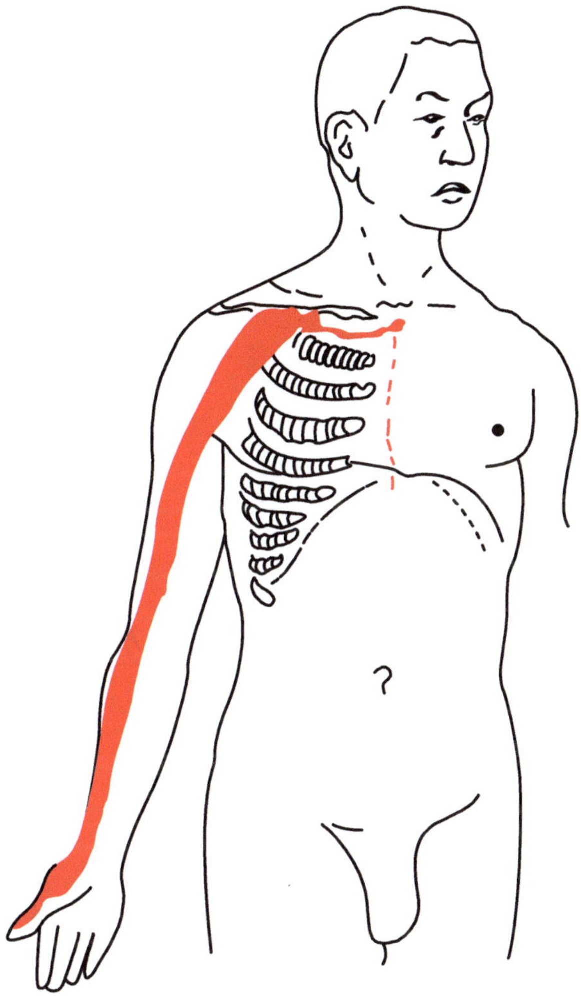

Fig. 36.10 Starts at the inner corner of the thumb nail, goes up to the thenar eminence, passes the external side of the wrist (L10), follows the forearm up to the center of the elbow, back along the medial surface of the arm, enters the armpit, goes to GB22, reappears in the supraclavicular fossa at St12, penetrates into the chest until the it reaches the cardias, goes deeper into the thorax up to the cardias, then reaches the ribs up to RM17 and then to the diaphragm and the cardias

36.2.11 Xin Bao

Disturbances of TMM of xin bao (Fig. 36.11) are chest pain, axillary pain, oppression, contracture and pain on the course of the meridian.

36.2.12 Heart

Disturbances of the TMM of the heart (Fig. 36.12) are the clogging syndrome of the energy at the navel, contractures and pain with a sense of snare at the elbow, contractures and pain in the chest with a painful contracture along the path.

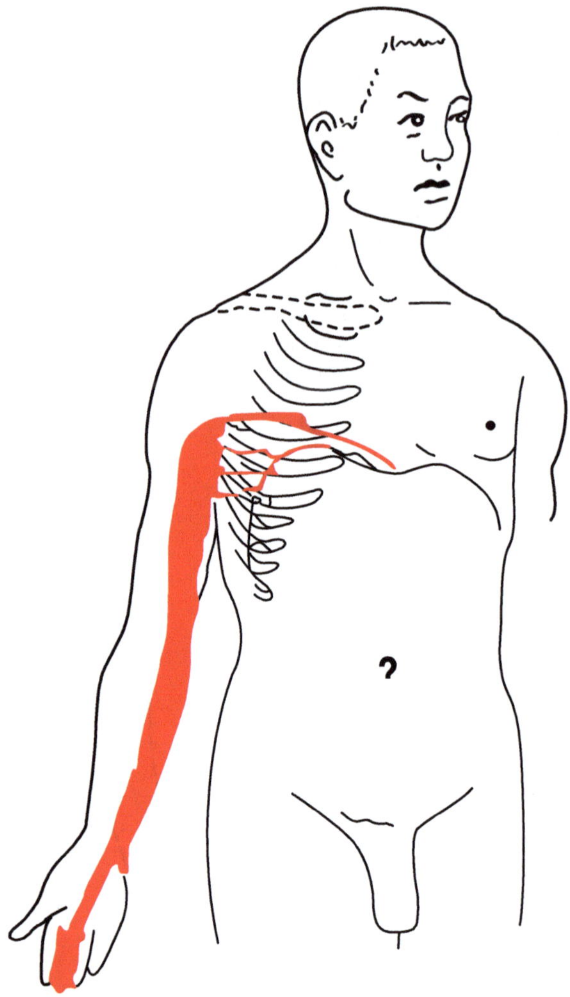

Fig. 36.11 Starts on the external corner of the nail of the middle finger, reaches the center of the elbow, follows the medial side of the arm, fits under the armpit and branches to the ribs. A vessel penetrates deep into the arm, arrives at the inner part of the chest and goes into the cardias

36.3 Whiplash-Associated Chronic Pain Treatment

Acupuncture is widely used for the treatment of neck and other musculoskeletal pain, and there is some evidence supporting its effectiveness for short-term pain relief. The effectiveness of acupuncture in the treatment of whiplash-associated disorders is not clear and, in my experience, the Quebec classification (orthopedic relevance, racture or dislocation of the vertebrae or intervertebral discs with spinal cord compression) and the outcome of whiplash to surgical procedure has to be considered in any way. Considering the classification of the Quebec Task Force, whiplash grade 0-1-2 can be combined and treated as a syndrome of TMM, while grade 3 is related to the Longitudinal Luo of Du Mai Syndrome, although symptoms may persist and then we can find a simultaneous involvement of TMM. We will not

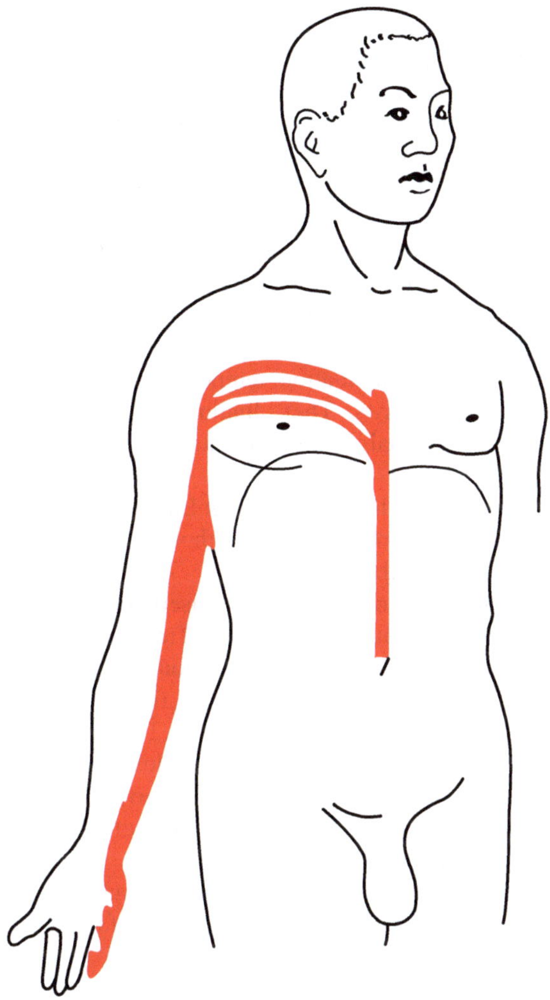

Fig. 36.12 Starts at the internal side of the little fingernail, goes to the styloid process of the ulna, up to the medial aspect of the forearm to the elbow, reaches the armpit and joins with TMM of the lung and SJ to 22GB. Penetrates into the chest and continues into the interior space of the breast, goes to RM17 and down to the cardias and then reaches the navel

consider level 4 in any way because it has to be dealt with in the vascular/orthopedics/surgical field.

When there are symptoms resulting from whiplash, we will certainly find the symptoms that usually accompany you when the tendino-muscular meridian (TMM) and the Luo of Du Mai are involved [2] – not only the path, but above all the special form of presentation (traumatic and therefore recently acquired) that characterize the pathology of this particular type of energies' pathways. That said, it is also necessary to make clear that if the treatment is not for a recent whiplash injury, but for a chronic form of symptoms, it may no longer reflect the pathology of these types of energetic pathways but would cover other types of them, which would better explain the chronic painful traumatic event [3].

Many patients with whiplash-associated chronic pain show features of central sensitization. Randomized trials examining whether treatments are able to influence the process of central sensitization in patients with chronic WAD are emerging. Acupuncture results in activation of endogenous analgesia and relief in symptoms in patients with chronic WAD Quebec 1-2-3.

Tobbackx et al. [4], through a randomized crossover pilot trial with blind assessors, that was performed on 39 patients, have recently shown that local baseline pressure pain sensitivity and during conditioned pain modulation decreased more significantly following acupuncture compared with simple aspecific relaxation, both in the neck and at a site distinct from the painful region. When comparing the long-term effects of acupuncture versus relaxation, no differences were observed in conditioned pain modulation, temporal summation of pressure pain, neck disability, or symptom severity. Their findings suggest that acupuncture treatment activates endogenous analgesia in patients with chronic WAD at least in the short-medium period [5].

The ancient texts of Nei Jing: Ling Shu, and Su Wen describe the treatment to be carried out according to the pathological state of the event, considering first of all the interest of the surfaces:

- Disease found in the skin: insert the needle into the distal jing points of the meridians Interested, jing jin. Treatment of jing distal point, toning point of the meridian, ashi point in dispersion; for the treatment of TMM.
- Disease is in the subcutaneous tissue: insert the needle into the Luo and Shu points of the meridians involved. For the treatment of Luo M.
- Disease is in deep tissues (muscles, bones and joints, after passing the surface layers and the subcutaneous): insert the needle into the Jing proximal points of the yin meridians and the He points of yang meridians. For the treatment of rheumatic disorders.
- Disease (humidity) is in the yin meridians of the lower: o needle the distal jing points and the ying points. For the treatment of rheumatic syndromes located at the bottom.

36.4 Clinical Practice

36.4.1 TMM

Observe whether the radiation of pain extends along the path of TMM.

Check if the point of union of the 3 TMM involved is painful on palpation.

Check the organ/bowels of the main meridian involved.

36.4.1.1 Needling – Declaration of Qi Bo

Needle the distal point jing.

Tonify the main meridian.

Puncture with a needle the point where the three TMM

Puncture with a needle the painful points (ashi) in dispersion, then continue using the stimulator.

Example 1:
Facial pain – TMM yang of the foot (meeting point SI18)

If the pain goes down to the lower jaw moving from the temporal area: facial point + tones the regular meridian of the gall bladder.

If the pain is associated with the inner corner of the eye: facial point + tones the regular meridian of the urinary bladder. If pains go to the wing of the nose, lips, inner corner of the eye: facial point + tones the regular meridian of the stomach.

(Points to tonify: GB43, B67, ST41; Shu points: GB41, B65, ST43.)

Example 2:
Migraine – TMM yang of the hand (meeting point St8-GB13)

If the pain goes to the outer corner of the eye, ear, jaw, neck, shoulder: painful point + tonify the regular meridian of the small intestine.

If the pain goes to the outside corner of the eye, neck, shoulder, and throat, with a contraction of the tongue: painful point + tonify the regular meridian of San Jiao.

If the pain goes to the cheekbone, if you feel the sensation of a helmet that surrounds the forehead and goes to the opposite side of the jaw: painful point + tones the regular meridian of the large intestine (Points to tonify: SJ3, SI3, LI11; Shu: SJ3, SI3, LI3).

Example 3:
Subaxillary pain – TMM yin of the hand (meeting point GB22)

Pain accompanied by a small pain in the shoulder, chest: painful point + tonify the regular meridian of lung.

If it is accompanied by oppression with pain in the hips and chest: painful point + tonify the regular meridian of Xin Bao. If it is accompanied by pain between the heart and navel: painful point + tonify the regular meridian of the heart: subaxillary pain.

(Points to tonify: PC9, Ht9, L9 Shu; PC7, HT7, L9)

36.4.2 Luo Vessel of Dumai-DU

This vessel starts from Changqiang (DU 1) located at the end of the coccyx and goes up to the heart where it branches toward the shoulder.

It communicates with the bladder meridian at the B10 point and penetrates deeply into the muscles. Symptoms may be divided into symptoms of fullness (stiffness of the spine) or symptoms of feeling empty (dizziness with a heavy head).

In the case of "fullness," the treatment is to disperse Changquiang (DU1), while in the case of the "empty feeling," it is necessary to tonify Changquiang (DU1).

Conclusions

Acupuncture is a well-tolerated treatment for people with chronic WAD pain. The main effects are more evident in the short and medium run, thus it is useful to combine Chinese medicine techniques with the traditional western medicine therapies. Findings suggest that acupuncture treatment activates endogenous analgesia in patients with chronic WAD, that acupuncture is more effective than no treatment, a sham, or alternative [6–8] interventions but also that it is often necessary to combine it with manual and supervised exercise interventions and low-level laser therapy.

For whiplash-associated chronic pain, without radicular symptoms, interventions that focused on regaining function as soon as possible are relatively more effective than interventions that do not have such a focus.

References

1. Nguyen-Van-Nghi, Fisch G, Kao J (1973) An introduction to classical acupuncture. Am J Chin Med (Garden City NY) 1(1):75–83
2. Rosted P, Jørgensen A (2009) Acupuncture for a patient with whiplash-type injury. Acupunct Med 28(4):205–206
3. Chen Y, Zheng X, Li H, Zhang Q, Wang T (2011) Effective acupuncture practice through diagnosis based on distribution of meridian pathways & related syndromes. Acupunct Electrother Res 36(1–2):1–18
4. Tobbackx Y, Meeus M, Wauters L, De Vilder P, Roose J, Verhaeghe T, Nijs J (2013) Does acupuncture activate endogenous analgesia in chronic whiplash-associated disorders? A randomized crossover trial. Eur J Pain 17(2):279–289
5. Cameron ID, Wang E, Sindhusake D (2011) A randomized trial comparing acupuncture and simulated acupuncture for subacute and chronic whiplash. Spine (Phila Pa 1976) 36(26):E1659–65. doi: 10.1097/BRS.0b013e31821bf674
6. Hurwitz EL, Carragee EJ, van der Velde G, Carroll LJ, Nordin M, Guzman J, Peloso PM, Holm LW, Côté P, Hogg-Johnson S, Cassidy JD, Haldeman S, Bone and Joint Decade 2000–2010 Task Force on Neck Pain and Its Associated Disorders (2008) Treatment of neck pain: noninvasive interventions: results of the Bone and Joint Decade 2000–2010 Task Force on Neck Pain and Its Associated Disorders. Spine (Phila PA 1976) 33(4 Suppl):S123–S152
7. Hurwitz EL, Carragee EJ, van der Velde G, Carroll LJ, Nordin M, Guzman J, Peloso PM, Holm LW, Côté P, Hogg-Johnson S, Cassidy JD, Haldeman S (2009) Treatment of neck pain: noninvasive interventions: results of the Bone and Joint Decade 2000-2010 Task Force on Neck Pain and Its Associated Disorders. J Manipulative Physiol Ther 32(2 Suppl):S141–S175
8. Bismil Q, Bismil M (2012) Myofascial-entheseal dysfunction in chronic whiplash injury: an observational study. JRSM Short Rep 3(8):57

Acupuncture and Chinese Medicine: Equilibrium Disorders

37

P.L. Ghilardi, C. Borsari, A. Casani, L. Bonuccelli, and B. Fattori

37.1 Introduction

Acupuncture [1] may be considered a valid and efficacious tool in the treatment of cervically originated vertigo, since it intervenes on a known physiopathological substrate [2]. It exerts its function through the activation of the transducers in the skin and in the surface and deep muscles in the neck, which are capable of affecting the vestibulospinal reflex arc [3, 4].

It is well known, in fact, that vestibulospinal reflexes play a fundamentally important role in the maintenance of posture [5].

The above-mentioned physiopathological considerations prompted us to apply acupuncture (particularly as reflex therapy) to disorders in which there is a prevalent alteration in the macular and cervical inputs; this is seen at its utmost in trauma from cervical torsion. In fact, in these patients particularly there is an alteration in the cervical proprioceptive inputs due to stretching of the neuromuscular spindles and the osteo-tendon articulation receptors in the neck [6]. In patients affected by balance disorders of cervical origin and particularly in those with whiplash injury (WI), there is a prevalence of postural disorders linked with alterations in the VSR (vestibulospinal reflex) over those related to VOR (vestibulo-ocular reflex). For this reason, posturographic examination appears to be the most appropriate method for both qualitative and quantitative clinical assessments of the alterations in the postural patterns of these patients and for monitoring their follow-up [7, 8].

P.L. Ghilardi • A. Casani • L. Bonuccelli • B. Fattori (✉)
Institute of Otorhinolaryngology, University of Pisa, Pisa, Italy
e-mail: bfattori@ent.med.unipi.it

C. Borsari
3rd Department of Anesthesiology, Santa Chiara Hospital, Pisa, Italy

D.C. Alpini et al. (eds.), *Whiplash Injuries*,
DOI 10.1007/978-88-470-5486-8_37, © Springer-Verlag Italia 2014

37.2 Methods

Posturographic examination is performed first of all in OE conditions (open eyes) with the patients gazing at an illuminated spot, then in CE (closed eyes). In this routine posture test, we also used sensitisation tests to eliminate and/or disturb one or two of the three sensitive entrances to the posture system (visual, proprio-exteroceptive and vestibular). Two of these tests which we routinely applied were the head retroflexion test (CER) and the head shaking posturography test (CE HST). The posturographic examination of the patient was performed, during the first session, with three investigations consisting each of four tests: OE, CE, CER and CEHST. The first investigation was performed in basal conditions. The second was carried out after simulating acupuncture, that is, by placing four needles on random points of the cervical region so that the patient could feel only subjective stimulation.

This simulation of acupuncture before the true acupuncture session served to exclude the presence of functional components. The third investigation was performed immediately after the actual acupuncture. Thereafter, further sessions were carried out once a week for 3–5 weeks according to the patient's clinical response, and they were always monitored with posturography.

We evaluated by computerised static posturography the postural changes after acupuncture treatment in a group of 27 patients (12 men and 15 women; mean age, 35.7±6.8 SD) having balance disorders caused by cervical torsion due to whiplash injury [9].

Acupuncture was performed by piercing deeply and bilaterally points 10 V (Tienn Chou) and 20VB (Fong Tcheou) with steel needles which were twirled manually for 20 s after insertion. Each session lasted 20 min. We chose these acupuncture points on the basis of the long-established Chinese experience in this field [10, 11].

However, other points may be used with equal results (17TR, 3IG, 62V, ear points, scalp puncture, etc.), though we have not used them in order to maintain uniformity in the investigation. The posturographic examination in our patients with WI confirmed alterations in both OE and CE in 45 % of the cases, though no specific pattern could be distinguished.

The control group consisted of 25 patients complaining of the same symptoms as those recorded by the study group due to whiplash injury but treated with nonsteroidal anti-inflammatory drugs and myorelaxation or with physiotherapy only.

The stabilogram gave a prevalence of wide and arrhythmic oscillations on both planes, though the sagittal plane prevailed over the other (Fig. 37.1). The statokinetic parameters showed an increase, particularly, in the surface. The centre of gravity often appeared shifted to one side (Fig. 37.2).

These findings were seen to be altered even more in the sensitisation tests, particularly, when the head was retroflexed (Fig. 37.3). In CE and CER, analysis peak on 0.1–0.2 Hz of the Fourier spectrogram revealed frequencies shifted towards 0.1–0.2 Hz (Fig. 37.4).

After the first acupuncture session in our experiment, we noticed an improvement in stance in 75 % of our patients. Nevertheless, this result was transient in the majority of cases; once the acupuncture sessions were repeated, this improvement tended to stabilise. After the three to five sessions of acupuncture on our group of

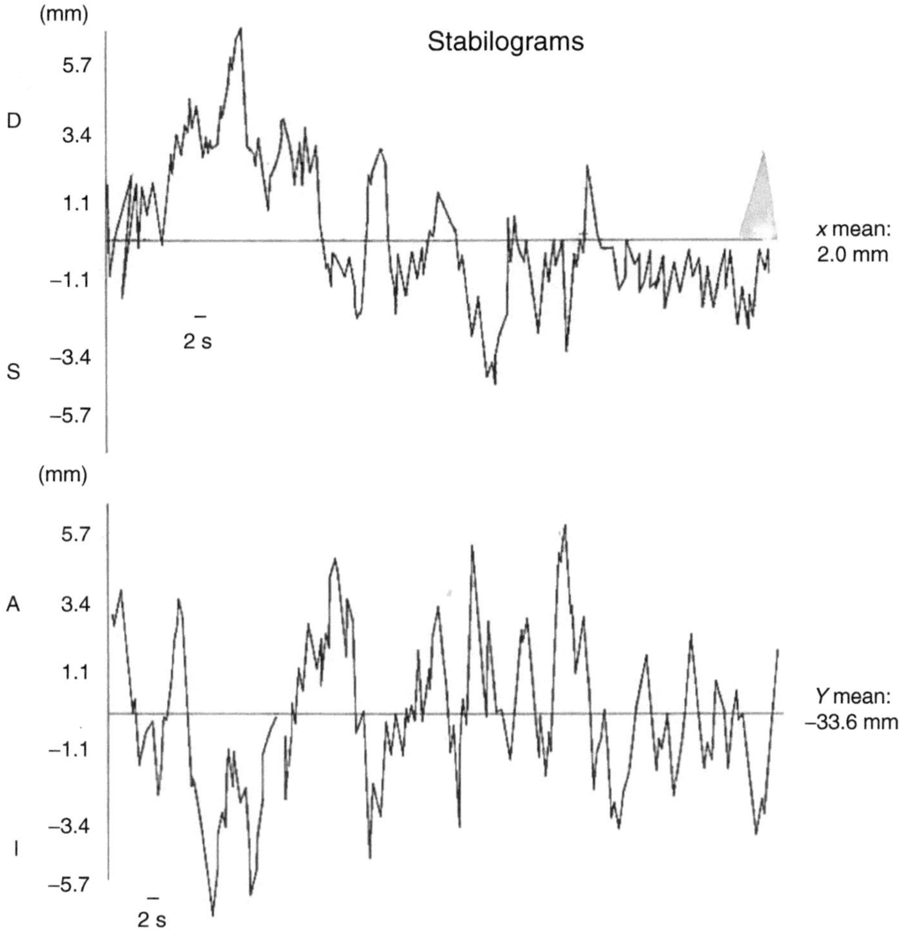

Fig. 37.1 Stabilograms: prevalence of wide and arrhythmic oscillations on both planes, with prevalence on sagittal plane

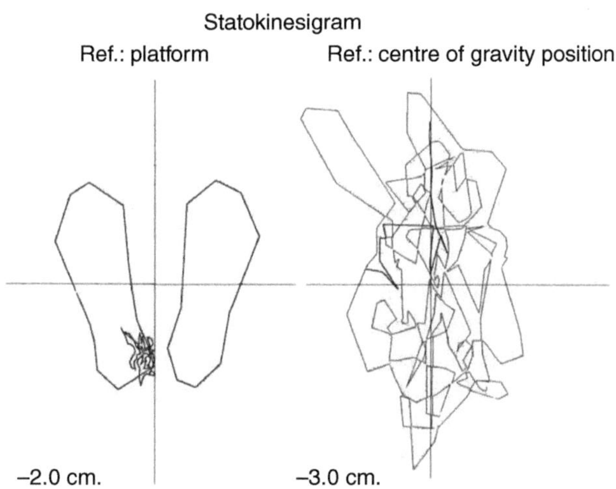

Fig. 37.2 Statokinesigram: the centre of gravity appears shifted to the left

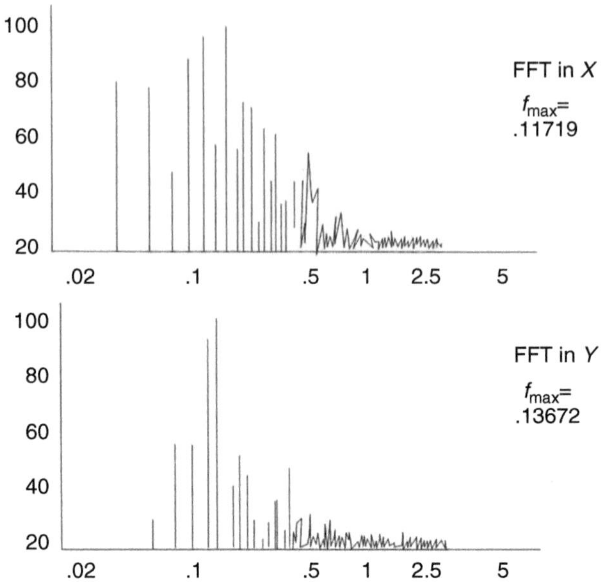

Fig. 37.3 Test performed in CE: the Fourier spectrogram shows a maximal frequency

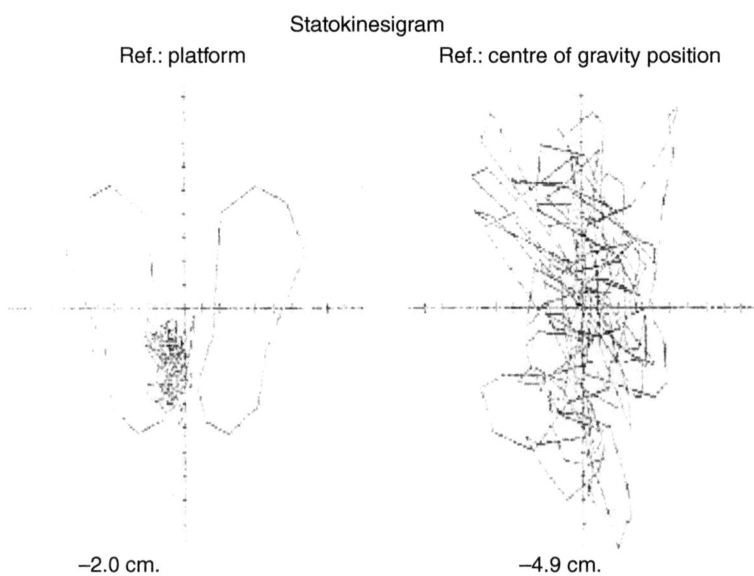

Fig. 37.4 CER test: the statokinesigram shows a remarkable increase of surface

patients with cervical torsion trauma, 60–70 % of the balance disorders were cured, whereas 20 % showed considerable improvement as compared with the initial conditions. The results were nonsatisfactory in only 10–20 % of the patients, either because of a lack of response to acupuncture treatment or due to rapid regression of the improvement achieved once the sessions were over. Cervical torsion trauma and balance disorders with cervical origin in general, such as those connected with pronounced antalgic contracture of the nape muscles due to cervical arthrosis, are the conditions which responded best to acupuncture. In fact, other groups of patients suffering from vertigo of other natures did not respond so well.

In central-type disorders (vasculopathies or neurodegeneration), we saw no positive response to acupuncture in any of the patients we treated and who were always submitted to posturography in the same manner as described before. In the cases of monolateral peripheral vestibular deficiency, we encountered positive responses to acupuncture in 35 %, while no statistically significant improvement ($p > 0.1$) was seen in the posturography performed n the group of patients with cupulolithiasis.

Conclusions

Posture study with the aid of a stabilometric platform can supply an objective assessment of acupuncture efficacy, particularly, in patients with balance disorders of cervical origin. In fact, the stabilometric examination permits quantifying the various postural parametres and gives a graphic description of any shifting in pressure centres on both sagittal and transversal planes; hence it is possible to perform a series of repeated tests which are perfectly comparable with each other. The patients suffering from central-type vertigo disorders, mainly vascular, showed very few variations in stance both before and after acupuncture. The most interesting results were accomplished in the group of patients with balance disorders of cervical origin; these cases showed satisfactory results right from the first acupuncture session, and the postural parametres of the four stabilometric tests became normal in 75 % of the cases. Even the patients with peripheral vestibular disorders, particularly monolateral vestibular damage, had interesting results with an improvement in posture performance in 35 % of the cases, which can very likely be attributed to a plastic and self-corrective rebuilding of the vestibulospinal reflex (VSR) arc produced by acupuncture. Acupuncture stimulation in these situations appears to activate the ascending reticulospinal cerebellar pathways and, therefore, the descending projections which, from the cortical vermis are of the basis of the VSR. There are many clinical reports which confirm the efficacy of acupuncture in balance disorders when performed according to the traditional methods established by ancient Chinese energetic medicine, but there are very few experimental data referring to the neurophysiological and/or neuroendocrinological mechanisms of action of acupuncture in vertigo of cervical origin. In recent years much progress has been accomplished regarding the anatomy and physiology of the acupuncture points, but, above all, modern acupuncture specialists have shifted their interest towards research into the physiological aspects of the points. Present-day research is still far from a thorough explanation of acupuncture, and many hypotheses have been pronounced on this matter: the mechanisms of action are quite definitely many. Acupuncture is certainly capable of interfering with the mechanism of action of numerous neurotransmitters (endogenous opioids, serotonin, P substance, catecholamine, GABA, cortisol, etc.), and it also provokes excitation reflexes and inhibition of the spinal cord (grey gel substance of the periaqueduct), of the bulbar areas (reticular substance) and of the thalamic and cortical regions. Another possible mechanism of action which must be considered, especially in cases of vertigo of cervical origin, is a sympathicolytic action exerted via inhibition of the brainstem reticular substance. These data indicate that this treatment is capable of directly modifying the reflexes which start from the cervical region and which are responsible for balance disorders. One must also take into account an antiedema activity, however, which can reduce the effects of pressure on the posterior roots of the cervical nerves and also a more generalised activity of stabilisation of the basilar vertebral system. The positive effects manifest immediately after even just one acupuncture session; nevertheless, in this experiment, we noticed a decrease in efficacy during the following days which required a series of further sessions of acupuncture in order to stabilise the results, as seen in the follow-up of these patients. The high percentage of positive responses, particularly in the cases of vertigo of cervical origin and less so in those with monolateral peripheral vestibular deficiency, leads us to advocate the therapeutic efficacy of acupuncture, at least in disorders in which it can be associated with or proven as a valid alternative to pharmacological treatment.

No statistically significant advantage of the acupuncture (or laser acupuncture) treatment was found [12] in the acute phase regarding mobility in all three planes, duration of pain and duration of use of a cervical collar, that to say problems regarding myofascial pain and headaches while, in our experience, in the chronic phase of whiplash associated vertigo and dizziness, a considerable reduction of the postural sway that can be obtained. In fact the frequency oscillation on the sagittal plane in CER was reduced in the study group, whereas we noticed a progressive increase of its values in the control group. The high percentage of positive results in whiplash injury patients leads us to advocate acupuncture for chronic balance disorders due to whiplash.

References

1. Chen Zheng Qiu (1993) Participation of GABA in sn emanating descending modulation on the nucleus centrum medianum in motor cortex in acupuncture analgesia. Word J Acupunct Moxibust 3:46–50
2. Coan RM, Wong G, Coan PL (1982) The acupuncture treatment of neck pain: a randomized controlled study. Am J Clin Med 9:327–332
3. Boyle R, Pompeiano O (1981) Convergence and interaction of neck and macular vestibular inputs on vestibulospinal neurons. J Neurophysiol 45:852–868
4. Han J (1988) Central neurotransmitters and acupuncture analgesia. In: Pomeranz B, Stux G (eds) Scientific bases of acupuncture. Springer, Berlin/Heidelberg/New York, pp 7–33, 195
5. Abrahams VC, Richmond FJR (1988) Specialization of sensorimotor organization in the neck muscle system. In: Pompeiano O, Allum JHJ (eds) Vestibulospinal control of posture and locomotion, vol 76, Progress in Brain Research. Eisevier, Amsterdam/New York, pp 125–135
6. Chan SHH, Fung SF (1975) Suppression of polysynaptic reflex by electro-acupuncture and a possible underlying mechanism in the spinal cord of the cat. Exp Neurol 48:336–342
7. Gurfmkel EV (1973) Physical foundation of stabilography. Agressologie 14C:9–14

8. Norré ME, Forrez G (1985) Application otoneurologiques cliniques de la posturographie. Les Cahiers d'ORL 20:255–273
9. Fattori B, Ursino F, Cingolani C, Bruschini L, Dallan I, Nacci A (2004) Acupuncture treatment of whiplash injury. Int Tinnitus J 10(2):156–160
10. Senelar R (1979) Les caractéristiques morphologiques des points chinois. In: Niboyet GEH (ed) Nouveau Traité d'Acupuncture. Maisonneuve, Moulins-Les-Metz, pp 249–277
11. Zhang S, Luo Y, Bo M (1991) Vertigo treatment with scalp acupuncture. J Tradit Chin Med 11:26–28
12. Aigner N, Fialka C, Radda C, Vecsei V (2006) Adjuvant laser acupuncture in the treatment of whiplash injuries: a prospective, randomized placebo-controlled trial. Wien Klin Wochenschr 118(3–4):95–99

Part V

Conclusive Remarks

Management and Treatment of WAD Patients: Conclusive Remarks

38

D.C. Alpini, G. Brugnoni, and A. Cesarani

38.1 Introduction

Whiplash-Associated Disorder (WAD) represents a significant public health problem, resulting in a substantial socioeconomic burden throughout the industrialised world, wherever costs are documented.

WAD is caused by an acceleration-deceleration mechanism of energy transfer to the neck, mainly, and the spine, generally. The most common cause of WAD is a motor vehicle collision (MVC), but sporting accidents or falls can also cause whiplash.

Under the point view of time course, whiplash may be classified as *acute* (less than 2 weeks), *subacute* (2–12 weeks) or *chronic* (longer than 12 weeks).

Under the point of view of lesion, WAD has been classified in 1995, by the Quebec Task Force (QTF) [1], in four progressive grades. According to the QTF, 'whiplash is an acceleration deceleration mechanism of energy transfer to the neck, which…may result in bony or soft tissue injuries (whiplash injury), which in turn may lead to a variety of clinical manifestations (whiplash-associated disorders, "WAD")' (Table 38.1).

D.C. Alpini (✉)
ENT-Otoneurology Service, IRCCS "Don Carlo C. Gnocchi" Foundation, Milan, Italy
e-mail: dalpini@dongnocchi.it

G. Brugnoni
Italian Academy of Manual Medicine, Italian Institute for Auxology, Milan, Italy
e-mail: guido.brugnoni@libero.it

A. Cesarani
Department of Clinical Sciences and Community Health, University of Milan, Milan, Italy

Audiology Unit, IRCCS "Ca' Granda" Ospedale Maggiore Policlinico, Milan, Italy
e-mail: antonio.cesarani@unimi.it

D.C. Alpini et al. (eds.), *Whiplash Injuries*,
DOI 10.1007/978-88-470-5486-8_38, © Springer-Verlag Italia 2014

Table 38.1 Quebec Task Force Classification of Grades of WAD

Grade	Classification
0	No complaint about the neck No physical signs
1	Neck complaint of pain, stiffness or tenderness only No physical signs
2	Neck complaint *and* musculoskeletal signs Musculoskeletal signs include decreased range of motion and point tenderness
3	Neck complaint *and* neurological signs Neurological signs include decreased or absent tendon reflexes, weakness and sensory deficit (e.g. hearing loss) Neck complaint *and* fracture or dislocation

Many treatments have been advocated for patients with WAD, and many diagnostic procedures have been proposed to document lesions or dysfunctions induced by whiplash, but the majority of therapeutic interventions used in the treatment of WAD had undergone little to no scientific investigation. Due to the paucity of scientifically rigorous studies, the QTF was forced to rely on consensus opinion for the majority of their mandated treatment recommendations, offering little in the way of evidence-based clinical guidelines.

The conclusive considerations and remarks presented into this chapters on one hand are based on the main reviews [2–9] and the published guidelines [9] and on the other hand on the personal experience in the field of diagnosis and treatment of WAD.

Under the point of view of symptoms, main WADs regard pain, especially but not uniquely neck pain, and unsteadiness. Thus, both management and treatment in this chapter will be focused on pain and vertigo/unsteadiness.

Management refers to the overall approach to care, or plan, formulated for individual patients; treatment refers to the therapeutic modalities utilised as part of the management approach, including advice and education, exercise, joint mobilisation, pharmacotherapy, etc.

38.2 Management

38.2.1 Acute and Subacute Phases

Neck symptoms, pain and stiffness, are the most common symptoms after a whiplash trauma. Pain often occurs soon, while stiffness can occur later.

Thus, a comprehensive assessment and physical examination of the patient is mandatory (see Chaps. 14 and 21).

The first aim of the assessment in the acute phase is a correct classification of the patient in the QTF WAD grade.

Neck symptoms may exist without objective findings during clinical examination (QTF WAD grade I). Tenderness at palpation over muscle attachments and over muscles in the cervical spine, the shoulder region and/or the back is common (QTF WAD grade II). Approximately 50–60 % of patients who present to emergency rooms have QTF WAD grade II.

It is very important to take in mind that prompt and adequate management of the acute pain reduces the risk of chronic pain.

History taking is a cornerstone of early management of WAD patients of all grades.

Personal and circumstances of the injury have to be carefully collected [10].

Radiological procedure is preferably based on Canadian C-spine rule [11, 12] (Table 38.2).

The most important element of initial assessment is the identification of patients who are at risk of developing serious consequences such as fractures, dislocations (QTF WAD grade IV) or significant neurological damage (QTF WAD grade III).

In QTF WAD grade III, specialised imaging techniques (CT scan and/or MRI) have to be used when nerve root compression or spinal cord injury are suspected.

QTF WAD grade III may be estimated to be documented in 2–6 % of patients even if 20 % of patients report neurological symptoms like paraesthesia, sensory deficit and weakness in an arm or hand.

Dizziness and unsteadiness are very common, while true vertigo is rare. However, when a patient complains vertigo that appears on moving the head or in postural changes, a paroxysmal positioning vertigo (PPV) has to be suspected and adequately treated (see Chaps. 14 and 23-I).

Tinnitus is common enough, while hearing loss is rare. However, when a patient complains of unilateral constant and continuous tinnitus and/or unilateral hypoacusia, a sensorineural sudden hearing loss (SSHL) has to be suspected and adequately investigated and treated (see Chaps. 11, 13, and 17).

In QTF WAD grade IV, when imaging confirms the existence of a fracture, the patient has to be immediately referred for a specialised management.

Table 38.2 Canadian C-Spine Rule

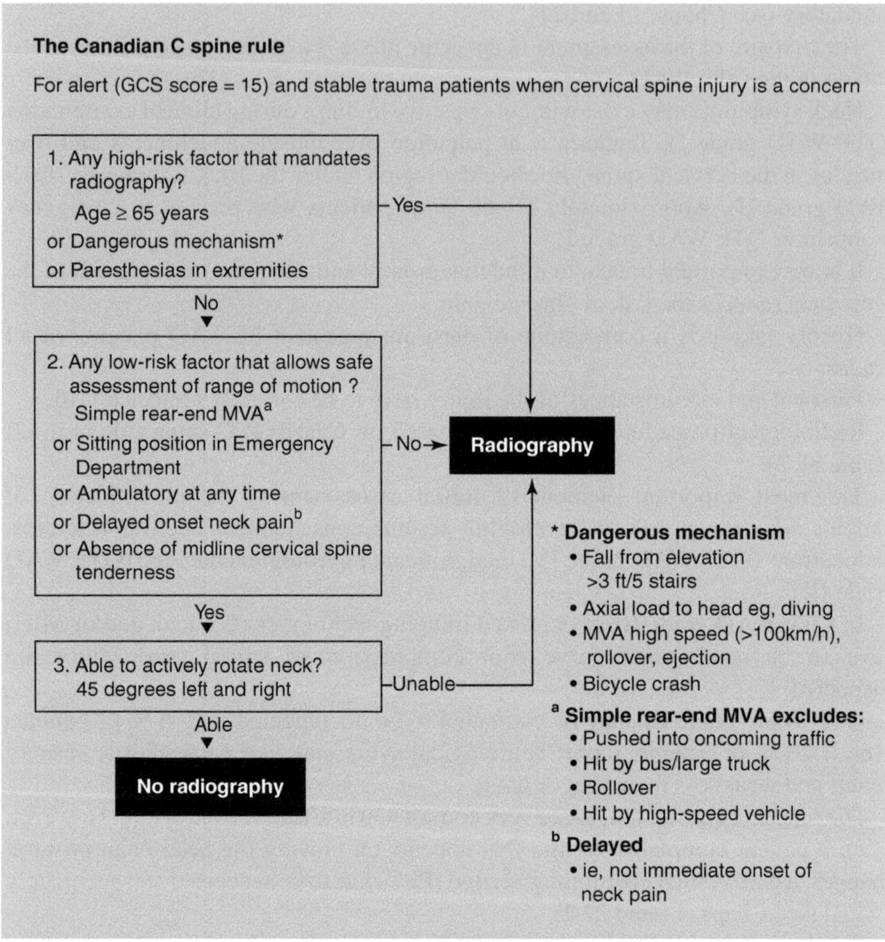

Pain intensity and disability may be quantified using the Visual Analogue Scale (VAS) and the Neck Disability Index [13] (NDI) respectively (Table 38.3).

Table 38.3 Neck Disability Index

Best practice management of whiplash-associated disorders: Clinical resource guide

The Neck Disability Index (NDI)

Instructions

This questionnaire has been designed to give your health practitioner information as to how your neck pain has affected your ability to manage in everyday life. Please answer every section and mark in each section only the ONE box which applies to you. We realise you may consider that two of the statements in any one section relate to you, but please just mark the box which most closely describes your problem.

Section 1 - Pain intensity

- ☐ I have no pain at the moment.
- ☐ The pain is very mild at the moment.
- ☐ The pain is moderate at the moment.
- ☐ The pain is fairly severe at the moment.
- ☐ The pain is very severe at the moment.
- ☐ The pain is the worst imaginable at the moment.

Section 2 - Personal care (washing, dressing etc)

- ☐ I can look after myself normally without causing extra pain.
- ☐ I can look after myself normally but it causes extra pain.
- ☐ It is painful to look after myself and I am slow and careful.
- ☐ I need some help but manage most of my personal care.
- ☐ I need help every day in most aspects of self-care.
- ☐ I do not get dressed, I wash with difficulty and stay in bed.

Section 3 - Lifting

- ☐ I can lift heavy weights without extra pain.
- ☐ I can lift heavy weights but it gives extra pain.
- ☐ Pain prevents me from lifting heavy weights off the floor, but I can manage if they are conveniently positioned, for example on a table.
- ☐ Pain prevents me from lifting heavy weights, but I can manage light to medium weights if they are conveniently positioned.
- ☐ I can lift very light weights.
- ☐ I cannot lift or carry anything at all.

Section 4 - Reading

- ☐ I can read as much as I want to with no pain in my neck.
- ☐ I can read as much as I want to with slight pain in my neck.
- ☐ I can read as much as I want with moderate pain in my neck.
- ☐ I cannot read as much as I want because of moderate pain in my neck.
- ☐ I can hardly read at all because of severe pain in my neck.
- ☐ I cannot read at all.

Table 38.3 (Continued)

Section 5 - Headaches

- □ I have no headaches at all.
- □ I have slight headaches which come infrequently.
- □ I have moderate headaches which come infrequently.
- □ I have moderate headaches which come frequently.
- □ I have severe headaches which come frequently
- □ I have headaches almost all the time.

Section 6 - Concentration

- □ I can concentrate fully when I want to with no difficulty.
- □ I can concentrate fully when I want to with slight difficulty.
- □ I have a fair degree of difficulty in concentrating when I want to.
- □ I have a lot of difficulty in concentrating when I want to.
- □ I have a great deal of difficulty in concentrating when I want to.
- □ I cannot concentrate at all.

Section 7 - Work

- □ I can do as much work as I want to.
- □ I can only do my usual work, but no more.
- □ I can do most of my usual work, but no more.
- □ I cannot do my usual work.
- □ I can hardly do any work at all.
- □ I cannot do any work at all.

Section 8 - Driving

- □ I can drive my car without any neck pain.
- □ I can drive my car as long as I want with slight pain in my neck.
- □ I can drive my car as long as I want with moderate pain in my neck.
- □ I cannot drive my car as long as I want because of moderate pain in my neck.
- □ I can hardly drive at all because of severe pain in my neck.
- □ I cannot drive my car at all.

Section 9 - Sleeping

- □ I have no trouble sleeping.
- □ My sleep is slightly disturbed (less than 1 hr sleepless).
- □ My sleep is mildly disturbed (1-2 hrs sleepless).
- □ My sleep is moderately disturbed (2-3 hrs sleepless).
- □ My sleep is greatly disturbed (3-5 hrs sleepless).
- □ My sleep is completely disturbed (5-7 hrs sleepless).

Section 10 - Recreation

- □ I am able to engage in all my recreation activities with no neck pain at all.
- □ I am able to engage in all my recreation activities, with some pain in my neck.
- □ I am able to engage in most, but not all of my usual recreation activities because of pain in my neck.
- □ I am able to engage in a few of my usual recreation activities because of pain in my neck.
- □ I can hardly do any recreation activities because of pain in my neck.
- □ I cannot do any recreation activities at all.

Poor prognosis is associated with a high pain score (*VAS*>*7/10*) *and/or high disability score* (*NDI*>*40/100*). The presence of either of these factors should alert to the potential need for more regular review of treatment or earlier referral to a specific specialist. Identification of poor prognosis patients is mandatory in order to provide adequate prevention of chronicisation.

Reassessment has to be planned at 7 days, 3 weeks, 6 weeks and 3 months for acute WAD.

At 3 months resolution has occurred in approximately 50 % of acute cases. Treatment should have ceased or, if the patient is still improving, self-management should be promoted.

Patients who still require treatment after 3 months are considered to have chronic WAD.

It could be useful to 'measure' the impact of WAD on patient health and lifestyle through the 'Core Whiplash Outcome Measure' [14] (Table 38.4), a five-item scale that is brief and user-friendly for clinicians. It measures several constructs of health including pain, function and well-being. In addition, it measures the days off work.

Table 38.4 Core Whiplash Outcome Measure

Date: ______________

1. During the past week, how bothersome have your whiplash symptoms been?

- ☐ 1 Not at all bothersome
- ☐ 2 Slightly bothersome
- ☐ 3 Moderately bothersome
- ☐ 4 Very bothersome
- ☐ 5 Extremely bothersome

2. During the past week, how much did your whiplash injury interfere with your normal work (including both work outside the home and housework)?

- ☐ not at all
- ☐ a little bit
- ☐ moderately
- ☐ quite a bit
- ☐ extremely

3. If you had to spend the rest of your life with the whiplash symptoms you have right now, how would you feel about it?

- ☐ very dissatisfied
- ☐ somewhat dissatisfied
- ☐ neither satisfied nor dissatisfied
- ☐ somewhat satisfied
- ☐ very satisfied

4. During the past 4 weeks, about how many days did you cut down on the things you usually do for more than half the day because of your whiplash symptoms?

________ number of days

5. During the past four weeks, how many days did your whiplash symptoms keep you from going to work or school?

________ number of days

Persistent or recurrent vertigo and/or persistent dizziness and unsteadiness have to be investigated.

Vestibular evoked potentials (see Chap. 17-II) are specific to detect vestibular lesion causing relapsing positioning vertigo. Posturography allows a precise documentation of stance control disturbances (see Chap. 15); Smooth Pursuit Neck Torsion Test (SPNTT) and Cranio-Corpo-Graphy (CCG) (see Chap. 16) allow accurate documentation of cervico-cephalic dynamic control disturbances either as oculomotor (SPNTT) and gait (CCG) disturbances.

Handicap induced by persistent dizziness may be quantified by means of the Dizziness Handicap Inventory [15, 16] (Table 38.5).

Table 38.5 Dizziness Handicap Inventory

Instructions: The purpose of this scale is to identify difficulties that you may be experiencing *because of* your dizziness or unsteadiness. Please answer 'yes', 'no' or 'sometimes' to each question. Answer each question as it pertains to your dizziness or unsteadiness problem only.
Does looking up increase your problem?
Because of your problem, do you feel frustrated?
Because of your problem, do you restrict your travel for business or recreation?
Does walking down the aisle of a supermarket increase your problem?
Because of your problem, do you have difficulty getting into or out of bed?
Does your problem significantly restrict your participation in social activities such as going out to dinner, going to movies, dancing or parties?
Because of your problem, do you have difficulties in reading?
Does performing more ambitious activities like sports, dancing and household chores such as sweeping or putting dishes away increase your problem?
Because of your problem, are you afraid to leave your home without having someone accompany you?
Because of your problem, have you been embarrassed in front of others?
Do quick movements of your head increase your problem?
Because of your problem, do you avoid heights?
Does turning over in bed increase your problem?
Because of your problem, is it difficult for you to do strenuous housework or yardwork?
Because of your problem, are you afraid people may think you are intoxicated?
Because of your problem, is it difficult for you to go for a walk by yourself?
Does walking down a sidewalk increase your problem?
Because of your problem, is it difficult to concentrate?
Because of your problem, is it difficult for you to walk around your house in the dark?
Because of your problem, are you afraid to stay at home alone?
Because of your problem, do you feel handicapped?
Has your problem placed stress on your relationships with members of your family or friends?
Because of your problem, are you depressed?
Does your problem interfere with your job or household responsibilities?
Does bending over increase your problem?

38.2.2 Chronic Phase

The prognosis for a whiplash injury is usually favourable, and 90–95 % of patients recover or have only minor remaining symptoms.

However, if symptoms persist more than 2 months after a whiplash injury, there is a considerable risk of long-term problems.

Symptoms such as sleep impairment or memory and concentration problems as well as signs of stress are reported approximately 25 % of the cases.

It is important to establish a correct diagnosis, both morphological (radiological) and functional (motor and neurophysiological). QTF WAD grade has to be reconsidered. For example, symptoms seen in rhizopathy are usually dominated by sensory symptoms in terms of pain and paraesthesia, while motor symptoms in terms of clinically demonstrable paresis are often missing because single muscles are usually innervated by neighbouring nerve roots as well even if EMG changes can be detected at the earliest within several weeks of the injury.

Recent studies focus on cervical ligament and facet joint lesions as specific factor of biomechanical chronicisation of WAD. It is uncommon that ligament injuries can be detected in the acute phase after whiplash trauma, and it is uncommon or radiologically verified instability to present later in the course.

MRI could be an important support to investigate patients developing WAD chronicisation even if pronounced cervical flexor muscles are uncommon.

The most important element of late assessment is thus the identification of patients who have developed serious consequences such as fractures, dislocations (QTF WAD grade IV) or significant neurological damage (QTF WAD grade III) or chronic pain or chronic functional disability.

Reduced cervical range of motion (ROM) is not necessarily associated with ongoing disability after whiplash. Flattened cervical lordosis on X-rays is NOT associated with ongoing pain.

Also crash aspects like direction of impact, speed of impact and seating position in the car are not necessarily associated with ongoing pain and/or disability.

Older age, >75, and gender are not associated, too.

Chronicisation is due to the several physiological changes that occur in both the peripheral and the central nervous system in acute and, when solved, long-term pain associated with whiplash injury. Peripheral sensitisation is characterised by the release of pain-producing substances, such as prostaglandins, bradykinins, cytokines and substance P. Central sensitisation is characterised by the activation of the NMDA receptor, decreased production of endogenous opioids, production of pain-producing substances in the spinal cord and in the brain and activation of a neuronal network that increases the pain impulse.

Although the same phenomena are observed in diffuse and chronic pain not associated with whiplash [17], central sensitisation mechanisms have to be taken in mind when planning the treatment of patient affected with WAD (see Chaps. 21 and 25) [18].

Chronic unsteadiness has to be extensively investigated. The background to the dizziness is usually unclear but, even if there are diagnostic tests that can demonstrate a connection between the dizziness and the whiplash trauma, extensive and specific tests have to be performed with the aim of patient's treatment. Posturography allows a precise documentation of stance control disturbances (see Chap. 15); Smooth Pursuit Neck Torsion Test (SPNTT) and Cranio-Corpo-Graphy (CCG) (see Chap. 16) allow accurate documentation of cervico-cephalic dynamic control disturbances either as oculomotor (SPNTT) and gait (CCG) disturbances.

Chronic dizziness requires also extensive investigation of eye movements (see Chap. 18); chronic tinnitus, which could mask a not-investigated hearing loss, requires an extensive audiological test battery (see Chap. 17).

Handicap induced by persistent dizziness may be quantified by means of the Dizziness Handicap Inventory [15, 16].

Reassessment has to be planned at 2 weeks, 6 weeks and 3 months. If at 6 weeks no significant improvement of pain or functional disability is noted despite multimodal therapeutic approach, the introduction of cognitive behavioural therapy (CBT) is appropriate. In fact several studies indicate an increased occurrence of post-traumatic stress disorder (PTSD) among people who have experienced a car accident. According to the DSM-IV psychiatric diagnostic manual, PTSD is the remaining condition that may follow acute stress disorder (ASD) that may occur after an individual has been exposed to a traumatic event, if the symptoms occur within 1–3 months. This remark highlights the importance of a correct management of WAD in the acute and subacute phases. Thus, it is therefore important during patient visit to gather information about previous conditions and examine the patient's current mental health. Psychiatric consultation is recommended in difficult and/or complicated cases to minimise the risk of long-term PTSD.

Also minor psychological disorders like sleep impairment and anxiety have to be adequately treated in WAD patients.

38.3 Treatment

38.3.1 Acute

Generally speaking, active exercise involving functional exercises and advice to 'act/as/usual' should be routinely undertaken. QTF WAD grade I and II patients should also be advised that voluntary restriction of activity may delay recovery and that it is important to focus on improvement in function.

In QTF WAD grade III, neurological and sensorial disorders have to be promptly treated. Regarding the sensorial and/or functional symptoms that could lead to a QTF WAD grade III classification, it is important to note that the QTF classification states 'symptoms and disorders that can be manifested in all grade include deafness, dizziness, tinnitus, headache, memory loss, dysphagia, and temporomandibular joint pain'.

Thus, for example, in the case of vertigo, positioning vertigo has to be diagnosed and treated by means of the appropriate manoeuvres (see Chap. 23-I). In the case of tinnitus and/or ear fullness, a hearing loss has to be immediately suspected and a complete audiological battery performed: Pure Tone Audiometry is not sufficient to exclude a hearing whiplash-associated damage (see Chap. 17).

38.3.1.1 Unsteadiness

Methylprednisolone, a drug with both neuroprotective and anti-inflammatory effects, is reported to be associated with a significant reduction in disabling symptoms, total number of sick days and sick leave profile at 6 months after injury.

In QTF WAD grades I and II, exercise and mobilisation programmes to improve kinaesthetic sensibility and coordination are indicated, together with educational interventions in which patients are instructed about the nature and course of WAD using personal communication: protect the neck from cold; walk daily; maintain good posture; avoid lifting; and refrain from collar use after the first 2 days.

38.3.1.2 Pain

The successful management of acute pain reduces the risk of chronic pain.

In patients complaining moderately severe pain (VAS scale 5–6), irrespectively of QTF WAD grade, paracetamol in combination with *nonsteroidal anti-inflammatory drug* (NSAID) is indicated.

When pain intensity is severe (>7 in the VAS scale), a central-acting analgesic combined with NSAID is necessary. They could be associated with an antihistamine for emesis even if the combination may improve central sedative effects. Intra-articular injections and intravenous methylprednisolone have no support to be used.

Severe pain in QTF WAD grade III has a very high risk of long-term symptoms. Patients should completely refrain from work for at least 1 week until making a return visit to the doctor for a strict and very careful follow-up.

Immobilisation with a soft collar is less effective than active mobilisation and no more effective than advice to act as usual. In contrast, there is strong evidence that active mobilisation is associated with reduced pain intensity and limited evidence that mobilisation may also improve ROM. Collar use could be suggested for the first 2 days, no more than that. Cervical pillows have to be avoided.

Simple exercise programme promoting mobilisation of the neck is an effective noninvasive intervention. Mobilisation programmes were differentiated from exercise programmes in that exercise programmes had specific treatment aims (e.g. strength and endurance), whereas mobilisation programmes were aimed at simply increasing or maintaining mobility. Although long-term recovery may be unaffected by either exercise or immobilisation in a soft collar during the acute phase of WAD, it appears that exercise programmes are significantly more effective in reducing pain intensity over both the short and medium term. Conversely, supplemental exercise programmes added to mobilisation programmes may not be any more beneficial than mobilisation programmes alone.

Multimodal therapy and active and passive repetitive movements (10 h over 6 weeks). Mobilisation (one 30 min session) has to be complemented with a home exercise programme consisting of arm and shoulder movements eventually while holding a 1.5 kg weight on the back in order to improve postural automatic alignment control (so-called torso weighting) and balance [19–21].

Patients who actually wore the collars as frequently as was stipulated had a significantly higher risk of being disabled and/or having altered work ability compared with patients in the mobilisation group. In terms of reducing pain at 2 months after injury, active therapy is significantly more effective than passive therapy.

Educational interventions are interventions in which patients are instructed about the nature and course of WAD using evidence-based pamphlets, videos or personal communication. Advice to remain active (act as usual) is associated with significantly better recovery in terms of a wide range of outcomes, including neck pain, headache, memory and concentration.

PEMT decreases pain intensity and increases cervical ROM over the short term; the evidence is insufficient to support the use of this treatment with confidence. Laser acupuncture does not appear to be any more effective than placebo in the treatment of acute WAD.

38.3.2 Subacute

Patients with whiplash do not constitute a homogeneous group; they do not have the same type of injury and the same underlying causes of persistent or long-term problem that can be treated according to a single, across-the-board programme. The hallmark should be the implementation of actions that promote rapid return to normal activity.

Interdisciplinary interventions may be more effective in reducing pain and sick leave than passive physiotherapy modalities, although it is not clear enough which components of such interventions are beneficial.

Patients who receive interdisciplinary treatment earlier are more likely to return to work, but it is uncertain whether this simply reflects natural history or is a consequence of the intervention.

Manipulation has short-term benefit to patients in the subacute stage of WAD I–II. Thoracic and cervical spinal manipulations are effective in reducing pain and improving cervical ROM (see Chap. 21).

The use of botulinum toxin injections during the subacute stage of WAD may have a small treatment effect, and it does not appear that botulinum toxin injections are any more effective than placebo.

The importance of physical therapy in patients with subacute whiplash injuries varies significantly in relation to outcome parameter. Thus, a referral for physical therapy may not be considered medically necessary for restoring range of motion, yet it would appear to be extremely important from an economic standpoint in reducing patients' period of disability. From the patients' point of view, however, reduction in pain intensity is the most important goal. Here, prescription of 'active' physical therapy should be preferred. Considering all these factors, active physical therapy is recommended for patients with QTF WAD grade II whiplash injuries as the best option for achieving both therapeutic and economic objectives.

The effect of botulinum toxin A injections suggests that earlier treatment may have some benefit in subacute WAD.

The serotonin-noradrenalin reuptake inhibitors (SNRIs) could be prescribed due to their positive effects on pain and dizziness perception.

38.3.3 Chronic

Generally speaking, advice to act as usual, adequate reassurance and active exercises involving functional exercises should be undertaken in QTF WAD grade I–II patients. In QTF WAD grade III patients, neurological involvement has to be specifically treated.

38.3.3.1 Unsteadiness

Vestibular rehabilitation has to be instituted for persons experiencing dizziness in the chronic phase. Planning the treatment requires subdividing patients into two main groups:

1. Equilibrium disorders are mainly caused by a ‘quantitative’ decreasing of the sensorial inputs or motor outputs or central integration of sensorimotor patterns.
2. Equilibrium disorders are mainly caused by a ‘qualitative’ decreasing of central sensorimotor integration in which the centre is not able to integrate sensorial inputs comparing different sensorimotor patterns.

The treatment of disorders grouped in the first condition is mainly based on neurorehabilitation. On the basis of responses to vestibular battery examination, excitatory (nicergoline, ginkgo biloba, piracetam) or inhibitory drugs (cinnarizine, flunarizine) may be employed, too. On the basis of general vascular conditions, some pathogenetic (aspirin, ticlopidine) drugs are associated.

In these patients neurorehabilitation (see Chap. 23) increases the activity of good peripheral inputs acting on sensorial and motor redundance. Prognostic evaluation is based on three specific goals: (1) the primary damage, the structural lesion of one or more equilibrium subsystem; (2) the secondary damage, functional imbalance of subsystems not directly involved by the lesion such as equilibrium disorders caused by post-lesional postural syndromes; and (3) the tertiary damage, the crystalisation of pathological sensorimotor patterns and/or psychological avoiding behaviours.

Rehabilitation is likely pointed toward limiting the primary damage, reducing the secondary damage and avoiding the tertiary damage.

Rehabilitation is based either on peripheral sensorial and motor redundance or on central spontaneous compensation mechanisms: functional sensorial substitution, structural reorganisation, recalibration of sensorimotor patterns and internuclear inhibition. Drugs are given to increase neural plasticity by means of axonal sprouting and reorganisation of neural networks.

Weakness of ankle joint muscles, loss of ankle sensation and reduced mobility of the ankles are contraindications for movement strategy training unless the underlying physiological factors are also addressed.

Contraindications to teaching appropriate use of hip movements might include weakness or loss of mobility about the hip joints. There is also clinical evidence suggesting that patients with profound loss of peripheral vestibular function cannot effectively coordinate hip movements and that training in these cases is ineffective.

The treatment of disorders grouped in the second condition is mainly based on combination of rehabilitation and drugs with the aim of regaining correct balance subsystem interconnection [22, 23].

The different behaviour of the two groups of equilibrium pathological systems is caused by the pre-lesional characteristics of the patient, the quantitative characteristics of the lesion, the qualitative characteristics of the disease and the side of lesion(s).

Chronic WAD and dizziness in a vestibular rehabilitation programme twice a week for 6 weeks and a 4-week home exercise programme consisting of slow eye-head-neck coordination exercises twice daily. Different balance measures (tandem standing and standing on one leg, both performed with eyes open and eyes closed) and the Dizziness Handicap Inventory have to be assessed at baseline, 6 weeks and 3 months.

A 6-week programme aimed at stimulating the vestibular system is significantly more effective than no treatment in increasing postural control and reducing self-perceived handicap. Physiotherapy programme consists of soft tissue treatment, isometric and isotonic exercises and advice regarding relaxation techniques, posture and home exercise.

38.3.3.2 Pain

Collar immobilisation, cervical pillows and prescribed rest have to be avoided. Intra-articular steroid injections and analgesic injections are not recommended.

Different treatments may be considered: exercise programmes, interdisciplinary interventions, manipulations, pharmacological interventions and alternative treatments (including myofeedback training and other alternative therapies).

Graded exercise with advice in a 4-week exercise programme has significantly greater gains in pain intensity and pain bothersomeness, and functional ability exercise programmes provided during the chronic phase of WAD are effective in relieving pain, although it does not appear that these gains are maintained over the long term.

The programme consists of learning basic and applied skills and application and generalisation of those skills in everyday activities with exercises to enhance muscular stabilisation of the neck, shoulder mobility, body posture and arm muscle strength.

In the case of temporomandibular disorders, therapeutic jaw exercises are substantially ineffective in reducing pain (see Chap. 11) if not combined with adequate dentistry treatment such as stabilisation splint.

Changes in self-rated pain is significantly greater for patients treated by multimodal physiotherapy group in a 10-week intervention consisting of either a self-management programme (education and information about exercise) or a multimodal physiotherapy programme (including low-load exercises, low-velocity mobilising techniques and education and assurance).

Groups that receive also home training report significantly less pain during rest and less fatigue in the final week of treatment.

Trigger point treatment is effective in reducing pain. Injection-based interventions may use both sterile water and saline. Sterile water injection or simple dry needling results in significantly less mean pain distress and greater cervical mobility immediately postinjection.

In selected subjects Botox may be used in order to obtain significant improvements in terms of both pain intensity and cervical ROM.

Cognitive behavioural therapy (CBT) is aimed at promoting the acceptance of pain and distress, when combined with physiotherapy. In severe disabling WAD, CBT allows greater improvements in terms of pain disability, life satisfaction, kinesiophobia, depressive symptomology and psychological flexibility.

Melatonin may be particularly useful in the treatment of chronic whiplash-related sleep disturbance especially in older subjects [24]. Melatonin is involved in synchronising circadian rhythms, and in healthy individuals, melatonin levels begin to rise between 20:00 and 21:30. Treatment is not associated with reductions in pain or any of the cognitive deficits associated with delayed melatonin onset but with improvement of balance dizziness and tinnitus [25, 26].

In chronic QTF WAD grade III, fluoroscopically guided cervical selective nerve root blocks using the corticosteroid solution or 'joint regeneration' (dextrose and lidocaine intra-articular) therapy may reduce whiplash-related pain and disability, in addition to physical therapy.

In shoulder chronic pain with both a positive impingement sign and a positive analgesic block response of a painful shoulder, the programme is subacromial space corticosteroid (40 mg methylprednisolone acetate) injections in conjunction with physiotherapy programme designed to correct scapulothoracic rhythmic dysfunction and strengthen the rotator cuff muscle. This approach may be effective for patients with late-onset shoulder pain.

For patients with chronic WAD who do not respond to conventional treatments, it appears that radiofrequency neurotomy (RFN) may be the most effective treatment option, lesioning the cervical medial branches or third occipital nerve for headache. Complications are lasting pain and/or numbness following surgery; ataxia was a regular side effect of third occipital neurotomy. Pain refractory to the initial treatment (less than 30 days relief) did not respond to a second treatment.

Epidural blood patch (EBP) is the therapy of choice in patients with chronic WAD with a suspected cerebrospinal fluid (CSF) leak. Suspecting symptoms are headache, memory, dizziness, visual impairment, cervical pain, nausea and auditory symptoms. They may be significantly reduced 1 week following treatment. However, the association of a CSF leak with chronic WAD has never been established.

References

1. Spitzer W, Skovron M, Salmi L, Cassidy J, Duranceau J, Suissa S, Zeiss E (1995) Scientific monograph of Quebec Task Force on whiplash associated disorders: redefining "whiplash" and its management. Spine 20:1–73
2. Teasell RW, McClure JA, Walton D, Pretty J, Salter K, Meyer M, Sequeira K, Death B (2010) A research synthesis of therapeutic interventions for whiplash-associated disorder: part 1 – overview and summary. Pain Res Manag 15(5):287–94
3. Teasell RW, McClure JA, Walton D, Pretty J, Salter K, Meyer M, Sequeira K, Death B (2010) A research synthesis of therapeutic interventions for whiplash-associated disorder (WAD): part 2 – interventions for acute WAD. Pain Res Manag 15(5):295–304
4. Teasell RW, McClure JA, Walton D, Pretty J, Salter K, Meyer M, Sequeira K, Death B (2010) A research synthesis of therapeutic interventions for whiplash-associated disorder (WAD): part 3 – interventions for subacute WAD. Pain Res Manag 15(5):305–12
5. Teasell RW, McClure JA, Walton D, Pretty J, Salter K, Meyer M, Sequeira K, Death B (2010) A research synthesis of therapeutic interventions for whiplash-associated disorder (WAD): part 4 – noninvasive interventions for chronic WAD. Pain Res Manag 15(5):313–22
6. Teasell RW, McClure JA, Walton D, Pretty J, Salter K, Meyer M, Sequeira K, Death B (2010) A research synthesis of therapeutic interventions for whiplash-associated disorder (WAD): part 5 – surgical and injection-based interventions for chronic WAD. Pain Res Manag 15(5):323–34
7. Sterling M (2004) A proposed new classification system for whiplash associated disorders-implications for assessment and management. Man Ther 9(2):60–70, Review
8. Conlin A, Bhogal S, Sequeira K, Teasell R (2005) Treatment of whiplash-associated disorders–part I: non-invasive interventions. Pain Res Manag 10(1):21–32
9. Conlin A, Bhogal S, Sequeira K, Teasell R (2005) Treatment of whiplash-associated disorders–part II: medical and surgical interventions. Pain Res Manag 10(1):33–40
10. Clinical guidelines for best practice management of acute and chronic whiplash associated disorders: Clinical resource guide. TRACsa: Trauma and Injury Recovery, South Australia. Adelaide 2008. www.mac.sa.gov.au
11. Pope MH (2010) The Canadian C-spine rule safely reduces imaging rates for cervical spine injuries. J Physiother 56(1):59
12. Michaleff ZA, Maher CG, Verhagen AP, Rebbeck T, Lin CW (2012) Accuracy of the Canadian C-spine rule and NEXUS to screen for clinically important cervical spine injury in patients following blunt trauma: a systematic review. CMAJ 184(16):E867–76. doi: 10.1503/cmaj.120675
13. Vernon H (2008) The Neck Disability Index: state-of-the-art, 1991–2008. J Manipulative Physiol Ther 31(7):491–502
14. Rebbeck TJ, Refshauge KM, Maher CG, Stewart M (2007) Evaluation of the core outcome measure in whiplash. Spine (Phila Pa 1976) 32(6):696–702
15. Jacobson GP, Newman CW (1990) The development of the Dizziness Handicap Inventory. Arch Otolaryngol Head Neck Surg 116(4):424–7
16. Tesio L, Alpini D, Cesarani A, Perucca L (1999) Short form of the Dizziness Handicap Inventory: construction and validation through Rasch analysis. Am J Phys Med Rehabil 78(3):233–41
17. DeSantana JM, Sluka KA (2008) Central mechanisms in the maintenance of chronic widespread noninflammatory muscle pain. Curr Pain Headache Rep 12(5):338–343
18. Giordano J (2005) The neurobiology of nociceptive and anti-nociceptive systems. Pain Physician 8:277–290
19. Widener GL, Allen DD, Gibson-Horn C (2009) Randomized clinical trial of balance-based torso weighting for improving upright mobility in people with multiple sclerosis. Neurorehabil Neural Repair 23(8):784–91
20. Widener GL, Allen DD, Gibson-Horn C (2009) Balance-based torso-weighting may enhance balance in persons with multiple sclerosis: preliminary evidence. Arch Phys Med Rehabil 90(4):602–9

21. Willigenburg NW, Kingma I, van Dieën JH (2012) Precision control of an upright trunk posture in low back pain patients. Clin Biomech (Bristol, Avon) 27(9):866–71
22. Perna G, Alpini D, Caldirola D, Raponi G, Cesarani A, Bellodi L (2003) Serotonergic modulation of the balance system in panic disorder: an open study. Depress Anxiety 17(2):101–6
23. Cesarani A, Meloni F, Alpini D, Barozzi S, Verderio L, Boscani PF (1998) Ginkgo biloba (EGb 761) in the treatment of equilibrium disorders. Adv Ther 15(5):291–304
24. Alpini D, Cesarani A, Fraschini F, Kohen-Raz R, Capobianco S, Cornelio F (2004) Aging and vestibular system: specific tests and role of melatonin in cognitive involvement. Arch Gerontol Geriatr Suppl (9):13–25. PubMed PMID: 15207391
25. Fraschini F, Cesarani A, Alpini D, Esposti D, Stankov BM (1999) Melatonin influences human balance. Biol Signals Recept 8(1–2):111–9
26. Cesarani A, Fraschini F, Alpini D (2009) Melatonin in patients with chronic tinnitus. Audiol Med 3(4):243–244

Index

D.C. Alpini et al. (eds.), *Whiplash Injuries*,
DOI 10.1007/978-88-470-5486-8, © Springer-Verlag Italia 2014

MIX
Papier aus verantwortungsvollen Quellen
Paper from responsible sources
FSC® C105338

If you have any concerns about our products,
you can contact us on
ProductSafety@springernature.com

In case Publisher is established outside the EU,
the EU authorized representative is:
Springer Nature Customer Service Center GmbH
Europaplatz 3, 69115 Heidelberg, Germany

Printed by Libri Plureos GmbH
in Hamburg, Germany